RSSDI Atlas of
Diabetic Foot

RSSDI Atlas of Diabetic Foot

Editor-in-Chief
Vijay Viswanathan MD PhD FRCP (London, Glasgow)
Honorary President—D-Foot International
Immediate Past National Vice President—RSSDI
Head and Chief Diabetologist
MV Hospital for Diabetes and Prof. M. Viswanathan Diabetes Research Centre
Chennai, Tamil Nadu, India

Assistant Editor
Ashu Rastogi MD DM MNAMS FACE FRCP (Edinburgh)
Associate Professor
Department of Endocrinology and Metabolism
Postgraduate Institute of Medical Education and Research (PGIMER)
Chandigarh, India

Associate Editors

BM Makkar MD FIAMS FICP
FRCP (Glasgow, Edinburgh) FACP (USA)
FACE (USA) FRSSDI
President—RSSDI
Diabetologist and Bariatric Physician
Director, Dr Makkar's Diabetes and
Obesity Centre
Paschim Vihar, New Delhi, India

Sanjay Agarwal MD FACE FACP FRSSDI
Secretary General—RSSDI
Director, Aegle Clinic–Diabetes Care Head,
Department of Medicine and Diabetes
Ruby Hall Clinic
Senior Consultant in Diabetes and
Medicine Jehangir Hospital
Pune, Maharashtra, India

Ch Vasanth Kumar MD
Immediate Past President – RSSDI
Senior Consultant Physician
Apollo Hospitals
Hyderabad, Telangana, India

Rakesh Sahay MD DNB DM
President Elect—RSSDI
Professor and Head
Department of Endocrinology
Osmania Medical College
Hyderabad, Telangana, India

Ghanshyam Goyal MD (Medicine)
Director, Consultant Diabetologist and
Diabetic Foot Specialist
SK Diabetes Research and
Education Centre
Kolkata, West Bengal, India

Ashok Damir MD
Head of Diabetic Foot and
Wound Care Management
Fortis Super Specialty Hospital
Patel Nagar, New Delhi, India

Pratap Jethwani MD PG Dip
Diab FRSSDI FDiab India
Joint Secretary—RSSDI
Director and Consultant
Diabetes Specialist
Jethwani Diabetes Care Center
Jethwani Hospital
Rajkot, Gujarat, India

Forewords
BM Makkar
Sanjay Agarwal
Ch Vasanth Kumar

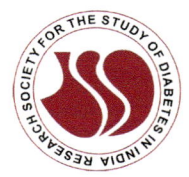

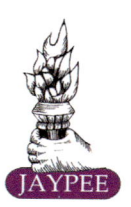

JAYPEE BROTHERS MEDICAL PUBLISHERS
The Health Sciences Publisher
New Delhi | London

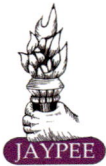 **Jaypee Brothers Medical Publishers (P) Ltd**

Headquarters
EMCA House
23/23-B, Ansari Road, Daryaganj
New Delhi 110 002, India
Landline: +91-11-23272143, +91-11-23272703
+91-11-23282021, +91-11-23245672
E-mail: jaypee@jaypeebrothers.com

Corporate Office
Jaypee Brothers Medical Publishers (P) Ltd.
4838/24, Ansari Road, Daryaganj
New Delhi 110 002, India
Phone: +91-11-43574357
Fax: +91-11-43574314
E-mail: jaypee@jaypeebrothers.com

Overseas Office
JP Medical Ltd.
83, Victoria Street, London
SW1H 0HW (UK)
Phone: +44-20 3170 8910
Fax: +44(0)20 3008 6180
E-mail: info@jpmedpub.com

Website: www.jaypeebrothers.com
Website: www.jaypeedigital.com

© 2024, Jaypee Brothers Medical Publishers

The views and opinions expressed in this book are solely those of the original contributor(s)/author(s) and do not necessarily represent those of editor(s) or publisher of the book.

All rights reserved. No part of this publication may be reproduced, stored or transmitted in any form or by any means, electronic, mechanical, photocopying, recording or otherwise, without the prior permission in writing of the publishers.

All brand names and product names used in this book are trade names, service marks, trademarks or registered trademarks of their respective owners. The publisher is not associated with any product or vendor mentioned in this book.

Medical knowledge and practice change constantly. This book is designed to provide accurate, authoritative information about the subject matter in question. However, readers are advised to check the most current information available on procedures included and check information from the manufacturer of each product to be administered, to verify the recommended dose, formula, method and duration of administration, adverse effects and contraindications. It is the responsibility of the practitioner to take all appropriate safety precautions. Neither the publisher nor the author(s)/editor(s) assume any liability for any injury and/or damage to persons or property arising from or related to use of material in this book.

This book is sold on the understanding that the publisher is not engaged in providing professional medical services. If such advice or services are required, the services of a competent medical professional should be sought.

Every effort has been made where necessary to contact holders of copyright to obtain permission to reproduce copyright material. If any have been inadvertently overlooked, the publisher will be pleased to make the necessary arrangements at the first opportunity.

Inquiries for bulk sales may be solicited at: jaypee@jaypeebrothers.com

RSSDI Atlas of Diabetic Foot / *Vijay Viswanathan*

First Edition: **2024**

ISBN: 978-93-5465-956-0

Printed at Replika Press Pvt. Ltd.

RSSDI Current Executive Committee Members 2023

President
BM Makkar

Immediate Past President
Ch Vasanth Kumar

President Elect
Rakesh Sahay

Secretary General
Sanjay Agarwal

Vice President
Sujoy Ghosh
L Sreenivasa Murthy

Honorary Joint Secretary
Pratap Jethwani

Honorary Treasurer
JK Sharma

All India Member
Aravinda J
Manoj Chawla
NK Singh
M Shunmugavelu

Zone-wise Committee
Amit Gupta - North Zone
Jothydev Kesavadev - South Zone
Rakesh Parikh - West Zone
Anil Virmani - East Zone

Co-opted Member
Vijay Viswanathan
Anuj Maheshwari
Sunil Gupta

Diabetic Foot Task Force
Vijay Viswanathan
Sharad Pendsey
Ghanshyam Goyal
Ashok Damir
Sujith Kumar

RSSDI Past Executive Committee Members 2022

President
Ch Vasanth Kumar

Immediate Past President
Banshi Saboo

President Elect
BM Makkar

General Secretary
Sanjay Agarwal

Vice President
Anuj Maheshwari
Vijay Viswanathan

Joint Secretary
Sujoy Ghosh

Treasurer
Sunil Gupta

Executive Member
JK Sharma
L Sreenivasa Murthy
Pratap Jethwani
Sanjay Reddy
Shalini Jaggi
Anand Moses
Bikash Bhattacharjee
Sudhir Bhandari
Vijay Panikar
Rakesh Sahay
Amit Gupta

CONTRIBUTORS

EDITOR-IN-CHIEF

Vijay Viswanathan MD PhD FRCP (London, Glasgow)
Honorary President—D-Foot International
Immediate Past National Vice President—RSSDI
Head and Chief Diabetologist
MV Hospital for Diabetes and Prof. M. Viswanathan Diabetes Research Centre
Chennai, Tamil Nadu, India

ASSISTANT EDITOR

Ashu Rastogi MD DM MNAMS FACE FRCP (Edinburgh)
Associate Professor
Department of Endocrinology and Metabolism
Postgraduate Institute of Medical Education and Research (PGIMER)
Chandigarh, India

ASSOCIATE EDITORS

BM Makkar MD FIAMS FICP FRCP (Glasgow, Edinburgh) FACP (USA) FACE (USA) FRSSDI
President—RSSDI
Diabetologist and Bariatric Physician
Director, Dr Makkar's Diabetes and Obesity Centre
Paschim Vihar, New Delhi, India

Sanjay Agarwal MD FACE FACP FRSSDI
Secretary General—RSSDI
Director, Aegle Clinic–Diabetes Care
Head, Department of Medicine and Diabetes
Ruby Hall Clinic
Senior Consultant in Diabetes and Medicine Jehangir Hospital
Pune, Maharashtra, India

Ch Vasanth Kumar MD
Immediate Past President—RSSDI
Senior Consultant Physician
Apollo Hospitals
Hyderabad, Telangana, India

Rakesh Sahay MD DNB DM
President Elect—RSSDI
Professor and Head
Department of Endocrinology
Osmania Medical College
Hyderabad, Telangana, India

Ghanshyam Goyal MD (Medicine)
Director, Consultant Diabetologist and Diabetic Foot Specialist
SK Diabetes Research and Education Centre
Kolkata, West Bengal, India

Ashok Damir MD
Head of Diabetic Foot and Wound Care Management
Fortis Super Specialty Hospital
Patel Nagar, New Delhi, India

Pratap Jethwani MD PG Dip Diab FRSSDI FDiab India
Joint Secretary—RSSDI
Director and Consultant
Diabetes Specialist
Jethwani Diabetes Care Center
Jethwani Hospital
Rajkot, Gujarat, India

CONTRIBUTING AUTHORS

Amit Gupta MBBS DNB (General Medicine) MNAMS FICP FACE FRCP (Glasgow, Edinburgh) FACP PGD-Diab DFID F-Diab (Diab India) FGSI FIMSA FIACM
Director
Department of Internal Medicine and Diabetes
Centre for Diabetes Care
Greater Noida, Uttar Pradesh, India

Ashu Rastogi MD DM MNAMS FACE FRCP (Edinburgh)
Associate Professor
Department of Endocrinology and Metabolism
Postgraduate Institute of Medical Education and Research
Chandigarh, India

Jayaditya Ghosh MD
Senior Resident
Department of Endocrinology
Postgraduate Institute of Medical Education and Research
Chandigarh, India

Manisha Singh Jadaun MS
Additional Professor
GRD Medical College
Gwalior, Madhya Pradesh, India

Ragghuraman Soundararajan MD
Senior Resident
Department of Radiodiagnosis
Postgraduate Institute of Medical Education and Research
Chandigarh, India

R Ravikumar DMRD DNB (RadioDiagnosis) PhD FIAMS FICS
Consultant Interventional Radiologist
MV Hospital for Diabetes
Chennai, Tamil Nadu, India

Bamila Selvaraj MPT (Neurology) MIAP Dip in Podiatry
Senior Physiotherapist and Podiatrist
MV Hospital for Diabetes and
Prof. M. Viswanathan Diabetes Research Centre
Chennai, Tamil Nadu, India

Sanjay Agarwal MD FACE
Director, Aegle Clinic–Diabetes Care
Head, Department of Medicine
Ruby Hall Clinic
Senior Consultant in Diabetes and Medicine
Jehangir Hospital
Pune, Maharashtra, India
Secretary General—RSSDI

Seena Rajsekar Msc (Psychology) Dip in Podiatry
Senior Podiatrist and Diabetic Foot Counsellor
MV Hospital for Diabetes and
Prof. M. Viswanathan Diabetes Research Centre
Chennai, Tamil Nadu, India

Senthil Govindan MS (General Surgery) MCh (Plastic Surgery)
Consultant Podiatric, Plastic and Reconstructive Surgeon
MV Hospital for Diabetes
Chennai, Tamil Nadu, India

Sivashankari SelvaElavarasan MDS APGDipCRM
Medical Writer and Clinical Research Associate
MV Hospital for Diabetes
Prof. M. Viswanathan Diabetes Research Centre
Chennai, Tamil Nadu, India

Ch Vasanth Kumar MD
Senior Consultant Physician
Apollo Hospitals
Hyderabad, Telangana, India
Immediate Past President—RSSDI

Vibhakar R Vachhrajani MS
Consultant, Vijay Vachhrajani Memorial Diabetic Foot Hospital and Wound Management Center
Rajkot, Gujarat, India

Vijay Viswanathan MD PhD FRCP (London, Glasgow)
Honorary President—D-Foot International
Immediate Past National
Vice President—RSSDI
Head and Chief Diabetologist
MV Hospital for Diabetes and
Prof. M. Viswanathan Diabetes Research Centre
Chennai, Tamil Nadu, India

FOREWORD

India is considered the diabetes capital of the world with currently 74 million people living with diabetes according to International Diabetes Federation 2021. It is also considered a chronic disease that can have serious microvascular as well as macrovascular complications. This has put a tremendous burden on the healthcare sectors, society, and the nation to handle and take the essential endeavors, which are indispensable to reduce the burden of the disease. The diabetic foot is one of the major and most neglected health problems, which can have dreadful potential complications like amputation. Lower limb amputations are found to affect the patient's quality of life, which can affect their psychological and functional well-being.

The RSSDI has taken up enormous initiatives in the field of diabetes for its prevention and management and has received worldwide recognition for its extraordinary contributions. A book is a great platform or medium through which we can connect to healthcare professionals as well as students. One such incredible accomplishment is the *"RSSDI Atlas of Diabetic Foot"*, which has stupendous efforts compiled by stalwarts in this field. This book has concise chapters on the epidemiology of foot infections, essential elements of foot examination, the quintessential steps necessary to reduce the rate of amputations and a distinct chapter on a campaign conducted by the RSSDI. The authors have provided us with incredible insights into the management of peripheral arterial disease, surgical aspects of foot infections, and the concept of angiosomes. It has some dedicated sections on the role of imaging, orthotics, and wound dressing which are of paramount importance in the management of diabetic foot infections.

This book, written by *Dr Vijay Viswanathan* who is a pioneer in the field of research and diabetic foot, is indeed a comprehensive and remarkable contribution for the benefit of numerous readers, which gives them insights into the various aspects of diabetic foot and the most frequent clinical problems encountered. We would like to congratulate *Dr Vijay Viswanathan* along with the other coauthors for their earnest, sincere, and outstanding efforts in compiling this book and would also like to wish them success in launching this wonderful book.

Dr BM Makkar
President—RSSDI

Dr Sanjay Agarwal
Secretory-General—RSSDI

Dr Ch Vasanth Kumar
Immediate Past President—RSSDI

PREFACE

"A good book is a man's best friend" is a famous saying, which means that good books enrich our knowledge, enlighten the mind, and are therefore considered the best company a man can always have. It is with immense pride and pleasure that we bring out this *"RSSDI Atlas of Diabetic Foot"*, which can help us to increase our knowledge and understanding of diabetic foot.

This book provides us with exhaustive and extensive information about the various aspects of diabetic foot. We have fourteen unique and distinct chapters with a special emphasis on *Diabetic Foot Infections in India* enlightening us about the epidemiology, risk factors, pathogenesis, and preventive strategies to identify high-risk patients and also prevent dreadful complications like amputations. Special attention has been given to a wonderful and distinct initiative—*"Save the Feet and Keep Walking Campaign,"* which was launched by the RSSDI to train healthcare professionals and create more awareness among the people to prevent and manage diabetic foot infections in India. A separate chapter emphasizes the significance of a *Three-minute Foot Examination*, which is simple, less time-consuming yet effective in the identification of high-risk patients to prioritize them and treat them accordingly. We have some lucid and concise chapters enlightening us about the ominous association between Peripheral Artery Disease and Diabetic Foot Infections and the role of orthotics, wound dressings, and imaging in the integrated management of foot infections. We have incorporated some of our invaluable experiences on the basic concept of angiosomes and surgical approach of foot infections which are both considered indispensable for every diabetic foot care specialist. The uniqueness of this book lies in our best efforts to include high-resolution clinical photographs of the common diabetic foot problems encountered with a short narrative that can help the readers to learn, understand, and enhance their existing knowledge about diabetic foot.

We have made sure that we have used simple language and well-referenced chapters illustrated with flowcharts, and photographs of clinical cases to make it very appealing and interesting for our wide range of readers like diabetologists, physicians, and even students. This book can also be used as a comprehensive guide for updating our current concepts to identify and treat patients with diabetic foot problems in the most appropriate manner because it is well-known that *"The eyes do not see what the mind does not know."*

We have indeed taken a strenuous effort in compiling all the chapters and photos for the benefit of our readers and matching the quality of standards set by the RSSDI.

Vijay Viswanathan

ACKNOWLEDGMENTS

We would like to acknowledge the entire RSSDI Executive Committee members under the able guidance of the President Dr BM Makkar and the Secretary-General Dr Sanjay Agarwal. We would also like to acknowledge Dr Ch Vasanth Kumar (Immediate Past President), Dr Rakesh Sahay (President-Elect), Dr Sujoy Ghosh (Vice President), Dr L Sreenivasa Murthy (Vice President), Dr Pratap Jethwani (Joint Secretary), Dr JK Sharma (Treasurer), Dr J Arvinda, Dr Manoj Chawla, Dr NK Singh, Dr M Shunmugavelu, Dr Amit Gupta, Dr Jothydev Kesavadev, Dr Rakesh Parikh, Dr Anil Virmani, Dr Anuj Maheshwari, and Dr Sunil Gupta who have been providing us extraordinary support to launch this wonderful and prestigious *RSSDI Atlas of Diabetic Foot*. We would like to acknowledge the past Executive Committee members of RSSDI who have provided us with immense support and encouragement. We would like to express our sincere thanks to all the RSSDI members who have contributed to this remarkable project. We would like to acknowledge Dr Sivashankari SelvaElavarasan, medical writer, and Jaypee Brothers Medical Publishers (P) Ltd for their tremendous effort and excellent work contributed towards writing, editing, compiling and publishing this book. We would also like to thank Dr Leela Baid, Dr Milind Ruke, and Dr Amit Naghate who assisted us in compiling the photos of the campaign for better comprehension of diabetic foot. We acknowledge the help rendered by USV for the logistic support of this project.

Acknowledgment for "Common Diabetic Foot Problems Encountered"

We would like to thank and acknowledge all the RSSDI members who participated in the "Save the Feet and Keep Walking campaign" and provided their valuable contributions for photographs of the common diabetic foot problems encountered.

- Aakanksha Pathria
- Aashna Patil
- Aastha Kansal
- Abani Patra
- Abdul Azeez
- Abdulhalim Khan
- Abha Gupta
- Abha Mahajan Chandwani
- Abhash Jain
- Abhaydeep Arage
- Abhay Kumar Srivastava
- Abhay Tirki
- Abhigan Ghosh
- Abhijeet Namde
- Abhijit Jadhav
- Abhijit Moullick
- Abhisekh Raha
- Abhishek Arun
- Abhishek Das
- Abhishek Jain
- Abhishek Rath
- Abhishek Sharma
- Abhishek Shrivastava
- Abirami Abirami
- Absar Ahmad
- Abuzar Dakhni
- Achyut Adhikary
- Adhiraj Barman
- Aejaz Ali Qadri
- Aiswarya Yalamanchi
- Ajay Joshi
- Ajay Kukreja
- Ajay Mishra
- Ajinkya Mhase
- Ajit Kulkarni
- Ajit Kumar Panda
- Ajoy Tewari
- A Kalaiselvan
- Akash C
- AK Bali
- AK Bhalla
- Akeel Khan
- Akil Memon
- AK Satsangi
- Akshay Kothari
- Akshaykumar Doshi
- Akshay Saha
- Akshay Shirsath
- Alan Soares
- Alka Bhefi
- Aloke Kumar Gupta
- Alok Saxena
- Aman Gaonkar
- Amar Buduk
- Amar Jagtap
- Amar Mandol
- Amarnath Har
- Ameet Chordiya
- Amey Veer
- Amina Bharvin
- Ami Sanghvi
- Amita Baghchi
- Amitabha Chattaraj
- Amitabh Jain
- Amit Bedi
- Amit Dey
- Amit Goyal
- Amit Gupta
- Amit Kale
- Amit Khan
- Amit Kothari
- Amit Mane
- Amit Palange
- Amit Ray
- Amit Saraf
- Amit Shah
- Amit Singh
- Amit Taneja
- Amod Borkar
- Amol Kulkarni
- Amol Nanaware
- Amol Pathak
- Anadi Bhusan Tarafdar
- Ana Monteiro
- Anand C
- Anandeep Agrawal
- Anand Nikalje
- Ananth Bandhu Nath

Acknowledgments

- Anasuyak Ray
- Anbuchelvan Chelvan
- Anil Gupta
- Anil Kulsesthra
- Anil Kumar Sahu
- Anilkumar Undhad
- Anil Kumar Upadhyay
- Anilmathew Philip
- Anil Pisharody
- Anil Shrivstav
- Anirban Das
- Anirban Mitra
- Aniruddha Bhattacharya
- Aniruddha Tongaonkar
- Anirudh Raghavendra
- Anish Thakur
- Anita Nambiar
- Anitha Moorthy
- Anjali Nakra
- Ankan Pathak
- Ankita Aneja
- Ankita Gupta
- Ankita Tiwari
- Ankit Jain
- Ankur Patel
- Ankush Gupta
- Annamma Chako
- Anoosha Bhandarkar
- Anthony D Souza
- Antonio Rodrigues
- Anubha Srivastava
- Anuja Phalak
- Anuj Bansal
- Anuj Maheshwari
- Anupam Goel
- Anupam Mondal
- Anuradha HS
- Anurag Agarwal
- Anurag Chawla
- Aparna Kodre
- Aparna More
- Aparna Zaveri
- A Prabhavathy
- AP Sonawar
- Apurba Jana
- Apurva Kulkarni-Patil
- Arabinda Nayak
- Arati Shahade
- Archana Kabara
- Arijit Samanta
- Arijit Sen
- Arindam Nandi
- Arnab Kar
- Arokiya Jai A
- Arpan Bhattacharya
- Arpan Kumar Ghosh
- Arpan Kumar Ghoswami
- Arti Dharaskar
- Arunava Pal
- Arun Chander Krishnamurthy
- Arun Darna
- Arun Dhawale
- Arun Kedia
- Arun Kumar Pande
- Arun Patil
- Arun Shinde
- Arvind Ghongane
- Arvind Gupta
- Arvind Pandit
- A Seshadhri
- Asgerali Mahamed
- Asha Ahuja
- Ashish Ashish
- Ashish Gautam
- Ashish Kakaria
- Ashish Kansal
- Ashok Bamoriya
- Ashok Damir
- Ashok Doshi
- Ashok Kamra
- Ashok Kumar
- Ashok Mittal
- Ashok Singh
- Ashu Rastogi
- Ashutosh Chaturvedi
- Ashutosh Das
- Ashutosh Kumar
- Ashwini Malhotra
- Ashwini V
- Ashwin Sadavarte
- Asish Kumar
- Asish Kumar Basu
- Asit Behera
- A Sukumar
- Aswathy Vijayakumar
- Atanu Chatterjee
- Athili Veeraja
- Atul Mehrotra
- Austin Philomena
- Avadhut Warake
- Avijit Ghosh
- Avinash Kharade
- Avishek Das
- AV Ramesh Babu
- Awadhoot Prabhudesai
- Ayush Chandra
- Badriprasad Ghuge
- Bahadur Singh
- Balagangadharao Meka
- Balaji Chidambaram
- Balamudra Sriniwas Rao
- Balasaheb Karad
- Balram Shivaiah
- Bana Bihari Sen
- Banumathy Srikant
- Basab Ghosh
- Basavaraj SK
- Basith Lateef
- Bellary Srinivas
- Bhagatram Somani
- Bhagirathi Parida
- Bharat Lahane
- Bhargava Dinni
- Bhaskar Anand
- Bhaskar Kamat
- Bhaskar Rao
- Bhaskar Sinare
- Bhavani Prasad
- Bhavatharini Aruyerchelvan
- Bhumika Vaishnav
- Bhupesh Mehta
- Bhushan Itkelwar
- Bhuvaneswari Subrahmanyam
- Bibek Ananda Mohanty
- Bijal Kapadia
- Bijaya Ketan Dash
- Bijaya Kumar Mishra
- Bikram Banerjee
- Binday Kumar
- Bipul Ghosh
- Birendrakishore Nayak
- Birendra Kumar Singh
- Biswanath Agrawal
- Bivash Banerjee
- BK Malik
- BK Singh
- BM Makkar
- B Nagarajan
- BN Singh
- Brij B Gupta
- Brijendra Srivastava
- Brijesh Aggarwal
- B Tamil Azhagan
- Buddhadeb Mukherjee
- Buddhiraj Patil
- Budhadev Dey
- Chakkarai Muralidharan
- Chandni Radhakrishnan
- Chand Patel
- Chandragiri Abhinay
- Charanjit Singh
- Chetan Haria
- Chirag Aghara
- CR Anand Moses
- Dakshata Padhye
- Dantam Bheema Rao
- Darpan Suchak
- Dasharath Prajapati
- Dattatraya Patil
- Dayanand BS
- Dayanand Dhekane
- Dayanidhi Jena
- Debashis Basak
- Debashis Das
- Debashish Chakraborty
- Debasis Chakrabarti
- Debasish Chattoapadhya
- Debmalya Sanyal
- Debobrata Roy
- Deepak Agarwal
- Deepak Girdhar
- Deepak Lotalikar
- Deepak Manhans
- Deepak Morey
- Deepak Munshi

Acknowledgments — xv

- Deepika
- Devasish Gupta
- Devendra Ahirwar
- Devidas Chavan
- Dharmendrakumar Mavani
- Dharmik Soni
- Dheeraj K Bahua
- Dhiraj Gandhi
- Dhiraj Jadhav
- Dhiren Joshi
- Dhruvi Hasnani
- Dhruv Patel
- Dibyajyoti Karmakar
- Dilip Padghan
- Dilip Shirsath
- Dinakar Kumar
- Dinanath Chatterjee
- Dinesh Agarwal
- Dinesh Gangwani
- Dinesh Moda
- Dinesh Singh
- Dipak Aghara
- Dipak Chudasama
- Dipankar Ghosh
- Dishank Patel
- Diwashish Bishwas
- DN Das
- DN Sarangi
- Drnikhil Upadhyay
- Drsuguna Priya
- Drvijayarani Govindarajan
- D Senthil Kumar
- DS Satiar
- DT Gaikwad
- Durai Samy
- Durga Murmu
- Eage Priyatam Reddy
- Ekta Bharathi
- Gajanan Hegde
- Gajjala Srikant Reddy
- Gana Sekaran
- Ganesh Dahale
- Ganesh Dahiwal
- Ganeshkumar Satpute
- Ganesh Raja
- Gangakishan Chandak
- Ganga Vashy
- Gangumalla Bharati
- Gaurav Bhambhani
- Gaurav Chhaya
- Gaurav Kesar
- Gaurav K Sisodia
- Gaurav Sahastrabudhe
- Gaurav Subhedar
- Gayatri Harshe
- GC Patni
- GD Ramchandani
- Ghanshyam Goyal
- Girija Nair
- Girish Rajadhyaksha
- Girja Shankar Sinha
- Gladys V
- GN Singh
- Gobharsni Gopalsn
- Gopalakrishnan M Manakiveetil
- Gopal Kedia
- Gour Goswami
- Govind Vyas
- GR Ravi
- GS Mahapatra
- GS Sandeep
- Gulshran Singh Sethi
- Gurmeet Kundi
- Gurpreet Singh
- Gurunath Katkar
- Gurusamy Kirubakaran
- Hakeem Uddin Malvi
- Hanumant Gorad
- Hardik Thakker
- Haresh Udani
- Hariballav Mahapatra
- Hariom Gupta
- Hariprasad Iyer
- Hari Shankar Kosta
- Harish Chaudhari
- Harsha Master
- Harsha Vardhana
- Harsh Shah
- Harvinder Singh
- Hasmukh Jain
- Hemanth Sangamesh
- Hemant Kumar Kumar
- Hemant Mundhe
- Hemant Nagda
- Hemant Salve
- Hemant Waghmare
- Hema V Hema
- H Gokula Krishnan
- Himangshu Nagar
- Himanshu Sekhar Behera
- Himanshu Sekhar Nanda
- Hiranmoy Paul
- Hiten Barot
- Hiten L Furia
- Hitesh Patel
- Hitesh Punyani
- Honey Evangelin
- Honey Savla
- HS Jadhav
- Hussain Nulwala
- Immanuvel Moses
- Imran Ghanchi
- Inder Raj Singh
- Indrajit Banerjee
- Indrajit Gupta
- Indranil Ghoshdastidar
- Indu Panda
- Irshad Ahaned
- Jagdip Nanavati
- Jagdish Paduthur
- Jagdish Shah
- Jagjit Singh Sethi
- Jagmohan Singh Rana
- Jami Bharatudu
- Jaminikant Mishra
- Janakiraman Chandrasekar
- Janak Shah
- Janavi Gangadar
- J Appa Rao
- Jasbir Singh
- Jaya Bhanu Kanwar
- Jayachadran V
- Jayakrishnan B
- Jayandhi Anbu Chelvam
- Jayanta Rana
- Jayant Rath
- Jayant Shelgikar
- Jaydeep Shinde
- Jayendra Maoo
- Jayesh Balsara
- Jayesh Boricha
- Jeet Singh
- Jenish J Vira
- Jessica Pereira
- Jignesh Lodhari
- Jigyasu Singh
- Jitenda Saraf
- Jitendra Lahamge
- Jitendra Patel
- J Manickavasagam
- JN Sarengi
- Joel Nesaraj
- Jogendra Patra
- John Peter
- Jothydev Kesavadev
- Jotideb Mukhopadhyay
- Joy Sanariya
- J Sagar Prusty
- J Selvakumar Jayavel
- Jyothi Gupta
- Jyoti Gayal
- Jyoti Kale
- Jyoti Mannari
- Jyoti Ranjan Dash
- Kaggalgoudar SM
- Kailash Chandra Lohani
- Kailash Meghwal
- Kakasaheb Gandal
- Kalavathy Ramesh
- Kali Varthan
- Kalpana Pattabiraman
- Kalpesh Kavar
- Kamal Krishna Aich
- Kamal Shah
- Kannan Alagarsamy
- Kannan Natarajan
- Kannathasan Kannathasan
- Kanniappan Mathew
- Kapil Mahajan
- Kapil More
- Karthic Sonai
- Karthikeyan Selvan
- Karunesh Kumar HS
- Kaushik Banerjee
- Kaushik Melawane
- Kaustav Kumar Das
- Kavya Jonnalagadda

Acknowledgments

- Kayalvizhi Sivakumar
- K Bala Subramanian
- KC Jana
- Kedar Deodhar
- Keshu Jindal
- Ketan Pakhale
- Ketan Shah
- Khaja Mohiuddine MK
- Khushal Ram Choudhary
- Killivalavan Dhanasekaran
- Kinnary Shah
- Kiran Somkuwar
- Kishore Boral
- Kishore Verlekar
- KK Parouha
- KK Sinha
- K Mahesh Kumar
- KM Mohan
- KN Sree Sai Gayathri Sree
- Kollal Sinha
- Komal Totala
- Krishna Karekar
- Krishnanjan Chakraborty
- Krishna Prasanthi Penna
- Krunal Chandarana
- K Saravanan
- KS Dhanyakumar
- Kshitij Masani
- Kulbhushan Gangwani
- Kuldeep Dutta
- Kumarprafull Chandra
- Kumar Pushpal
- Kunal Mehta
- Kundan Chaurasia
- Kushal Samani
- K Vijay Kumar
- Lakshmi Prapulla
- Lal Babu Tudu
- Lalit Chandwani
- Lalji Tanna
- Laly Monson
- Lavanya Yogi
- Laxmidhar Sendha
- Laxmikant Dasari
- Leela Pahurkar
- Leena Chauhan
- Lekshmi Sudhan
- L Gopal Naik
- Lily Rodrigues
- L Karpagavel Karpagavel
- Lokesh Goyal
- Lotika Purohit
- Lovelena Munawar
- LP Chaudhari Gavali
- L Sreenivasa Murthy
- Lucky Doshi
- MA Bhat
- Madhavi Ukalkar
- Madhav Lavte
- Madhura Parvatkar
- Madhuri Beloskar
- Madhu Sudan Senapati
- Madhusudan Yemul
- Madhusudhan Reddy
- Mahadev Banerjee
- Mahadev Das
- Mahalingam PL
- Mahendra Deshmane
- Mahendra Singh Suri
- Mahendra Sonwane
- Mahesh Baheti
- Mahesh More
- Mahesh Talegaonkar
- Mahuya Sikdar
- Malay Parekh
- Mallam Srikanth Goud
- Malobika Das
- Mamta Garg
- Manas K Das
- Maneesh Jain
- Mangala Devi KR
- Mani Kandan
- Manish Ghuge
- Manish Kumar Singh
- Manish Sachdev
- Manish Shrivastav
- Manju Sivaraj
- Manohar Nageshappa
- Manoj Chawla
- Manoj Indurkar
- Manoj Kumar
- Manoj Kumar Jha
- Manoj Kumar Srivastava
- Manoj Lokhande
- Manoj Sharma
- Manu Suresh
- Marconi Corriea
- Maulita Kapadia
- Mayuri Date
- Mayya SV
- MB Thangavelu
- Md Dilawez Shamim
- Md Habibur Rahaman
- Meenakumari
- Meghana Barve
- Mehul Rathod
- Melvin Gonsalves
- MH Sanwarwallla
- Milan Lekhadia
- Milind Chaudhari
- Millind Choudhary
- Mittakola Bharathpraveen
- MK Singh
- MM Agarwal
- MM Ahsan
- MN Noorjahan Beevi
- Mohammad Arif Khan
- Mohammad Gani
- Mohammed Dohadwala
- Mohan Bhat
- Mohan Sampath Kumar
- Mohan Tewari
- Mohd Khalid
- Mohd Yusuf Ansari
- Mohit Garg
- Mohit Goyal
- Mohit Lathar
- Molcymol Abraham
- Monivannan Doctor
- Mouli Madhab Ghatak
- Mounika Anitha Chintala
- MR Gupta
- Mrinmayi Sonwane Gavali
- M Sreekath Reddy
- MU Ahmed
- Mudrik Pateo
- Mugish Ahmed
- Mukesh Bhagat
- Mukesh Pednekar
- Mukul Borah
- Mukulesh Gupta
- Mukund Pujari
- Mukund Sasturkar
- Murari Mohan Mondal
- Murugesan Arumugham
- Murugesa Pandian Nagarajan
- Mushtaque Nizami
- Mustufa Rangwala
- Muthukumar Subramaniam
- Mythili Ayyagari
- Mythili Krishnan
- Naaz Inamdar
- Naganjaneyulu Doctor
- Naganna Jilla
- Nagaraj Rao
- Nagendra Hebbar
- Nagendra Kumar Singh
- Nageswara Rao
- Namdev Hendge
- Namrata Singh
- Nandan Karn
- Narayan Choudhari
- Narendra Dara
- Narendra Javadekar
- Naresh Bansal
- Naresh Kanojia
- Narsingh Verma
- Nasim Ahmed
- Naveen Kumar RA
- Navin Chandra
- Navinchandra Shah
- Neelambar Bhatt
- Neha Patel
- Nijagunasivayogappa Javali
- Nikhil Gupta
- Nikhil Khot
- Nikhil Sarkar
- Nikita Bothra
- Nilanjana Patra
- Nilay Bhatt
- Nilesh Agrawal
- Nilesh Bhatt
- Nilesh Sinhal
- Nilima Pawar
- Nimai Dutta

Acknowledgments

- Nirmal Chaudhari
- Nirmal Mukherjee
- Nirmalya Ghosh
- Nirmalya Mangal
- Nirodhbaran Debnath
- Nirupam Prakash
- Nishant Kanodia
- Nishikant A Sharma
- Nita Patnaik
- Nitesh Kumar
- Nitin Dour
- Nitin Jain
- Nitin Ranjan Gupta
- Nitin Varshney
- N Rama Jagannath Rao
- Nripen Tarafdar
- NS Prasad
- Nupur Das
- Obydul Khan
- Omkar Gavali
- Omkarr De Hazra
- Ompraksh Bhosle
- Onkar Talkokul
- Pabitra Kumar Mandal
- Padmashri Gulati
- Padmnabh Zinjuwadia
- Palanikumaran Vasudevan
- Pankaj Agarwal
- Pankaj Birari
- Pankaj Desai
- Pankaj Kharapkar
- Pankaj Kumar
- Pankaj Mahajan
- Pankaj Punjot
- Paras Doshi
- Paresh Banerjee
- Parikshit Goswami
- Parmanand Mishra
- Parmeshwar Kale
- Parthasarathy Balasubramanian
- Parul Jain
- Parveen K Gupta
- Patan Gulab Kasim Khan
- Pawan Begani
- P Bhavani Kala
- Pijush Kanti Pal
- Piyush Kanti Ghosh
- Piyush Kherde
- Piyush Lodha
- PK Das
- PK Gantayat
- PK Patra
- PL Jani
- PMR Subudhi
- Pooja Motimath
- Pooja Pardhi
- Prabhat Agrawal
- Prabhat Soni
- Prabhu S Prabhu
- Pradeep Bhattacharya
- Pradeep C
- Pradeep Kumar
- Pradeep N Shantagiri
- Pradeep Patel
- Pradeep Sardar
- Pradip Bhattarcharya
- Pradip Ganguly
- Pradip Kumar Majumder
- Pradipta Mahapatra
- Pradnya Kamble
- Pradyot Kumar Tripathy
- Prafulla Bramhe
- Prafullata Patel
- Prafull Pande
- Praful Pagare
- Praful Pandit
- Prahlad Chawla
- Prakash Gada
- Prakash Gandhi
- Prakash Jambulkar
- Prakash Jhurani
- Prakash Kanade
- Prakash Patil
- Prakash Prabhudesai
- Prakash Raut
- Pramod Chirania
- Pramod D Paritekar
- Pramod Gangurde
- Pramod Hiremath
- Pramod Sibbal
- Prantick Bhunia
- Prasad Gaikwad
- Prasanna Kumar Gupta
- Prasanna Kumar Rathor
- Prasanna Kumar VM
- Prasanta Paul
- Prasanth Sankar
- Prashant Chaudhary
- Prashanth Kumar M
- Prashant Mahandule
- Prashant Natu
- Prashant Patil
- Prashant Rane
- Prasin Pradeep
- Pratap Jana
- Pratap Jethwani
- Pratap Mishra
- Pratim Roy
- Praveen Kumar
- Praveen Kumar Baghel
- Praveen Kumar GB
- Praveen Kumar Gupta
- Praveen Kumar Korde
- P Ravi Kumar
- Pravin Chavan
- Pravin Dungarwal
- Pravin Jain
- Pravin Rathi
- Preeti Gahlan
- Premananda Basak
- Premnaryan Vaish
- Pritam Narkhedkar
- Prithwijit Banerjee
- Prithy Bhama
- Priti Y Tandel
- Priya Bhate
- Priyadarshi Ghodke
- Priyanka Kukrele
- Priyank Jain
- Priya Ravi
- Promise Jain
- PS Chouhan
- P Sivram
- Puja Mahato
- Puneet Rijhwani
- Purneetha Singh
- Purnendu Kumar Behera
- Purvi Chawla
- Pushpashil Surlakar
- PV Swami
- Raghavan V
- Rahul Baste
- Rahul Jalgaonkar
- Rahul Maheshwari
- Rahul Patil
- Rahul Sathe
- Rahul Singh
- Rahul Sulakhe
- Rajanshu Tiwari
- Rajaprabhu Prabhu
- Rajashekar MB
- Rajdeep Saha
- Rajeev Goyal
- Rajendra Atre
- Rajendra Auti
- Rajendra Bhalode
- Rajendra Chowda
- Rajendra Dhawle
- Rajendra Gondhali
- Rajendran MK
- Rajendra Waghadkar
- Rajesh Balar
- Rajesh Binyala
- Rajesh Chavhan
- Rajesh Jain
- Rajesh Kesari
- Rajesh Kumar Tiwari
- Rajesh Maheshwari
- Rajesh Parvadiya
- Rajesh Singh
- Rajesh Singhal
- Rajiv Anand
- Rajiv Awasthi
- Rajiv Bankar
- Rajiv Chaudhary
- Rajiv Dhokiya
- Rajiv Verma
- Rajnish Saxena
- Rajshekar JV
- Raju Kanak
- Rajul Mesvani
- Raka Sheohare
- Rakesh Grover
- Rakesh Parikh
- Rakesh Patel
- Ramakrishnan
- Rama Murthy P

- Ramanai L
- Ramasamy Vijayakumar
- Rameez Athar Falke
- Ramen Sinharoy
- Ramesh Bhoi
- Ramesh Kapadia
- Ramesh Pandey
- Ramesh P Jain
- Ram Kishore Dixit
- Ramnath Raut
- Ramya Ramakrishnan
- Ranga Ranjan
- Ranjan Bhattacharya
- Ranjith V
- Ranjitsinh Rajput
- Rashmi Sinha
- Ratnabharati Singh
- Ravi K
- Ravi Kant Saraogi
- Ravinder Pash
- Ravindra Gaikwad
- Ravindra Modi
- Ravindranath Venkatesan
- Ravindran Ravindran
- Ravindra Pagare
- Ravindra Parmar
- Ravi Ramteke
- Ravi Sankar Reddy Janga
- Ravi Shinde
- Ravisuthan Kannan
- RC Gupta
- RD Anand
- Rekha Mane
- Rekha R
- Renukaprasad AR
- Reshma Kaushik
- Revathy Sathis
- Ricardo Teles
- Rikin M Shah
- RK Luthria
- RK Marya
- RL Tiwari
- R Manjunath
- Rohan Patil
- Rohit Kaku
- Rohit Kasat
- Rohit Singh Chadha
- RP Sharma
- RS Giri
- RS Jagat
- Rudrajit Pal
- Rudra Prasad Sahu
- Rupesh Agrawal
- Rupinder Kaur
- Rutul Gokalani
- R Vijaya Kumar
- Sabyasachi Mukherjee
- Sachin Bhandare
- Sachin Mutalik
- Sachin Puranik
- Sachin Shelke
- Sachin Shendge
- Sadanand Sawant
- Sadasivarao Yalamanchi
- Sadika Kapadwala
- Sagar Bhalchandra Patil
- Sagar Kamble
- Sagar Pogul
- Saikat Ghosh
- Sai Krishna
- Sailaja Sailaja
- Saiyadali Allisabanavar
- Sajad Qadir Bhat
- Sajid Ansari
- Sakshi Baizal
- Salil Patil
- Samarth Sangamesh
- Sambit Das
- Sameer Doshi
- Sameer Gupta
- Sameer Pekhale
- Samira Patel
- Samir Nayak
- Sampat Sawant
- Samuel Sathweek
- Sandeep Desai
- Sandeep Naik
- Sandeep Rayavarapu
- Sandeep Sanap
- Sandeep Suri
- Sandhya Gautam
- Sandip Chaudhari
- Sandip Shravasti
- Sandip Taraphdar
- Sandip Thorat
- Sangeeta Aher
- Sangita Ghanate
- Sanhita Walawalkar
- Sanjay Agarwal
- Sanjay Agrawal
- Sanjay Arora
- Sanjay Chinchole
- Sanjay Gandhi
- Sanjay Gulhane
- Sanjay Gupta
- Sanjay Kambar
- Sanjay K Diwan
- Sanjay Kumar Panda
- Sanjay Mane
- Sanjay Reddy
- Sanjay Shah
- Sanjay Warude
- Sanjay Zacharia
- Sanjib Lenka
- Sanjoy George
- Sannaullah Khan
- Santanu Banerjee
- Santhini Bishal
- Santosh Chandekar
- Santosh K Dheer
- Santosh Mote
- Saptarshi Mandal
- Saravanan Rajaram
- Saravanan Sivagnanam
- Sarfaraj Majid
- Sarfaraz Malik
- Sasikala Ramakrishnan
- Saswata Achrya
- Satish Chandra Joshi
- Satish Galhotra
- Satish Gupta
- Satish Kumar
- Satish Raikar
- Satish Rao
- Satis Lalit
- Satyabrata Bute
- Satyajeet Shirale
- Satyajit Maity
- Satyaki Roy
- Satya Ranjan Sethy
- Satyendra Kumar Sonkar
- Saurabh Srivastava
- SA Vaidya
- Sayan Chatterjee
- Seema Bagri
- Seema Jashnani
- Sekhar Mandal
- Selvaraj Durairaj
- Sendhil E Doctor
- Senthil Kumar
- Shachin Gupta
- Shailaja Kale
- Shailja Rao
- Shaji Khan
- Shalin Bharat Shah
- Shalini Santhos
- Shalin Shah
- Shankar Patil
- Shankar R Prasad
- Shantanu Nandi
- Shanti Ahir
- Sharad Dhawde
- Sharad Garg
- Sharad Tripathi
- Sharanbasu Diggi
- Sharath Kumar
- Shaumil Waghela
- Shawinder Bansal
- Shaymsundar Bajaj
- Sheetal Aversekar
- Sheetal Mehta
- Shefali Karkhanis
- Sheilja Sudhir Singh
- Sheshman Pandey
- Shiek Mohamed Riyaz
- Shiju SS
- Shikha Agrawal
- Shilpa Paranjape
- Shirish Dehankar
- Shital Rathod
- Shivam Talwar
- Shivani Sidana
- Shivendra Sinha
- Shiv Kumar

Acknowledgments

- Shivkumar Mishra
- Shivraj Uthnur
- Shobhit Shakya
- Shraddha Dhawale
- Shreyas Despande
- Shrikant Jategaonkar
- Shrikant Magar
- Shrikant Shinde
- Shrikant Thanedar
- Shrikant Wasavade
- Shrishail Kannure
- Shubhangi Ghule Khedkar
- Shubhangi Munoli
- Shubhda Garg
- Shunmugavelu Minakshisundaram
- Shyamal Kumar Hazra
- Sibaprakash Mukherjee
- Sibi NS
- Siddhardha Varma
- Siddhnath Shinde
- Sidhartha Dash
- Sidharth Bhalerao
- Simit Jadia
- Sirajunisha Fiaz
- Sirh Fiaz
- Sivaji Chatterjee
- Sivakumar Krishnamoorthy
- Sivaram R Konduru
- SK A Ahmad
- SK Babul
- SK Gautam
- SK Maity
- S Krishna Priya
- Smita Swami
- Snehal Doshi Madhekar
- Sneha Nikte
- Snehlata Verma
- Sobhan Biswas
- Soma Chakraborty
- Somnath Bhattacharya
- Somnath Gaikwad
- Somnath SM
- Soorneedi Krishna Kumar
- Soumyabrata Roy Chaudhuri
- Soumyaranjan Mohanty
- Sourabh Sethi
- Souvik Paul
- Souvik Saha
- SP Garg
- S Rajkumar
- Srinivas Nagaraj
- SR Josephine
- SS Maniyar
- Subhash Kumar
- Subhasis Ganguly
- Subhodip Pramanik
- Subir Ghosh
- Subir Swar
- Subrahmanyam RV
- Subrata Bhattacharya
- Subrata Chakraborty
- Suchir Khetrapal
- Sudhakar Manoharan
- Sudipta Kumar Dey
- Sugata Roy Chowdhury
- Suhas Mote
- Suhas Ranjan Mandal
- Sujata Khatal
- Sujay Kotpalliwar
- Sujit Kadam
- Sujoy Panchadhaye
- Suman Ramachandra
- Sumedh Dhuldhule
- Sumit Lavania
- Sumit Patra
- Sumit Shrivastav
- Sumon Ghosh
- Sundar Rao
- Suneel Bharadwaj
- Sunil Bakshi
- Sunil Bansal
- Sunil Bhojane
- Sunil Deshpande
- Sunil Gupta
- Sunil Kota
- Sunil Kulkarni
- Sunil Mundhe
- Sunil Shanbaug
- Sunil Sharma
- Sunil Shinde
- Suparna Nirgudkar
- Supriya Mani
- Supriya Patil
- Supriyo Pramanik
- Suraj Dhainje
- Surajeet Patra
- Surajit Banerjee
- Surajit Manna
- Surendranath Das
- Suresh Acharya
- Suresh Khatod
- Suresh Kore
- Suresh Kumar
- Suresh Kumar Bhagra
- Suresh Kumar Pichakacheri
- Suresh Purohit
- Suresh Singla
- Susanta Sengupta
- Sushant Yadav
- Sushila Gambhir
- Sushil Kumar Agarwal
- Sushil Kumar Chauhan
- Sushil Patel
- Sushil Saini
- Sushil Shinghavi
- Swapnil Bhawsar
- Swapnil Deshmukh
- Swapnil Lahole
- Swarna Khanra
- Swarna Walia
- Swarup Verma
- Swati Naik
- Swati Srivastava
- Swetabh Roy
- Sweta Sharma
- Taiyab Shaikh
- Tajinder Pal Singh
- Tamal Taru Adhikary
- Tamoghna Maiti
- Tanveer Akram
- Tapan Halder
- Tapobrata Chowdhury
- T Arun Kumar
- Tarun Nigam
- TC Raja Sakkarapani
- Teesta Shah
- Tejas Khopkar
- Tejpal Shah
- Thammegowda SK
- Thangavelu Easwaran
- Thirupathi Rao
- Tirthankar Chatterjee
- TK Gyanchandani
- Trilochan Barik
- T Sanath Kumar
- T Sivakumar Thiruvengadam
- Tushar Doshi
- Tushar Gaikwad
- Tushar Kanti
- Uday Karan Singh
- Uday Kshatriya
- Uddhav Khaire
- Udit Thakker
- Umashankar Mishra
- Umesh Kapuskar
- UP Gupta
- Uthra Subash Chandra Bose
- Utsav Sahu
- Uttam Biswas
- Uvaraj MG
- Vaibhavi Patil
- Vaibhav Nautiyal
- Vaijanath Swami
- Vaiyamalai S Doctor
- Vamsi Krishna Kedarisetti
- Vandana RK
- Vani G
- Varalakshmi Muthukrishnan
- Vasantlal Kasundra
- Vasant Mungara
- Vasundaradevi Ragu
- V Deepak Kumar
- Vella Visweswara Rao
- Venkateswarlu Tirunamalli
- Venkat Tadwalkar
- Verghese Cherian
- Vibhav Tiwari
- Vidya Bhosale
- Vidya Sagar Kulshrestha

- Vignesh Jayaprakash
- Vijaya Kumar P
- Vijay Baghel
- Vijay Chile
- Vijay Katekhaye
- Vijay Kumar
- Vijay Mandora
- Vijay Naik
- Vijay Viswanathan
- Vikas Goel
- Vikas Ratnaparkhi
- Vikas Srivastava
- Vikas Tajane
- Vikkarmaditya Shinde
- Vikram Khurud
- Vikrant Chouhan
- Vikrant Khullar
- Vilas Panchbhai
- Vimal Kabra
- Vinanti Pol
- Vinayak Hiremath
- Vinayak Khedkar
- Vinay Dhandhania
- Vinay Malavade
- Vineet Wankhede
- Vinod Kumar
- Vinod Mishra
- Vinod Mittal
- Vinod Pawar
- Vipin Mehra
- Vipul Boda
- Vipul Chavda
- Vipul Rastogi
- Virupakshi Kothiwale
- Vishal Chaudhari
- Vishal Chougale
- Vishal Dhakre
- Vishal Phade
- Vishav Bandhu Jindal
- Vishvesh Rothe
- Vitrag Shah
- Vitthal Mardolkar
- Vivechana GB
- Vivek Anand
- Vivekananda Reddy
- Vivek Bhalerao
- Vivek Patil
- V Manakavala Perumal
- VM Laxmi
- VP Anandan
- Vrind Bhardwaj
- V Sudarsan
- VVLN Rao
- VV Rama Kumar
- Yaqub Ali
- Yash Gosavi
- Yasir Husain
- Yoganand Tangaraj
- Yogen Thakkar
- Yogesh Dahifale
- Yogesh Shetye
- Yogesh Velaskar
- Yuraj Bende
- Zia Ul Haq
- Zuber Khan

CONTENTS

Chapter 1: **Epidemiology of Diabetic Foot Infections in India** — 1
Vijay Viswanathan, Sivashankari SelvaElavarasan

Chapter 2: **Save the Feet and Keep Walking Campaign by the RSSDI** — 6
Sanjay Agarwal, Ch Vasanth Kumar, Amit Gupta, Vijay Viswanathan

Annexure 1: Patient Registration Form — 9

Chapter 3: **Three-minute Foot Examination** — 11
RSSDI Diabetic Foot Task Force

Chapter 4: **Reduction of Lower Limb Amputations among People with Diabetes in India** — 14
Vijay Viswanathan

Chapter 5: **Management of Peripheral Artery Disease in Diabetes** — 17
R Ravikumar

Chapter 6: **Surgical Approach to the Management of Diabetic Foot Infections and Complex Diabetic Foot Wounds** — 24
Senthil Govindan

Chapter 7: **Angiosome Concept: The Basics for Every Diabetic Foot Care Specialist** — 38
Sivashankari SelvaElavarasan, R Ravikumar

Chapter 8: **An Insight into the Radio Imaging of Diabetic Foot Infection** — 50
Senthil Govindan, Sivashankari SelvaElavarasan, Vijay Viswanathan

Chapter 9: **The Indispensable Role of Orthotics in the Prevention and Management of Diabetic Foot** — 61
Sivashankari SelvaElavarasan, Bamila Selvaraj, Seena Rajsekar, Vijay Viswanathan

Chapter 10: **Wound Dressings in the Management of Diabetic Foot Infections** — 68
Senthil Govindan, Vijay Viswanathan

Chapter 11: **Peripheral Arterial Disease and Diabetic Foot: Clinical Cases and Management Strategies** — 76
Vibhakar R Vachhrajani, Ashu Rastogi

Chapter 12: **Charcot Neuroarthropathy of the Foot** — 83
Jayaditya Ghosh, Ashu Rastogi

Chapter 13: **Infected Diabetic Foot Ulcer: Case Scenario and Management Considerations** — 90
Manisha Singh Jadaun

Chapter 14: **Imaging of Diabetic Foot** — 106
Ragghuraman Soundararajan, Ashu Rastogi

Common Diabetic Foot Problems Encountered 113

1. Gangrene *113*
2. Small Muscle Atrophy *113*
3. Callus *114*
4. Dry Feet with Fissure *114*
5. Charcot Neuroarthropathy *115*
6. Swelling of the Feet and Ankle *115*
7. Curved Corners of the Toenail *116*
8. Hallux Valgus Deformity *116*
9. Flatfoot *117*
10. Onychomycosis *117*
11. Toe Rings *118*
12. Clawing of Toenails *118*
13. Below-Knee Amputation *119*
14. Foot Examination in a Person with Diabetes *119*
15. Great Toe Amputee *120*
16. Intertrigo *120*
17. Healing of the Stump Wound *121*
18. Offloading of Foot Ulcer by Felted Foam Dressing *121*
19. Improper Footwear *122*
20. Diabetic Neuropathy *122*
21. Plantar Psoriasis *123*
22. Screening for Sensory Loss with 10 g Monofilament *123*
23. Ankle Callosity and Hyperkeratosis *124*
24. Eschar *124*
25. Hallux Varus *125*
26. Cellulitis with Blister *125*
27. Ankle-brachial Pressure Index Testing *126*
28. Probe-to-bone Test *126*
29. Ingrowing Toenails *127*
30. Offloading of Heel Ulcer *127*
31. Varicose Veins *128*
32. Pitting Edema *128*
33. Classification of Ulcer on the Basis of Depth *129*
34. Negative Pressure Wound Therapy *129*
35. Hyperbaric Oxygen Therapy *130*
36. SINBAD Classification *130*

37. Dry Skin *131*
38. Onychauxis *131*
39. Wet Gangrene *132*
40. Body and Mind *132*
41. Offloading for Charcot Foot *133*
42. Biofilm *133*
43. Slough *134*
44. Granulation Tissue *134*
45. Importance of Vascular Assessment *135*
46. Skin Grafts *135*
47. Necrotizing Fasciitis *136*
48. Toenail Injury *136*
49. Osteomyelitis *137*
50. Eczema *137*
51. Cracked Heels *138*
52. Amputation of Foot *138*
53. Bilateral Great Toe Amputee *139*
54. Maceration of Feet Due to Keeping the Feet Wet for a Long Time *139*
55. After Removing the Macerated Skin *140*
56. Angiosome *140*
57. Partial Gangrene of the Toe *141*
58. Cellulitis of Left Leg *141*
59. Recurrent Pressure Ulcers *142*
60. Self-treated Callus *142*
61. Abscess in the Right Leg with Typical Neuropathic Feet *143*
62. Hammer Toes *143*
63. Unilateral Pedal Edema *144*
64. Diabetic Dermopathy *144*
65. Diabetic Foot Infection *145*
66. Prick Injury *145*
67. Callus Debridement *146*
68. Callus in the Forefoot *146*
69. Wound with Healthy Granulation Tissue *147*
70. Diabetic Foot Ulcer in the Heel Region—Heel Wounds are Difficult to Heal *147*
71. Sausage Toe/Dactylitis *148*
72. Amputation of Second, Third, and Fourth Toes on the Right Foot *148*
73. Loss of Skin Elasticity in Autonomic Neuropathy *149*

74. Diabetic Foot Ulcer on the Medial Aspect 149
75. Diabetic Ulcer in the Forefoot Region 150
76. Foot Examination using A Biothesiometer 150
77. Skin Lesions on the Plantar Aspect of the Foot 151
78. Interdigital Infections 151
79. Plantar Foot Ulceration in a Person with Deformities 152
80. Treatment of Cellulitis 152
81. Importance of Foot Exercises in Diabetic Neuropathy 153
82. Recurrent Pressure Ulcer after Amputation 153
83. Left Foot Charcot with an Ulcer 154
84. Intertrigo 154
85. Skin Diseases in the Feet Like Psoriasis 155
86. Exostectomy (Resection of Bony Protrusion) 155
87. Right Foot Infection from the Stump of the Great Toe up to the Heel 156
88. Bilateral Bunion 156
89. Heel Ulcer Over Tendon Achilles 157
90. Pus Discharge from Abscess Over the Lateral Malleolus 157
91. Friction Blister 158
92. Monofilament 158
93. Ulcer Over the Base of the Great Toe 159
94. Deformed Nails in Fungal Infection 159
95. Examination of Peripheral Pulses 160
96. Ischemic Wound of the Forefoot with Extensive Necrosis or Gangrene 160
97. Clawing of Toes 161
98. Middle Toe Amputee with an Ulcer Over the Dorsum of the Foot 161
99. Skin Prone to Infection Due to Aging 162
100. Midfoot Infected Callus 162

Index **163**

Epidemiology of Diabetic Foot Infections in India

Vijay Viswanathan, Sivashankari SelvaElavarasan

INTRODUCTION

Diabetes mellitus is a serious and debilitating condition worldwide and is also considered a global epidemic of the 21st century. The incidence of diabetic foot infections (DFI) has increased due to the extensive prevalence of diabetes throughout the world and the prolonged life expectancy of these patients, which in turn, increases the burden of the disease. DFI is one of the most common causes of hospitalization and lower extremity amputation (LEA) contributing to significant morbidity and mortality.

EPIDEMIOLOGY OF DIABETES

According to the International Diabetes Federation (IDF), 537 million people worldwide aged between 20 and 79 years are affected by diabetes mellitus and it is also estimated that there will be more than 700 million people affected globally by the disease by the year 2045. With the world's population expected to increase by 20%, the number of people living with diabetes is also expected to increase by 46%.[1] These numbers are more likely to multiply rapidly, especially in developing countries like India. India is considered the diabetes capital of the world with the largest number of people living with diabetes. Unfortunately, the burden of the disease is going to increase due to the increase in the prevalence of obesity, the exponential increase in population size, and the recent trends in lifestyle modifications as well as urbanization.[2] This, in turn, will have a significant socioeconomic impact both on the individuals as well as our nation.

PREVALENCE OF DIABETES IN SOUTHEAST ASIA

The IDF estimates that the total number of people living with diabetes in the Southeast Asian region will reach 152 million by the year 2045. India accounts for one in seven adults living worldwide with diabetes. Over one in two (50.2%) adults living with diabetes are undiagnosed. The total number of deaths reported was 747,000.[3] The age-adjusted prevalence for people living with diabetes in the age group of 20–79 years was estimated for the countries in the Southeast Asian region, which was found to be approximately around 10% in India (**Fig. 1**).[3] India is one of the leading countries in terms of population affected by diabetes in the age group of 20–79 years, which is around 74.2 million in 2021 when compared to 61.3 million in 2011 (**Table 1**).[3] The prevalence of diabetes was also found to be higher in the age group of 45–79 years in Southeast Asian region (**Fig. 2**).[3]

EPIDEMIOLOGY OF DIABETIC FOOT INFECTIONS WORLDWIDE

It is estimated that people with diabetes have a 40% increased risk for LEA and the lifetime risk of developing diabetic foot ulcer (DFU) appears to be around 25%.[2] Around 67% of amputations in the United States and 90% of amputations in the United Kingdom that occur annually are found to be associated with diabetes.[3] The highest and lowest prevalence of DFU was found in Belgium (16%) and Australia (1.2%), respectively. The overall prevalence of DFU worldwide was found to be 6.3%. Globally, the risk of recurrence of DFU is around 50% and it is also projected that 33% of all the expenses related to diabetes are due to DFI.[4]

In high and middle-income countries worldwide, there is an exponential increase in DFU-related expenditure due to advances in treatment options and resources available to them. However, developing countries like India and China are more likely to spend less when compared to developed countries due to treatment with antibiotics and inaccessibility to novel technology for limb salvage procedures. Developed countries spend 10% of their gross domestic product (GDP) for healthcare expenditure when

2 Epidemiology of Diabetic Foot Infections in India

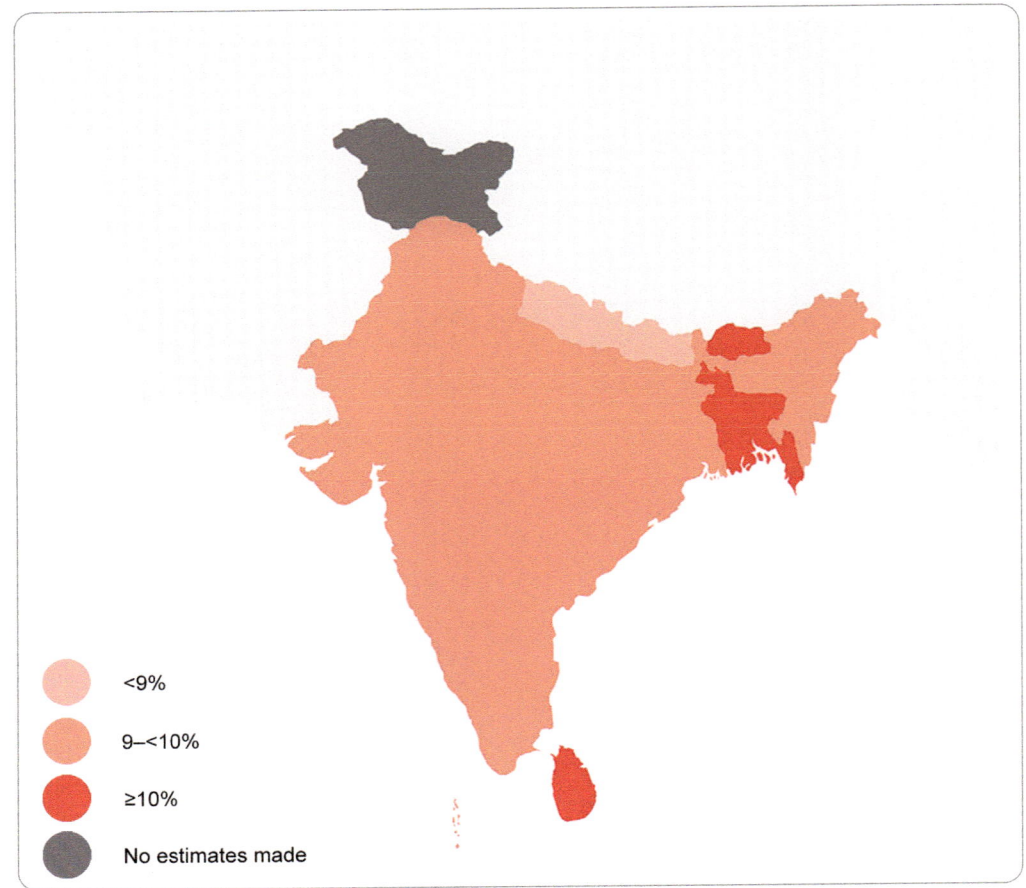

Fig. 1: The age-adjusted comparative prevalence (%) of diabetes (20–79 years) in the International Diabetes Federation (IDF) Southeast Asia Region in 2021.[3]

TABLE 1: The top five countries in Southeast Asia for people living with diabetes (20–79 years).[3]		
Country	2011	2021
India	61.3 million	74.2 million
Bangladesh	8.4 million	13.1 million
Sri Lanka	1.1 million	1.4 million
Nepal	488,200	1.1 million
Mauritius	138,200	250,400

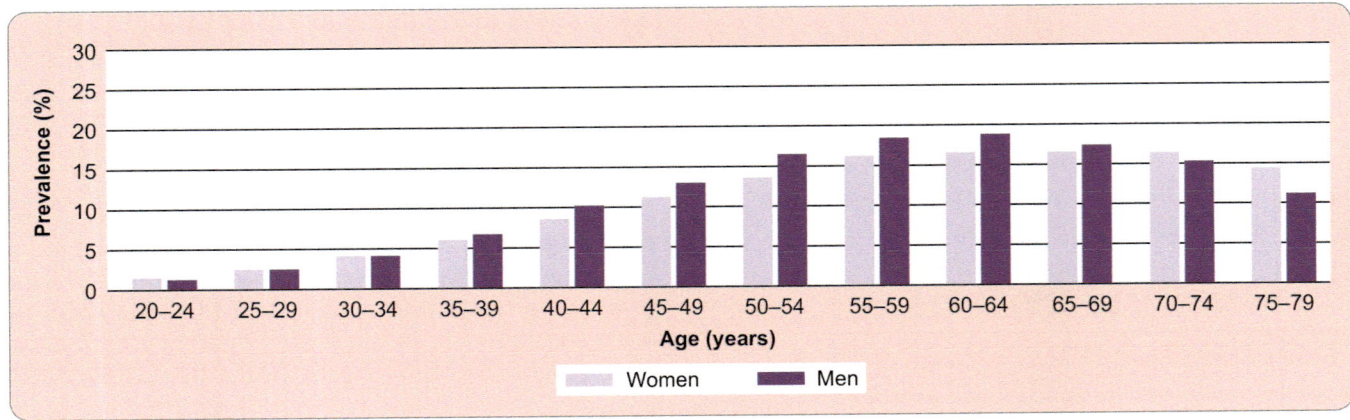

Fig. 2: Prevalence (%) estimates of diabetes by age and sex, International Diabetes Federation (IDF) Southeast Asia region in 2021.[3]

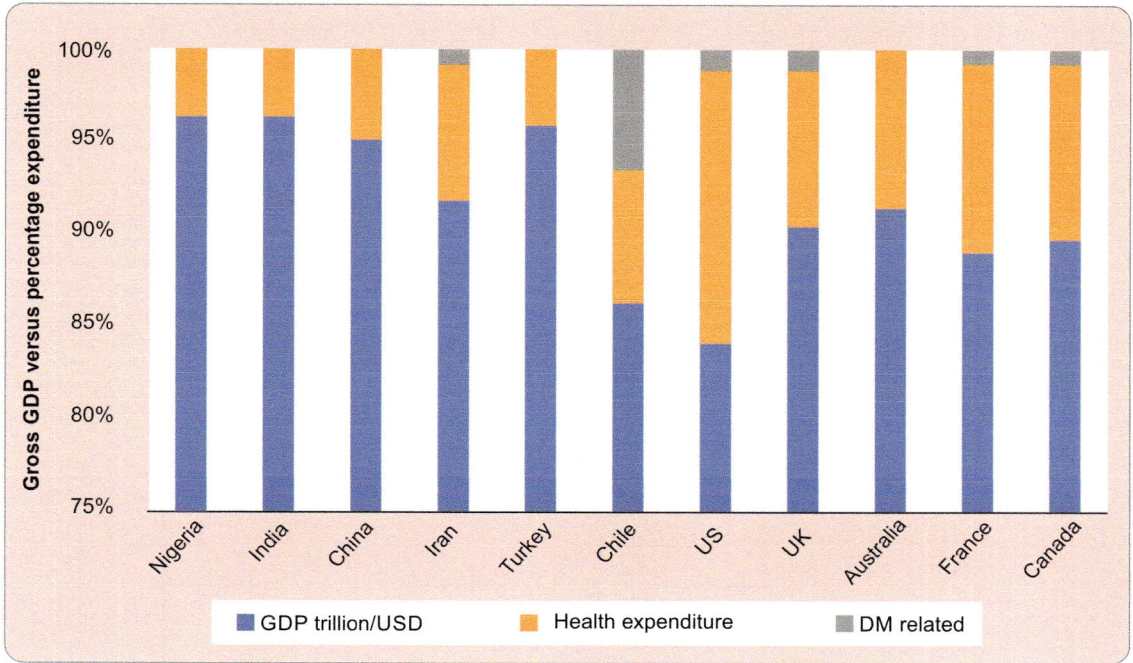

Fig. 3: Country-based comparison of diabetes-related expenditure (2016–2017).[4]
(DM: diabetes mellitus; GDP: gross domestic product)

compared to poorly developed or developing countries who spend less than 6% **(Fig. 3)**.[4]

EPIDEMIOLOGY OF DIABETIC FOOT INFECTIONS IN INDIA

In developing countries like India, diabetes mellitus is associated with high rates of mortality and morbidity as well as macrovascular and microvascular complications. In a study by Vijay et al., the prevalence of DFI was found to be between 6 and 11% in India and neuropathy was recognized as the predominant factor causing DFI.[5] In another study from North India, the prevalence of DFI was reported to be between 12.6 and 31.6% with one-third of patients with peripheral neuropathy, two-thirds of patients "at-risk" for foot ulcers and 9% had prevalent ulcers of which 20.2% required amputation.[6] Among the newly diagnosed cases of diabetes, the prevalence of DFI was found to be between 3 and 4.5% and this could be attributed to the reporting younger age, and shorter duration of diabetes among the Indian population.[7] In a study by Viswanathan et al., on the prevalence of diabetic foot complications, it was estimated that that infection was the major reason for amputation. Major amputation was done in 29.1% and minor amputation in 70% of the total amputations.[8] Moreover, it is also estimated that around 50% of diabetic patients with DFU, who get amputated once, are susceptible to another amputation in consecutive years.

In India, DFU affects 15% of diabetic patients in their entire lifespan. It is also found that DFU is seen in 25% of all adults living with diabetes in India with 50% of them requiring hospitalization and 20% of them requiring amputation. It is alarming to understand that DFUs are responsible for 80% of all nontraumatic amputations in India every year and patients with a history of DFU have a 40% higher 10-year death rate than those without the complication.[9] India is also considered the most expensive country in terms of care related to DFU because we spend 5.7 years of an average's patient income for its complete treatment. Two studies (Satyavani et al. and Shobhana et al.) are suggestive of the same idea that patients with DFU spend four times more than those without complications.[10,11] The lifetime risk of a diabetic person with a foot infection is as high as 25% which, in turn, contributes to 20% of the total healthcare costs that are spent for diabetes. In a developing nation like India, it puts a heavy burden on the shoulders of healthcare professionals and educators for its effective management.

RISK FACTORS FOR FOOT INFECTION

The pathophysiological process of DFI usually arises as a combination of several risk factors, which can be classified into first-degree, second-degree, and third-degree risk factors, as shown in **Table 2**.[12]

Neuropathy is a major risk factor responsible for DFI in 50% of cases, peripheral arterial occlusive disease is seen in 15% of cases, and in 35% of cases, it is a combination of both neuropathy and angiopathy, which seem to play a pivotal role in DFI.[12] This is in accordance with a multicentric study across India by Vijay et al., which states that the prevalence of neuropathy was 65% and that of peripheral vascular disease (PVD) was 35%.[8] Similarly, in a study from South India it is apparent that peripheral neuropathy is seen in

TABLE 2: Risk factors of diabetic foot ulceration.[12]	
First-degree risk factors	• Presence of sensorimotor polyneuropathy • History of previous ulcers • Age of the patient
Second-degree risk factors	• Peripheral arterial occlusive disease (PAOD) • Structural deformities in the skeleton of the foot

Third-degree risk factors	• Duration of diabetes
	• Male gender
	• Late complications of diabetes mellitus:
	  ○ Retinopathy
	  ○ Nephropathy

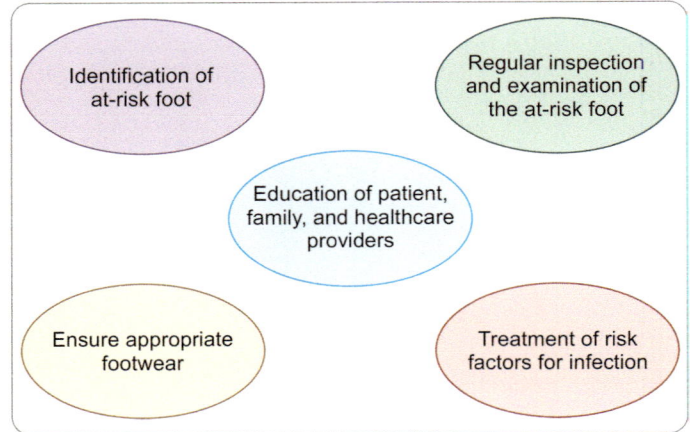

Fig. 4: The five cornerstones for prevention of diabetic foot infections (DFI) based on International Working Group on the Diabetic Foot (IWGDF) guidelines 2019.[18]

49.5% of cases and nonhealing ulcers in 41.51% of patients with DFI.[13] In another multicentric study by Vijay et al., the prevalence of neuropathy was found to be higher among southern Indians (15%) than northern Indians (9%).[5] It becomes imperative to assess patients for DFI and treat them appropriately because DFI in India are the second most common reason for infection-related mortality in hospitalized patients.[14] In a prospective study by Ashu et al., it is established that people with diabetes in India are at five times higher risk for mortality after the occurrence of DFU than those without foot infections. The 5-year mortality rate after a neuropathic DFU in this study was found to be 22% and limb amputation following the foot ulcer was considered to be the most important predictor for subsequent mortality.[15]

Improper footwear, lack of footwear, and burns were found to be the primary precipitating factors for foot infections in India.[16] High barefoot pressure can be linked to ulceration, which is evident in a South Indian study for diabetic patients where a higher F/R ratio (Forefoot pressure/Rearfoot pressure) was found to be associated with neuropathy, limited joint mobility, and ulceration.[17]

STRATEGIES TO MANAGE DIABETIC FOOT INFECTION

A multidisciplinary approach is required to prevent as well as treat patients with DFI. In a resource-constraint country like India, a thorough history and clinical examination need to be done to assess the severity of any potential DFI.

An initial relevant antibiotic regimen must be chosen based on the patient's severity of the foot infection, which should be modified later to a more specific therapy after tissue culture and antibiotic sensitivity reports.[14]

The microbial profiles from DFI showed a high prevalence of gram-negative bacteria. In a study by Viswanathan et al., among the aerobes causing DFI, it was found that the Enterobacteriaceae family was the most prominent (48%) followed by *Staphylococcus* (18.2%), *Streptococcus* (16.8%), and *Pseudomonas* (17%). Among anaerobes, *Peptostreptococcus* and *Clostridium* (69.4%) and gram-negative anaerobes like *Bactericides* and *Fusobacterium* (30.6%) were present among people with DFI. The most important inference was that the healing times were longer when the strict aerobic pathogen *Pseudomonas* and strict anaerobic pathogens were present.[2]

The five key elements for the prevention of DFI based on International Working Group on the Diabetic Foot (IWGDF) guidelines are given in **Figure 4**.[18]

CONCLUSION

It is imperative to understand that diabetes in India is rampantly increasing along with the population and DFI also seems to be a very important complication that puts a huge economic burden, which in turn affects the quality of life of patients. Regular screening along with effective strategies plays a very significant role in preventing as well as managing DFI in India.

TAKE-HOME MESSAGE
There is a need to promote awareness about diabetic foot infections and also implement strategies to reduce the burden of diabetic foot and its associated complications in India.

REFERENCES

1. International Diabetes Federation. (2021). IDF Diabetes Atlas, 10th edition.. [online] Available from https://www.diabetesatlas.org [Last accessed March, 2023].
2. Viswanathan V. Epidemiology of Diabetic Foot and Management of Foot Problems in India. Int J Low Extrem Wounds. 2010;9(3):122-6.
3. Magliano DJ, Boyko EJ; IDF Diabetes Atlas 10th edition Scientific Committee. IDF Diabetes Atlas [Internet]. 10th edition. Brussels: International Diabetes Federation; 2021. Chapter 5: Diabetes by region. [online] Available from https://www.ncbi.nlm.nih.gov/books/NBK581937/ [Last accessed March, 2023].
4. Jodheea-Jutton A, Hindocha S, Bhaw-Luximon A. Health economics of diabetic foot ulcer and recent trends to accelerate treatment. Foot (Edinb). 2022;52:101909.
5. Viswanathan V, Thomas N, Tandon N, Asirvatham A, Rajasekar S, Ramachandran A, et al. Profile of diabetic foot complications and its associated complications: a multicentric study from India. J Assoc Physicians India. 2005;53:933-6.
6. Jayaprakash P, Bhansali S, Bhansali A, Dutta P, Ananthraman R. Magnitude of foot problems in diabetes in the developing world: a study of 1044 patients. Diab Med. 2009;26(9):939-42.
7. Sinahary K, Paul UK, Bhattacharyya AK, Pal SK. Prevalence of diabetic foot ulcers in newly diagnosed diabetes mellitus patients. J Indian Med Assoc. 2012;110(9):608-11.
8. Vishwanathan V, Kumpatla S. Pattern and causes of amputation in diabetic patients – A multicentric study from India. J Assoc Phys India. 2011;59:148-51.
9. Ghosh P, Valia R. Burden of Diabetic Foot Ulcers in India: Evidence Landscape from Published Literature. Value in Health. 2017;20(9):A485.
10. Kumpatla S, Kothandan H, Tharkar S, Viswanathan V. The costs of treating long-term diabetic complications in a developing country: a study from India. J Assoc Physicians India. 2013;61(2):102-9.
11. Shobhana R, Rao PR, Lavanya A, Vijay V, Ramachandran A. Cost burden to diabetic patients with foot complications--a study from southern India. J Assoc Physicians India. 2000;48(12):1147-50.
12. Volmer-Thole M, Lobmann R. Neuropathy and Diabetic Foot Syndrome. Int J Mol Sci. 2016;17(6):917.
13. Jyothylekshmy V, Menon AS, Abraham S. Epidemiology of diabetic foot complications in a podiatry clinic of a tertiary hospital in South India. Indian J Health Sci Biomed Res. 2015;8(1):48-51.
14. Rastogi A, Bhansali A. Diabetic Foot Infection: An Indian Scenario. J Foot Ankle Surg Asia-Pacific. 2016;3(2):71-9.
15. Rastogi A, Goyal G, Kesavan R, Bal A, Kumar H, Mangalanadanam, et al. Long-term outcomes after incident diabetic foot ulcer: Multi-center large cohort prospective study (EDI-FOCUS investigators) epidemiology of diabetic foot complications study: Epidemiology of diabetic foot complications study. Diabetes Res Clin Pract. 2020;162:108113.
16. Morbach S, Lutalet JK, Viswanathan V, Möllenberg J, Ochs HR, Rajashekar S, et.al. Regional differences in risk factors and clinical presentation of diabetic foot lesions. Diabet Med. 2004;21(1):91-5.
17. Viswanathan V, Sivagami M, Seena R, Snehalatha C, Ramachandran A, Veves A. Increased forefoot to rearfoot plantar pressure ratio in South Indian patients with diabetic foot ulceration. Diabet Med. 2004;21:396-7.
18. Bus SA, Lavery LA, Monteiro-Soares M, Rasmussen A, Raspovic A, Sacco ICN, et al.; International Working Group on the Diabetic Foot. Guidelines on the prevention of foot ulcers in persons with diabetes (IWGDF 2019 update). Diabetes Metab Res Rev. 2020;36 Suppl 1:e3269.

Save the Feet and Keep Walking Campaign by the RSSDI

Sanjay Agarwal, Ch Vasanth Kumar, Amit Gupta, Vijay Viswanathan

INTRODUCTION

Diabetes mellitus is a chronic metabolic condition due to increased blood glucose levels with significant microvascular as well as macrovascular complications. India is often considered "The Diabetes Capital of the World" due to the alarming increase in the number of patients living with diabetes along with the rapidly increasing size of the population. Diabetes is also considered one of the four noncommunicable diseases targeted for prevention and control by leaders across the world. According to International Diabetes Federation (2021), diabetes is found to be associated with 745,000 deaths, and approximately 1 in 11 individuals (around 90 million) were found to be associated with diabetes in the South-East Asian region.[1]

BURDEN OF THE DISEASE

Diabetes is associated with severe complications, which can affect the heart, eyes, kidneys, as well as feet. These complications when not treated appropriately can lead to an increase in mortality rate and can put a huge burden on the patient as well as the healthcare professionals. In India, we face numerous challenges such as lack of awareness among the people and a lack of access to basic healthcare facilities for the management of diabetes and its complications. One of the most important complications is diabetic foot infection (DFI), which when left untreated can result in amputations or sometimes even death.

DIABETIC FOOT INFECTIONS AND THEIR RISK FACTORS

Neuropathy, vasculopathy, and immunopathy are considered three important reasons for developing DFI. Peripheral neuropathy is one of the major predisposing factors involved in the pathogenesis of diabetic foot. Diabetic angiopathy is a predominant reason for mortality and morbidity in patients with diabetes. A patient's innate susceptibility to infection and inflammation (immunopathy) also plays a pivotal role because people with diabetes have poor tolerance to infection which, in turn, can have an unfavorable effect on the glycemic control of the patient.[2] The various risk factors associated with DFI are the age of the patient, duration of diabetes, any history of foot ulcers, structural foot deformities, smoking, poor socioeconomic status, and other systemic conditions such as poor glycemic control, nephropathy, retinopathy, and peripheral vascular disease (PVD).[3]

Management of these risk factors requires a multidisciplinary and systematic approach to treat them effectively, to reduce the rate of amputations as well as deaths related to DFI, and to educate the patients to promote lifestyle modifications regarding glycemic control and self-foot care practices. This requires the immense support of organizations such as Research Society for the Study of Diabetes in India (RSSDI), which can help us to tackle the burden of the disease.

RESEARCH SOCIETY FOR THE STUDY OF DIABETES IN INDIA

The RSSDI was founded by Professor MMS Ahuja in 1972. It is the largest body of professional doctors and researchers in Asia, working in the area of diabetes and is the National Body recognized by IDF currently with around 8,054 life members from 21 Indian States and Union Territories.

The RSSDI has been conducting and promoting research related to diabetes in India which, in turn, helps in the effective prevention and management of the disease. Apart from facilitating research at the national level, the RSSDI also encourages the promotion of various research activities related to diabetes and organizes awareness programs for people living with diabetes at state-level chapters also. The

RSSDI has accredited 22 institutions until now for pursuing certificate courses in diabetology across India.[4]

The RSSDI has been supporting several state-level chapters since 2003, which are considered regional wings of RSSDI to conduct and promote educational and awareness programs among the people to prevent and effectively manage diabetes. This includes conducting several continuing medical education (CME) programs for physicians for enhanced comprehension of diabetes and its complications. The RSSDI also encourages research scholars to develop new ideas and implement them which, in turn, can help us in developing novel strategies for the appropriate management of diabetes. It provides numerous research grants and also accepts proposals from budding scientists to promote original research related to diabetes in India. It also emphasizes the need to develop several trained Health Care Personnel (HCP) who can help reduce the burden of this disease and its complications.

The RSSDI had also initiated an effective Learning Management Program, which comprised excellent courses under the able leadership of prominent senior diabetologists across India for the benefit of healthcare professionals. Digital workshops were conducted in 2020 and 2021 for doctors to enhance the knowledge and standard of treatment for type 1 diabetes mellitus. This helped to create a better apprehension of the updated technology in diabetes and enabled them to train district coordinators who are ultimately responsible for the execution of the ideas and guidelines.

In 2021, RSSDI launched the *Defeat Diabetes Campaign* with the key message of *"Test, Track, and Treat"* with a wonderful objective of reaching out to 100 million people in 100 days. This campaign was an extraordinary accomplishment as the RSSDI received The Asia Book of Records certificate for screening 106 million people in more than 10,000 locations all over India.[5]

In 2022, RSSDI initiated the *"Save the Feet and Keep Walking Campaign"* to examine patients, stratify them based on risk, as well as promote awareness about the prevention and management of DFIs.

SAVE THE FEET AND KEEP WALKING CAMPAIGN

A larger campaign was organized by the National RSSDI among its members mainly to create awareness of diabetic foot problems and also to determine the prevalence of high-risk feet [loss of protective sensation (LOPS)] among people with diabetes.

The diabetic foot screening camps were conducted across 29 states of India covering 10,000 clinics. People with diabetes who visited the outpatient department of these clinics from 10th July 2022 to 10th August 2022 were screened for high-risk diabetic foot **(Fig. 1)**. A three-minute foot examination tool (please refer to Chapter 4) was prepared and shared with the RSSDI members to identify the foot at high risk of amputation. A validated

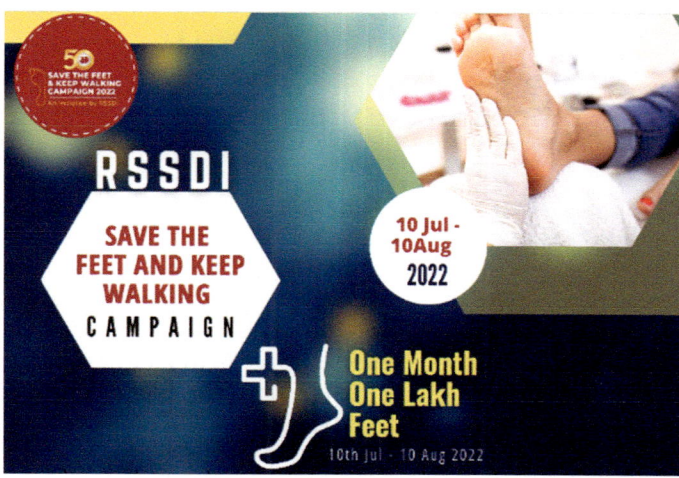

Fig. 1: The pamphlet designed for the "Save the Feet and Keep Walking Campaign" program organized by Research Society for the Study of Diabetes in India (RSSDI).

monofilament for the detection of LOPS was provided to all the members as part of the three-minute foot examination and also a video was shared with them demonstrating the foot examination. The RSSDI also conducted several online training programs for its members so that the diabetic foot examination will be standardized across India. Around 54,000 people with diabetes participated in the screening across the clinics in India.

A questionnaire for foot examination was prepared to standardize the procedure all over India, which is as follows: (Refer to **Annexure 1** for the questionnaire).

The examiner enquired the patient about a history of foot ulcers, lower limb amputation due to diabetes, and any burning or tingling sensation or numbness and pain while walking. A thorough examination of the toe's nails was done to report any discolored, disfigured, or ingrowing nails. It included inspection for any hardened skin, callus, or corns in the feet, especially on the plantar aspect, or any signs of fungal infections between the toes. Open wounds, heel fissures, signs of cellulitis, and a decrease in hair growth on the feet were also noted. A detailed record of the deformities in the feet which could be minor deformities like claw toes or major ones like Charcot's foot was also maintained. The dorsalis pedis and posterior tibial arterial pulses were also palpated and the findings were recorded.

The patient also underwent a 10-g monofilament test to detect diabetic neuropathy. It was decided to assign points to the patients based on the findings. Finally, we arrived at a diagnosis of high-risk feet if there was a positive answer to all the above mentioned questions.

IMPORTANCE OF SELECTING DIABETIC FOOT

One of the most common complications and one of the most important causes of hospitalization among people living with diabetes in India is DFI. Inappropriate treatment can lead to septic gangrene, amputations, and sometimes even death. A stepwise multipronged approach is, thus, advised for treating DFI.[6] In a study by Armstrong et al., it was observed that noncompliant patients were 54% more likely to develop foot ulcers and 20 times more liable to undergo amputations than compliant patients.[7] In India, due to practices like walking barefoot, poor diabetic care facilities, and low socioeconomic status, the magnitude of the problem has increased rampantly.[8] In a study by Viswanathan et al., it was found that infection was the major reason for amputations in India.[9] In another multicentric study, it was found that appropriate foot care practices were found to be lacking in 65% of patients, which was also considered one of the predominant reasons for the development of foot infections.[10] Intensive counseling and education on foot care practices were found to create a positive impact on decreasing the number of amputations.[11] A patient with DFI should be evaluated using the three most important criteria, namely assessing the extent and severity of infection, recognizing the risk factors that can promote infection, and interpreting the microbiological culture report and treating patients accordingly.[12]

CONCLUSION

Prevention of DFIs could be very challenging because it involves a complete evaluation of the patient's history along with comprehensive foot examination and intensive education about appropriate foot care. Thus, the "*Save the Feet and Keep Walking Campaign*" initiated by the RSSDI is a novel strategy initiated for the effective prevention of DFIs in India.

TAKE-HOME MESSAGE

Prevention and management of DFI require the implementation of new ideas and initiatives to create more awareness among the people and also provide adequate training among healthcare professionals to identify, stratify, and appropriately manage patients with DFI.

ACKNOWLEDGMENTS

We would like to acknowledge **Mr Mayank**, National Secretariat who helped us with data collection and in the preparation of the link. We would also like to acknowledge **Dr Sivashankari SelvaElavarasan** for the editorial support provided.

REFERENCES

1. International Diabetes Federation. (2021). IDF Diabetes Atlas, 10th edition. [online] Available from https://www.diabetesatlas.org [Last accessed April, 2023].
2. Hobizal KB, Wukich DK. Diabetic foot infections: current concept review. Diabetic Foot Ankle. 2012;3.
3. Sharma R, Kapila R, Sharma AK, Mann J. Diabetic Foot Disease—Incidence and Risk Factors: A Clinical Study. J Foot Ankle Surg (Asia-Pacific). 2016;3(1):41-6.
4. RSSDI [Online]Available from https://www.rssdi.in/newwebsite/page.php {Last accessed April, 2023}
5. IDF South-East Asia. [online] Available from https://idf.org/our-network/regions-members/south-east-asia/welcome.html [Last accessed April, 2023].
6. Armstrong DG, Lipsky BA. Diabetic foot infections: stepwise medical and surgical management. Int Wound J. 2004;1(2):123-32.
7. Armstrong DG, Harkless LB. Outcomes of preventative care in a diabetic foot specialty clinic. J Foot Ankle Surg. 1998;37(6):460-6.
8. Viswanathan V, Rao VN. Managing diabetic foot infection in India. Int J Low Extrem Wounds. 2013;12(2):158-66.
9. Viswanathan V. The diabetic foot: Perspectives from Chennai, south India. Int J Lower Extrem Wounds. 2007;6:34-6.
10. Viswanathan V, Thomas N, Tandon N, Asirvatham A, Rajasekar S, Ramachandran A, et al. Profile of diabetic foot complications and its associated complications: a multicentric study from India. J Assoc Physicians India. 2005;53:933-6.
11. Viswanathan V, Sivagami M, Seena R, Snehalatha C, Ramachandran A. Amputation prevention initiative in south India: Positive impact of foot care education. Diabetes Care. 2005;28:1019-21.
12. Oliver TI, Mutluoglu M. Diabetic Foot Ulcer. In: StatPearls [Internet]. Treasure Island (FL): StatPearls Publishing; 2023. [online] Available from https://www.ncbi.nlm.nih.gov/books/NBK537328/ [Last accessed April, 2023].

ANNEXURE 1

Patient Registration Form

Patient Address*	
Patient Age*	
Gender*	Male ☐ Female ☐ Other ☐
Type of Diabetes	Type 2 ☐ Type 1 ☐ Other ☐
Duration of Diabetes	Less than 1 year ☐ 1-5 years ☐ 5-10 years ☐ More than 10 years
Level of HbA1c% (if tested within 3 months)	
Random Blood Sugar (mg/dL)	
Fasting Blood Sugar (mg/dL)	
Postprandial Blood Sugar (mg/dL) (2 hours after meals)	
Does the patients have a history of	
A. Leg/Foot Ulcer	☐ Yes ☐ No
B. Lower Limb Amputation or Surgery	☐ Yes ☐ No
C. Lower limb Angioplasty/ Stent or Surgery	☐ Yes ☐ No
D. Other diabetic complications-renal (dialysis/transplant):	☐ Yes ☐ No
Retinal (visual impairment):	☐ Yes ☐ No ☐ Not tested
Smoking Habit	☐ Yes ☐ No If Yes, Current ☐ Smoker ☐ Ex-Smoker
Do you have burning or tingling sensation in feet or leg?	☐ Yes ☐ No
Does your leg or foot pain while walking?	☐ Yes ☐ No
Are there changes in skin color or skin lesions?	☐ Yes ☐ No
Is there any loss of lower extremity sensation in the leg or foot?	☐ Yes ☐ No
Dermatologic Exam	
Does the patient have discolored, ingrown, or elongated nails?	☐ Yes ☐ No
Are there signs of fungal infection especially in between the toes?	☐ Yes ☐ No
Does the patient have discolored and or hypertrophic skin lesions, calluses, or corns?	☐ Yes ☐ No
Does the patient has open wound or heel fissure?	☐ Yes ☐ No
Is there any warmth/swelling/redness in the foot which is suggestive of cellulitis?	☐ Yes ☐ No
Neurologic Exam	
Is the patient responsive to 10 g monofilament?	☐ Yes ☐ No
Left foot (A, B, C points marked on foot diagram)	A: ☐ Yes ☐ No
	B: ☐ Yes ☐ No
	C: ☐ Yes ☐ No

10 Save the Feet and Keep Walking Campaign by the RSSDI

Right foot (A at big toe, B and C on sole)	A	☐ Yes ☐ No	
	B	☐ Yes ☐ No	
	C	☐ Yes ☐ No	

Musculoskeletal Exam		
Does the patient have obvious deformities in the feet?	☐ Yes ☐ No If yes, for how long?	
Vascular Exam		
Is the hair growth on the foot dorsum or lower limb decreased?	☐ Yes ☐ No	
Are the dorsals pedis and posterior tibial pulses palpable?	☐ Yes ☐ No	
Is the temperature of the skin cold/warm/normal?	☐ Cold ☐ Warm ☐ Normal	
Patient's Foot image (OPTIONAL—MAX size 1MB)	Choose file No file chosen	

Once the data is entered and submitted, it cannot be changed/edited/modified later. Therefore, please fill the data carefully and double check the form before submitting.

Reset All   Submit Form

Three-minute Foot Examination

RSSDI Diabetic Foot Task Force

INTRODUCTION

Diabetes is a chronic serious debilitating disease characterized by severe devastating and life-threatening complications. Diabetic foot infections (DFI) are one among those complications which affect the patient's physical quality of life and create a heavy economic burden on the nation as well as the society. According to International Diabetes Federation (IDF) 2021, 537 million people are living in this world with diabetes and these numbers are projected to increase to 784 million by 2045.[1]

DIABETIC FOOT INFECTION

Diabetic foot infections are one of the major complications of diabetes mellitus which also remains a major reason for prolonged hospital admissions, thereby causing a considerable socioeconomic burden. The overall lifetime risk for a person to develop a diabetic foot ulcer (DFU) appears to be between 19 and 34%.[2] There is 23 times higher risk for a person with diabetes to undergo lower limb amputation than for a person without diabetes.[3]

Pathway to Diabetic Foot Ulcers

The three main factors (or triad) that can contribute to foot ulcers related to diabetes are neuropathy, trauma, and deformity **(Fig. 1)**.[4] Apart from this, many risk factors can be attributed to foot ulcers which include visual impairment, peripheral arterial disease (PAD), diabetic nephropathy, smoking, poor glycemic control, and any previous history of foot ulcers or amputation.[4]

Drawbacks of Comprehensive Foot Examination

Identification of at-risk patients remains the principal component of the prevention of foot ulcers which demands a comprehensive foot examination. Individual risk assessment should be based on history as well as systematic and integrated foot examination. The pivotal components of foot examination require inspection and evaluation of dermatological, musculoskeletal, and neurological systems. This comprehensive foot examination is time-consuming and requires the assistance of certain equipment for the evaluation of neurological and vascular systems. This drawback makes it difficult for it to be used in all healthcare settings.

THREE-MINUTE FOOT EXAMINATION

The three-minute foot examination is brief, requires considerably less time, and also removes all the barriers that require persistent evaluation. The three essential components of the three-minute foot examination are obtaining the history of the patient, doing a physical examination of the patient, and educating the patient **(Fig. 2)**.

History of Patient

While taking the patient's history, the healthcare professionals should not forget to include the history of surgery which must also include the history of amputation

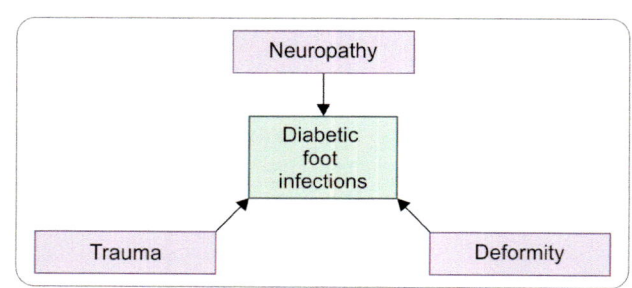

Fig. 1: Triad showing the pathway for diabetic foot infection.

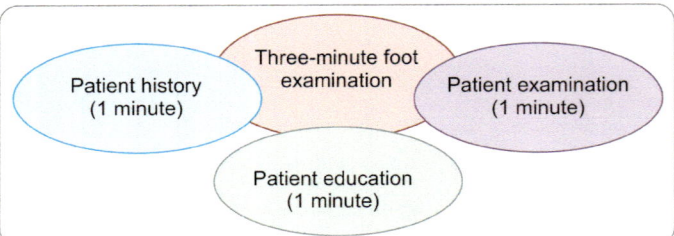

Fig. 2: Three-minute foot examination.

of limbs, if any, as well as glycemic control. This is because these patients have a greater predisposition to DFUs.[4] History of PAD and smoking or use of nicotine, which is considered a potential risk factor for PAD, should never be overlooked. The clinician must question the patient about the history of any complications encountered by the patient in the past due to diabetes.[5] He/she should also be questioned about any burning sensation or pain in the feet, any change in color of the skin of the feet, and regular podiatric visits.[6]

Physical Examination of the Patient

Careful inspection of the dermatological, vascular, musculoskeletal, and neurological systems of the patient plays a pivotal role in the physical examination of the patient.

Dermatological Examination

The clinician should look for signs of fungal infection, ulceration, skin discoloration, calluses, open wounds, or fissures in the feet of diabetic patients. Vascular insufficiency can be evaluated by inspecting the discoloration of the skin whereas, the presence of callus or hypertrophic skin is considered as a predisposition to the risk of developing foot ulcers.[4] The temperature of the skin of the diabetic foot should be assessed because it can help us to identify patients with neuropathic DFU. Interdigital foot examination should not be overlooked because it can help us to identify ingrown nails (onychocryptosis), dystrophy, or any inflammation of nails.[7]

Neurological Examination

Loss of protective sensation (LOPS) must be assessed in a patient with neuropathy as prompt and early intervention can prevent serious complications of the disease such as amputations. It is estimated that 75% of all nontraumatic lower limb amputations seem to be associated with neuropathic LOPS which explains the significance of this examination. Vibration perception threshold (VPT) can be evaluated by using devices such as the monofilament test (Semmes-Weinstein) and tuning fork which are more expensive, laborious, and time-consuming when compared to the Ipswich touch test (IpTT). In this test, the examiner touches the tips of the first, third, and fifth toes of both feet of the patient for 1–2 seconds with the tip of his/her index finger. When the light touch is not sensed in more than two sites, LOPS is more likely to be present. This is simple, sensitive, specific, quick, and reliable to be performed within 1 minute of neurological assessment.[8]

Musculoskeletal Examination

Musculoskeletal examination can help us to identify the deformities such as claw toe deformity, bunion, or rocker bottom deformity (seen in Charcot's neuroarthropathy) which are at a greater risk of developing DFU and eventually lower limb amputations.[4] If unidentified, these deformities can cause severe destruction to the associated bones and joints which, in turn, can affect the quality of life of the patients.[7]

Charcot's neuroarthropathy is considered a serious complication due to peripheral neuropathy and minor trauma that causes increased plantar pressure in the midfoot region, thereby creating a greater predisposition for the development of foot ulcers. Early identification of at-risk patients and referral to the most appropriate specialists can prevent further devastating complications such as amputations.[4]

Vascular Examination

Some of the important assessments that can be done within a minute in a 3-minute foot examination include palpation of pulses in the feet (a decrease can suggest vascular insufficiency), an inspection of the hair growth, and an examination of any change in temperatures of the feet to determine the risk of developing PAD.[6]

Patient Education

The education of patients and their family members regarding daily foot care practices plays a very significant role in reducing and preventing foot ulcers. It is imperative to make patients understand the importance of glycemic control, adherence to medication, and regular foot care practices to prevent and manage foot infections. Healthcare professionals share the responsibility of providing structured and individualized instructions for proper care and maintenance of patients' feet. Intensive patient education along with lifestyle modifications helps to prevent DFUs and lower the risk of amputation.

Within a minute, the patient can be given instructions to do regular inspection of feet, to keep the feet dry and clean, and to identify and reveal any new condition, swelling, or discoloration about the diabetic feet.

Ensuring Routine Wear of Appropriate Shoes

The choice of appropriate footwear for the prevention of DFUs as well as amputation is very essential. The patient should be adequately informed about the potential risks of walking barefoot which is a common practice seen in

India. The footwear should have a wide toe box and must be spacious with soft-cushioned soles, and Velcros or laces for adjustment.[9] The footwear should ideally be replaced within a year or sometimes more frequently if subjected to heavy wear and tear. In a study by Vijay et al., it was reported that there was a decrease in plantar pressure by 10–19% and a reduced risk of ulceration with the usage of therapeutic footwear.[10] Customized footwear was considered to be more beneficial for those with a history of previous foot ulcers and also for those who were considered to be at a higher risk for developing foot ulcers by Uccioli et al.[11] In a study by El-Nahas et al., he stated that lack of proper education regarding diabetic foot was responsible for almost 90% of recurrent ulcers in patients with diabetes.[12]

CONCLUSION

The 3-minute foot examination helps us to identify patients at risk and stratify as well as prioritize them based on the clinical findings obtained. Appropriate and timely referral to a specialist followed by consistent follow-up plays a very significant role in the prevention of these DFUs as well as subsequent complications such as amputation.

TAKE-HOME MESSAGE

The three-minute foot examination is simple, brief, less time-consuming and cost-effective, and does not require special equipment for assessment of the patient's history, inspection, examination, or education of the patient.

REFERENCES

1. International Diabetes Federation. IDF Diabetes Atlas, 10th edition, Brussels, Belgium, 2021. [online] Available from https://www.diabetesatlas.org [Last accessed March, 2023].
2. Edmonds M, Manu C, Vas P. The current burden of diabetic foot disease. J Clin Orthop Trauma. 2021;17:88-93.
3. Iversen MM, Tell GS, Riise T. History of foot ulcer increases mortality among individuals with diabetes: ten-year follow-up of the Nord-Trøndelag Health Study, Norway. Diabetes Care. 2009;32(12):2193-9.
4. Boulton AJ, Armstrong DG, Albert SF, Frykberg RG, Hellman R, Kirkman MS, et al.; American Diabetes Association; American Association of Clinical Endocrinologists. Comprehensive foot examination and risk assessment: a report of the task force of the foot care interest group of the American Diabetes Association, with endorsement by the American Association of Clinical Endocrinologists. Diabetes Care. 2008;31(8):1679-85.
5. Oliver TI, Mutluoglu M. Diabetic Foot Ulcer. [Updated 2022 Aug 8]. In: StatPearls [Internet]. Treasure Island (FL): StatPearls Publishing; 2022 Jan-. Available from https://www.ncbi.nlm.nih.gov/books/NBK537328/ [Last accessed March, 2023].
6. Miller JD, Carter E, Shih J, Giovinco N, Boulton AJM, Mills J, et al. The 3-minute diabetic foot exam. J Fam Practice. 2014;63:646-56.
7. Arsanjani Shirazi A, Nasiri M, Yazdanpanah L. Dermatological and musculoskeletal assessment of diabetic foot: A narrative review. Diab Metab Syndr. 2016;10:S158-64.
8. Rayman G, Vas PR, Baker N, Taylor CG Jr, Gooday C, Alder AI, et al. The Ipswich Touch Test: a simple and novel method to identify inpatients with diabetes at risk of foot ulceration. Diabetes Care. 2011;34(7):1517-8.
9. Viswanathan V, Rao VN. Managing diabetic foot infection in India. Int J Low Extrem Wounds. 2013;12(2):158-66.
10. Viswanathan V, Madhavan S, Gnanasundaram S, Gopalakrishna G, Das BN, Rajasekar S, et al. Effectiveness of different types of footwear insoles for the diabetic neuropathic foot: a follow-up study. Diabetes Care. 2004;27:474-7.
11. Uccioli L, Faglia E, Monticone G, Favales F, Durola L, Aldeghi A, et al. Manufactured shoes in the prevention of diabetic foot ulcers. Diabetes Care. 1995;18:1376-8.
12. El-Nahas M, Gawish H, arshoby M, State O, Boulton A. The prevalence of risk factors for foot ulceration in Egyptian diabetic patients. Pract Diab Int. 2008;25:362-6.

Reduction of Lower Limb Amputations among People with Diabetes in India

Vijay Viswanathan

INTRODUCTION

Nontraumatic lower limb amputations are one of the most serious and devastating complications of diabetes mellitus in India. Apart from increasing the mortality rates and affecting the quality of life of patient, amputations can cause heavy economic burden for the healthcare system of the entire nation. A comprehensive healthcare system with a multipronged approach becomes essential to reduce the amputations of lower limb extremities in diabetic patients in India.

EPIDEMIOLOGY

The prevalence of diabetes has been alarmingly increasing and is also expected to increase by 69% to around 152 million by the year 2045 in the Southeast Asian region.[1] One of the most common complications of diabetes is diabetic foot infections, which is the most important reason for nontraumatic lower extremity amputation (LEA). The Global Burden of Diseases (GBD), Injuries, and Risk Factors Study done in 2016 states that around 131 million people had lower extremity complications related to diabetes, which accounts to nearly 6.8 million amputations.[2] It is also estimated that nearly 1 million people undergo amputations due to diabetes and every 20 seconds a limb is being lost in this world.[3] LEA can cause significant increase in mortality, poor quality of life, and high rates of hospitalization due to readmission. It is very clear that LEA is one of the most dreadful complications of diabetic foot ulcers (DFUs) because it is estimated that around 85% of amputations in diabetic patients were preceded by DFU.[4]

CAUSES OF AMPUTATION

There could be several reasons for lower limb extremities amputation among diabetic people, the most common one being vascular or peripheral artery disease (PAD). The global prevalence of PAD in diabetic patients increased from 2001 to 2012 by 24% and approximately 11% could be attributed to critical limb ischemia (CLI). CLI is a condition in which loss of blood supply to the limb can result in pain, ulceration, and gangrene of the feet.[5] The trends in amputations have increased steadily over the years, which is evident from the fact that amputations related to diabetes have increased leaps and bounds when compared to nondiabetes-related amputations. Apart from vascular changes, bone and joint infections as well as soft tissue infections and ulcerations are the other major reasons for diabetes-related amputations (Fig. 1).[6]

Apart from this, there are several other reasons like neoplasm, sepsis, and other acute conditions, which were considered as rare or rather concomitant diseases and could not contemplated as a reason for amputation. The main reason for nondiabetes-related amputation could be associated with trauma. In a multicentric study in India by Vijay et al., the reasons for occurrence of LEAs were stated as infection, trauma, and frost bite.[7]

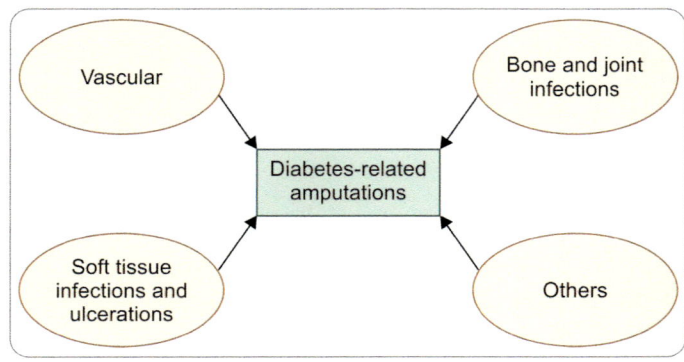

Fig. 1: The major reasons which can be attributed to the lower limb extremities-related amputation related to diabetes.[6]

PATHOPHYSIOLOGY AND RISK FACTORS

There are three factors namely, predisposing factors, triggering factors, and aggravating factors, which can contribute to the pathophysiology of DFUs, which in turn can lead to amputations that are best illustrated in **Figure 2**.[8] It becomes imperative to determine the various risk factors associated with DFUs ultimately leading to amputations, which is indispensable to appropriate management and prevention of amputations.

The risk factors and indicators for LEA are mentioned in **Table 1**.[9]

In a study from a South Indian tertiary hospital, the risk factors associated with amputation in diabetic foot disease patients were recognized to be neuropathy (36%), male predisposition, and associated with smoking and alcoholism as well as trauma, especially due to walking barefoot and inappropriate use of footwear.[10] This is in accordance with another multicentric study from South India in which 85% of them had neuropathy, 35% had peripheral vascular disease (PVD), and prevalence of claw deformities were seen in 64% of patients.[7] Some of the most common barriers for the management of foot infections and amputations in India are inappropriate usage of footwear or walking barefoot, accessibility to healthcare resources, and inadvertent use of antimicrobials to treat infections without obtaining the specific microbiological culture report.[11]

LEVELS AND TYPES OF AMPUTATION

Any partial amputation up to the level of the transverse tarsal joint (Chopart's joint) is considered as successful limb salvage and also defined as minor amputation. Amputations that involve the sacrifice of ankle joints are considered as major amputations.[12] If the amputations are done at the level of hip, hind quarter, above/through/below the knee, through tarus or ankle, they were considered as major amputation. Similarly, if the amputations are done through metatarsal bones, through tarsometatarsal joints, rays or toes, they were called minor amputations.[7]

In a multicentric study by Vijay et al., it was estimated that around 30% had undergone major amputations and the remaining 70% underwent minor amputations. Among the major amputations, more than 50% had encountered below knee amputations and around 12% had experienced above knee amputations.[7]

STRATEGIES TO REDUCE AMPUTATION

The American Heart Association (AHA) has developed key recommendations and policies to reduce the rate of nontraumatic lower limb amputations by 20% by the year 2030. A collaborative and comprehensive approach of the key contributors **(Fig. 3)** will play a significant role to reduce the amputations.[5]

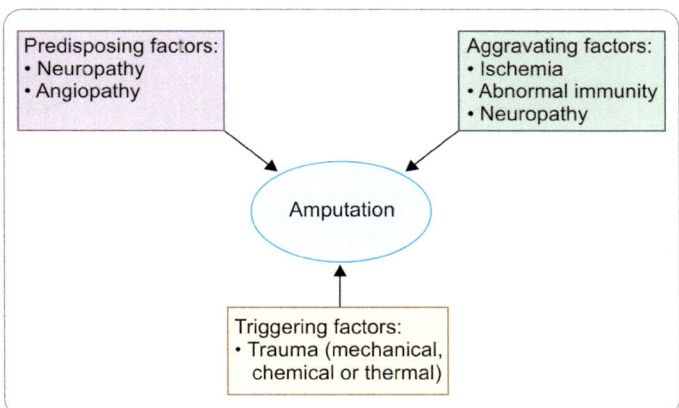

Fig. 2: Various factors associated with the pathophysiology of developing diabetic foot ulcers which in turn can lead to amputation.[8]

TABLE 1: Risk factors and indicators for lower extremity amputation (LEA).

Risk factors for diabetic feet amputation	Indicators for LEA amputation
Lower extremity ischemia	Peripheral arterial occlusion
History of foot ulcer	Septic gangrene nonhealing ulcer
Neuropathy	Severe soft tissue infection
Elevated HbA1c	Osteomyelitis
Retinopathy	Substantial necrosis of muscles and wet gangrene

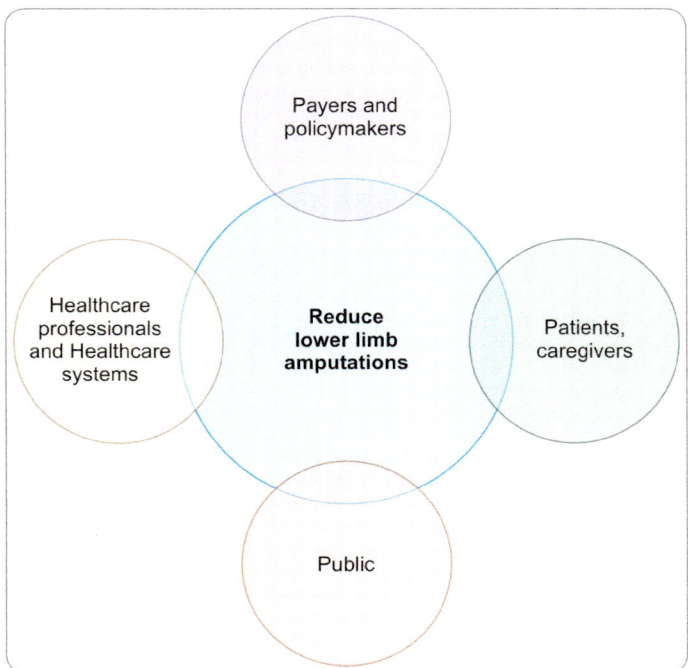

Fig. 3: The most significant contributors who can play a key role in reducing lower limb amputations.

The role of each of the key stakeholders must be established to improve the quality of treatment as well as to reduce the rate of amputations, which have been steadily increasing over the years.

The patients and caregivers must be adequately motivated and educated about adherence to the treatment and self-examination of feet, which is quintessential for prevention or reduction of amputations. Healthcare professionals must be given appropriate awareness about the evidence-based practical guidelines for comprehensive and imperative treatment. The payers can provide affordable risk-modifying measures for cessation of smoking and for treatment of PAD. The policy makers should provide preventive services to the patients at affordable costs and can also increase the funding toward research, which in turn will help us to treat patients in an efficient and effective manner. General awareness or education campaigns among the public and various lifestyle modifications to ensure and promote healthy life also play a very important role in reducing the levels of amputation in diabetes in India.[5] In a study on the amputation preventive initiative in South India by Vijay et al., it was concluded that strategies like intensive management and foot care education created a positive impact on the reduction of amputations.[11] The step-by-step project in developing countries like India, Nepal, Tanzania, Bangladesh, and Tanzania was a remarkable training program aimed at creating awareness among people to improve the diabetic foot care and sustainable training to the healthcare professionals to manage diabetic foot infections and reduce the lower limb amputations with the available human and financial constraints efficiently.[13]

A multidisciplinary approach is required for management of foot infections and prevention of amputations, which includes revascularization and appropriate surgeries, treatment of pain and infections, management of comorbidities, cautious wound control as well as biomechanical off-loading.[14]

CONCLUSION

Diabetes-related amputations are preventable to a great extent provided some simple effective strategies are followed to improve the quality of life of patients who are affected both economically as well as psychologically due to the loss of limbs. An integrated approach is thus recommended to reduce the lower limb amputations of diabetes in India.

TAKE-HOME MESSAGES

- Stratification of patients based on risk
- Identification of high-risk group
- Intensive education, motivation, and significant modification of lifestyle and behavior
- Appropriate treatment (wound care and off-loading)

REFERENCES

1. International Diabetes Federation. (2021). IDF Diabetes Atlas, 10th edition. [online] Available from https://www.diabetesatlas.org [Last accessed March, 2023].
2. Zhang Y, Lazzarini PA, McPhail SM, van Netten JJ, Armstrong DG, Pacella RE. Global disability burdens of diabetes-related lower-extremity complications in 1990 and 2016. Diabetes Care. 2020;43(5):964-74.
3. Putting feet first in diabetes. Lancet. 2005;366(9498):1674.
4. Apelqvist J, Larsson J. What is the most effective way to reduce incidence of amputation in the diabetic foot? Diabetes Metab Res Rev. 2000;16(Suppl 1):S75-83.
5. Creager MA, Matsushita K, Arya S, Beckman JA, Duval S, Goodney PP, et al. Reducing Nontraumatic Lower-Extremity Amputations by 20% by 2030: Time to Get to Our Feet: A Policy Statement From the American Heart Association. Circulation. 2021;143(17):e875-91.
6. Walicka M, Raczyńska M, Marcinkowska K, Lisicka I, Czaicki A, Wierzba W, et al. Amputations of Lower Limb in Subjects with Diabetes Mellitus: Reasons and 30-Day Mortality. J Diabetes Res. 2021;2021:8866126.
7. Viswanathan V, Kumpatla S. Pattern and causes of amputation in diabetic patients--a multicentric study from India. J Assoc Physicians India. 2011;59:148-51.
8. Ramirez-Acuña JM, Cardenas-Cadena SA, Marquez-Salas PA, Garza-Veloz I, Perez-Favila A, Cid-Baez MA, et al. Diabetic Foot Ulcers: Current Advances in Antimicrobial Therapies and Emerging Treatments. Antibiotics (Basel). 2019;8(4):193.
9. Calhoun JH, Overgaard KA, Stevens CM, Dowling JPF, Mader JT. Diabetic foot ulcers and infections: current concepts. Adv Skin Wound Care. 2002;15:31-45.
10. Nulukurthi TK, Kumar SR, Simhachalam Kutikuppala LV. A clinical study of risk factors associated with amputation in diabetic foot disease patients attending a tertiary care hospital in a rural setting. J Curr Res Sci Med. 2020;6:34-8.
11. Viswanathan V, Madhavan S, Rajasekar S, Chamukuttan S, Ambady R. Amputation Prevention Initiative in South India: Positive impact of foot care education. Diabetes Care. 2005;28(5):1019-21.
12. Choi MSS, Jeon SB, Lee JH. Predictive factors for successful limb salvage surgery in diabetic foot patients. BMC Surg. 2014;14:113.
13. Abbas ZG. Preventive foot care and reducing amputation: a step in the right direction for diabetes care. Rev Diabetes Manage. 2013;3(5):427-35.
14. Schaper NC, Apelqvist J, Bakker K. Reducing lower leg amputations in diabetes: a challenge for patients, healthcare providers and the healthcare system. Diabetologia. 2012;55(7):1869-72.

Management of Peripheral Artery Disease in Diabetes

R Ravikumar

INTRODUCTION

Peripheral artery disease (PAD) is the primary cause of lower limb amputation among people with diabetes. It refers to atherosclerosis of lower limb arteries causing partial or complete occlusion. Due to diabetic complications, more than one million patients undergo amputations approximately every 20 seconds; amputation is performed.[1] The prevalence of PAD among people with diabetes is continued to increase two-fold in the foreseeable future. The major complication of PAD is nonhealing ulcers, lower limb amputations, and physical disability. The incidence of PAD is higher in the age group above 60 years.[2] It is estimated that about half of the patients with diabetes and foot ulceration have underlying PAD in middle- and high-income countries. In contrast, neuropathic ulcers are more common in low-income countries. PAD remains underdiagnosed and undertreated as most patients lack the classic preceding clinical symptoms like claudication or rest pain. PAD significantly influences mobility and quality of life and is associated with increased morbidity and mortality. Thus, early diagnosis and management of patients with peripheral arterial disease can help to improve their quality of life, reduce the incidence of cardiovascular (CV) events, and thereby help save limbs.

PREVALENCE OF PERIPHERAL ARTERY DISEASE

The difference in the prevalence of PAD is observed among studies; the possible depending factors are the advanced age of study subjects and the prolonged duration of diabetes. In the Chennai Urban Population Study (CUPS), prevalence rates of peripheral vascular disease (PVD) were high in diabetes (6.3%) when compared to patients with normal glucose tolerance (2.7%) and impaired glucose tolerance (2.9%). Patients with known diabetes had a higher prevalence of PVD (7.8%) compared with newly diagnosed diabetic subjects (3.5%).[3] The prevalence of PVD in people with diabetes with age increased from 3.2% in those below 50 years to 33% in those above 80 years.[4] The prevalence of PVD in people with diabetes also increases with the duration of diabetes, from 15 to 45% 10 to 20 years, respectively after the diagnosis of diabetes.[5]

The overall prevalence of PVD among Indians is considerably low compared to Western patients. But, nowadays, a gradual increase in PVD is observed due to better disease care and longevity of people with diabetes. A prospective observational survey by Krishnan et al. showed an age-adjusted prevalence of PAD was 26.7%, with no difference between urban and rural populations.[6] A descriptive cross-sectional study showed the prevalence of PAD was 15.4%, asymptomatic claudication (8.5%), and claudication (6.9%) **(Box 1)**.[7]

BOX 1: Characteristics of peripheral artery disease (PAD) in persons with diabetes.

- More common
- Affects younger individuals
- Multisegmental and bilateral
- More distal
- More medial calcification
- Impaired collateral formation
- Faster progress with a higher risk of amputation

EARLY DETECTION OF PERIPHERAL ARTERY DISEASE

As a patient with PAD has two to four times more risk of CV events, early recognition of lower extremity peripheral arterial disease is of crucial importance. Most patients are asymptomatic and remain undiagnosed until they undergo proper foot examination and screening with special equipment. All bedside techniques should be performed by trained healthcare professionals in a standardized manner. No single modality is optimal, and there is no definite threshold value above which PAD can reliably be excluded.

History and Physical Examination

History taking in all patients with diabetes is essential to rule out the risk factors such as hypertension, obesity, dyslipidemia, smoking, and the duration of diabetes. The focus on other associated macrovascular complications should be evaluated as they are equally important. Early recognition and adequate treatment significantly decrease associated risks and mortality. International Working Group on the Diabetic Foot (IWGDF) recommends examining the feet of all patients with diabetes annually for the presence of PAD, even in the absence of foot ulceration.[8]

In addition, examining the feet for the signs of ischemia, such as dependent rubor, elevated pallor, shiny and hairless skin, and absence of foot pulses, alert the healthcare professional to the presence of PAD. To predict future ulceration symptoms and signs of PAD, such as claudication, absent pulses, and a low ABI should be identified.

Ankle–Brachial Index

Ankle–Brachial index (ABI) is a simple, noninvasive, and easily reproducible test for estimating the correct prevalence of PAD in diabetic patients. It is calculated by dividing the ankle systolic pressure by the brachial pressure. The European Society of Cardiology (ESC), the American Heart Association (AHA), and the American Diabetes Association (ADA) recommend the use of ABI to screen for PAD in all people with diabetes older than 50 years of age.[9] An ABI of <0.9 indicates obstructive disease and an ABI of >1.3 indicates arterial stiffening resulting from vascular calcification, which is also associated with an increased risk of mortality and amputation.[10] In patients with claudication symptoms, exercise treadmill ABI increases the test's sensitivity. A cross-sectional observational study by Mishra et al. showed the sensitivity of ABI measurement compared to Doppler ultrasound (DUS) was found to be 88.89% and specificity 90.48%.[11] ABI was found to be 95% sensitive and also 100% specific when validated against angiography.[12] However, in people with severe arterial calcification or vascular occlusion, the value of ABI may be abnormal.

Toe–Brachial index (TBI) compares the systolic toe pressure to the higher systolic brachial pressure. A TBI of >0.7 is generally considered to be normal. TBI is used in elderly patients or people with diabetes or chronic kidney disease (CKD) as ABI is often elevated due to medial calcification.[10]

Duplex Ultrasound

Duplex ultrasound is a combination of conventional and Doppler ultrasonography. Peak systolic velocity and waveform analyses are used to quantify and localize the extent of stenosis. It is indicated as a first-line imaging method, safe, cost-effective, and noninvasive adjust to physiologic testing. DUS helps detect the site and stenosis severity and length of stenosis or occlusion. It is two-dimensional imaging, along with color Doppler, which accurately assesses the lesion.

It is used in routine follow-up postprocedure for surveillance for recurrence of stenosis following endovascular or open revascularization. It gives additional knowledge of the stage and grade of the disease and helps in future management and treatment planning.[10]

Angiogram

Magnetic resonance angiography (MRA) or computed tomography angiography (CTA) provides high-quality results. Angiography is usually indicated in patients with planned revascularization to guide optimal revascularization strategies.

Computed tomography angiography is noninvasive imaging with high-resolution use of iodinated contrast agents to visualize lower extremity arteries. The major drawbacks include exposure to irradiation and a higher risk of contrast-induced nephropathy in patients with CKD and/or diabetes. Standard or dynamic CTA had good reliability and diagnostic specificity, ruling out false-negative PAD diagnoses of stenosis or occluded arteries verified by digital subtraction angiography (DSA).[13]

Magnetic resonance angiography noninvasive imaging study using magnetic resonance techniques with gadolinium contrast to visualize lower extremity arteries. The advantages of MRA include the ability to identify small runoff vessels and hemodynamically significant lesions. Compared with DSA, MRA has 90% sensitivity and 97% specificity, and 88.9% accuracy for diagnosing occluded or stenosed pelvis or femoral arteries, distal arteries, or collaterals and predicted endoscopic revascularization outcomes better than PAD determined by DSA.[14] A higher risk of contrast-induced nephropathy in patients with CKD and/or diabetes is acceptable in mild to moderate CKD.[15]

A DSA is the gold standard for diagnosing peripheral arterial disease. It locates the anatomy, flow dynamics, and perfusion of the foot at risk. In heavily calcified vessels, DSA scores better than computed tomography (CT)/MR angiograms. It is an invasive imaging technique where the blood vessel is accessed using the Seldinger technique and uses an X-ray and iodizing contrast agent to visualize lower extremity arteries **(Fig. 1)**. DSA helps detect arterial lesions, location, and severity and also helps to plan revascularization procedures **(Figs. 2A and B)**. It is associated with the risk of hematoma and other procedural complications.

MANAGEMENT

The management of PAD in diabetes includes lifestyle modifications such as regular physical exercise, promotion of a healthy diet, weight reduction and smoking cessation, symptomatic control, and reduction of the risk of CV events.

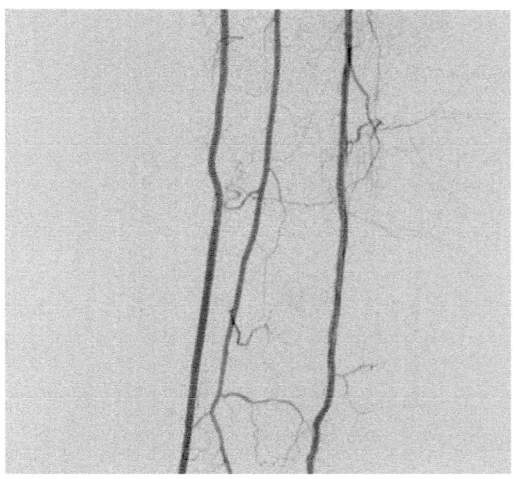

Fig. 1: Digital subtraction angiogram showing all the three infrapopliteal arteries and subtracting the bones and soft tissues.

Physical Activity

Regular physical activity improves the quality of life and claudication distance and reduces the risk of CV disease in PAD.[16] The American College of Cardiology (ACC)/AHA provides a class 1A recommendation for supervised therapy for patients with claudication.[17,18] Physical activity is recommended for a minimum of 30 minutes, at least 3 days a week. It is ideal to continue to exercise not for a discrete period (3–6 months) but throughout the patient's lifetime.[19] Randomized controlled trials in patients with PAD showed a better walking ability and improved 6-minute walk more than supervised treadmill exercise. Exercise of the lower extremity movement can increase the value of ABI in patients suffering from diabetes mellitus (DM) over 10 years.[20]

Managing the Associated Risk Factors

Therapies for patients with PAD are generally divided into noninvasive medical treatment, revascularization procedures, and critical stage lower limb amputation. Optimal medical therapy to control modifiable risk factors like smoking is of paramount importance. Followed by reducing premature adverse CVD events through pharmacological treatment (e.g., antiplatelet agents, statins, hypertension medications) is necessary. The treatment options for revascularization vary depending on the individual need like angioplasty with or without stenting and surgical bypass or hybrid procedures combining the two.

Revascularization

Surgical Bypass

Open surgical bypass is performed through the distal tibial or pedal vessels to restore blood flow to the foot. It helps the patient stands the best chance of wound healing with an 85% limb salvage rate in 1 year.[21] The longer term follow-up data for surgical bypass showed the limb salvage rates are superior to endovascular techniques. The disadvantage of surgical bypass management is extended hospital stay (5–10 days), postoperatively requiring extensive physiotherapy to regain lower limb functioning, and a greater chance of morbidity and mortality than endovascular intervention.[22] It is essential to follow-up with the patient regularly postoperatively for the early detection of hemodynamically significant graft-threatening stenosis.[23]

Endovascular revascularization interventions are a minimally invasive alternative to open peripheral bypass procedures. IWGDF recommends revascularization in a diabetic foot ulcer and PAD patient when the ulcer is not healing within 4–6 weeks despite optimal management.[8]

Indications for intervention include individuals who are unresponsive to risk factor modification, exercise, pharmacological therapy, claudication interfering with daily activity, and limb salvage in patients with critical limb ischemia. An interprofessional team approach involving a podiatrist, interventional radiologist, and vascular surgeon should be undertaken for personalized patient care to improve outcomes and patient satisfaction.[24]

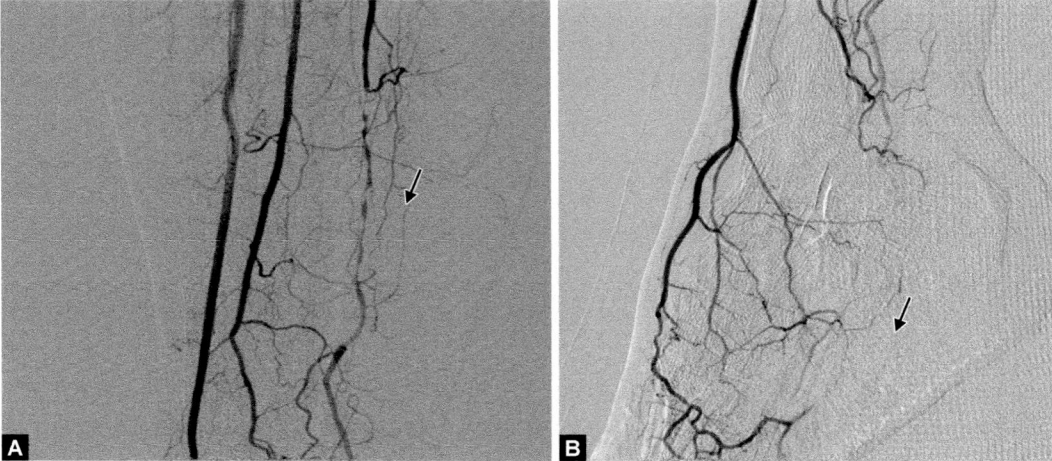

Figs. 2A and B: Digital subtraction angiogram shows distal posterior tibial artery >95% narrowing with nonopacification of plantar arteries.

Plain Balloon Angioplasty

Plain balloon angioplasty (POBA) remains the first-line endovascular treatment option in people with diabetes with a lesion on the infrapopliteal area. **Figure 3** shows POBA of the posterior tibial artery. The success rate of POBA ranges from 80 to 100%, with a satisfactory limb salvage rate. BASIL randomized trial showed a similar amputation-free and overall survival following vein bypass surgery or endovascular treatment after a follow-up period of 3 years. The main drawback of POBA is the development of neointimal hyperplasia, resulting in restenosis, low patency rates, and clinical relapse. To overcome the limitation of restenosis cryoplasty balloon catheter was introduced; it induces smooth muscle cell apoptosis and reduces neointimal hyperplasia. In a single-center randomized trial that included diabetic patients with femoropopliteal disease, compared cryoplasty and POBA after a 3-year follow-up, there were no significant differences in patient survival, and lower limb salvage with lower clinical relapse was observed in the cryoplasty subgroup.[25]

Pedal-plantar loop technique is useful and safe and could be essential for a specialist approaching below-the-knee artery disease **(Fig. 4)**. It helps improve the clinical results and local oxygen tension when PTA remains suboptimal or insufficient to achieve limb salvage. Due to advanced technology, low-profile long balloon catheters are highly conformable. These improvements have made percutaneous transluminal angioplasty for critical limb ischemia a reasonable alternative to the standard treatment, bypass surgery.[26]

Pedal Arch Angioplasty and the Angiosome

Pedal arch angioplasty is highly useful in people with diabetes, especially those with advanced renal disease, as they suffer from a diffuse steno-occlusive disease of the infrapopliteal and distal plantar vessels **(Fig. 5)**. The advantage of angioplasty is treating outflow plantar artery disease by reconstituting the pedal arch and the possibility of revascularizing more than one infrapopliteal artery, which is not amenable to surgical reconstruction. Following revascularization, adequate blood reperfusion is established, and blood flow to the ischemic tissue relieves ischemic symptoms and promotes wound healing **(Figs. 6 and 7)**.[25] Pre- and postoperative images of foot ulcer show improved healing achieved **(Figs. 8 and 9)**.

Percutaneous Deep Venous Arterialization

Percutaneous deep venous arterialization (pDVA) is considered in patients who lack viable target vessels for either bypass surgery or endovascular treatment. The technique is based on the concept that arterialization of the venous system could be considered an alternative source of perfusion of the distal foot. A fistula is created between a tibial artery and a tibial vein and provides pressurized arterial flow to the venous system of the foot **(Figs. 10A and B)**. In 2020, Schmidt et al. published the mid-term

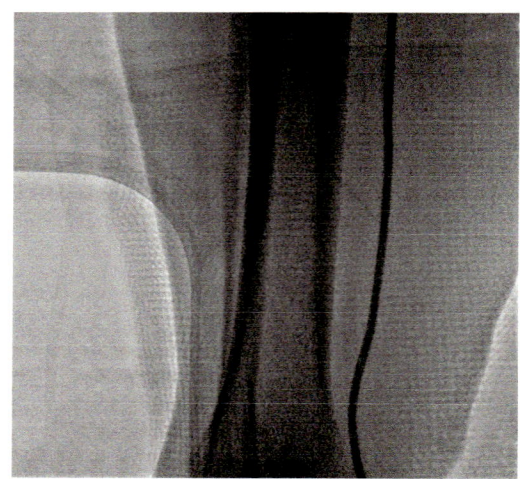

Fig. 3: Plain balloon angioplasty of posterior tibial artery.

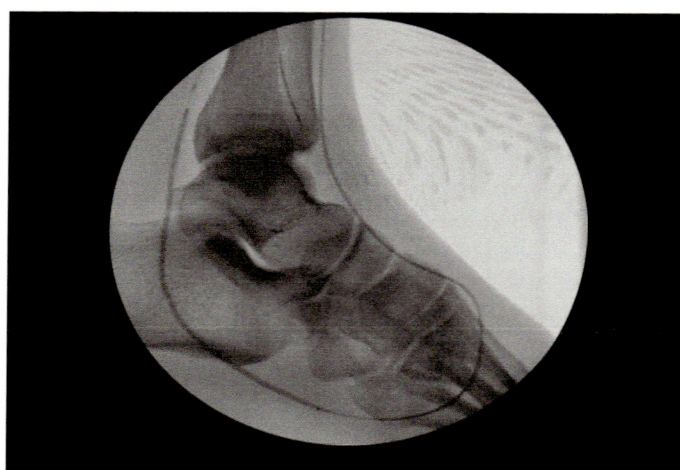

Fig. 4: Plantar loop technique: Guide wire is navigated through the anterior tibial artery along the plantar loop into distal segment of posterior tibial artery following which angioplasty is performed.

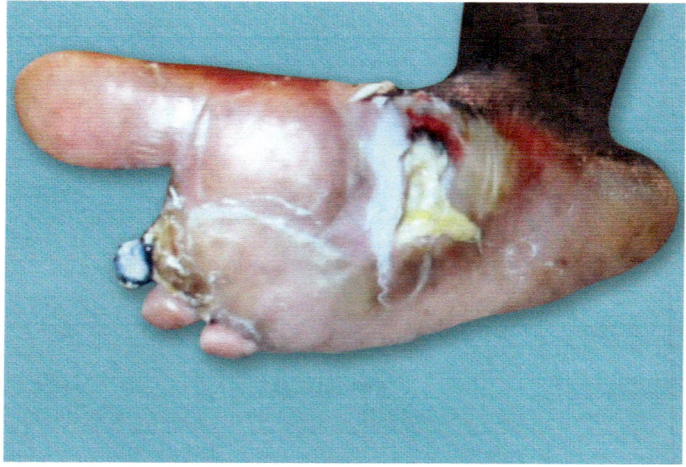

Fig. 5: Preangioplasty image showing nonhealing medial aspect foot ulcer.

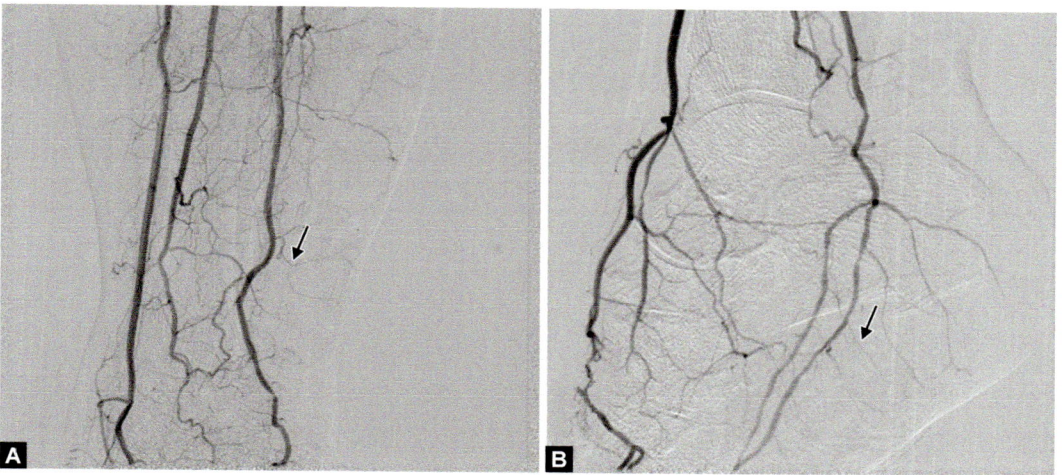

Figs. 6A and B: Postprocedure angiogram shows good flow through the posterior tibial artery with filling of plantar arteries.

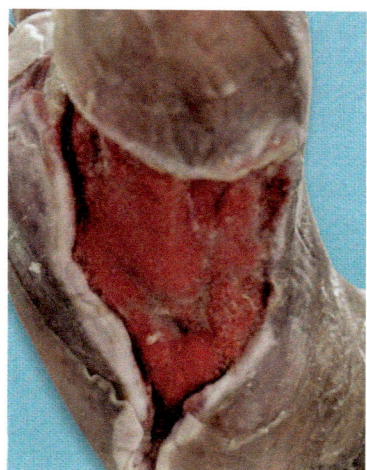

Fig. 7: Foot image showing granulation tissue and good healing of the wound 4 weeks after plain balloon angioplasty of posterior tibial artery.

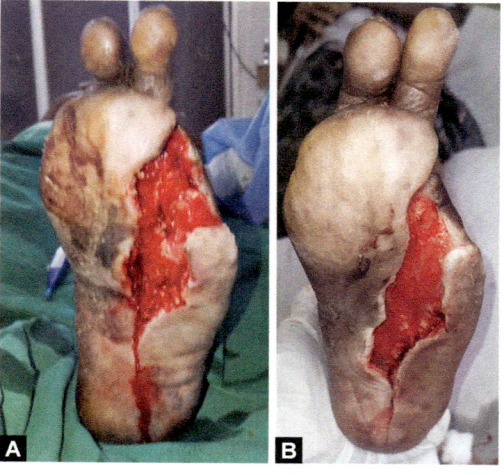

Figs. 9A and B: Postprocedure foot image showing improved healing.

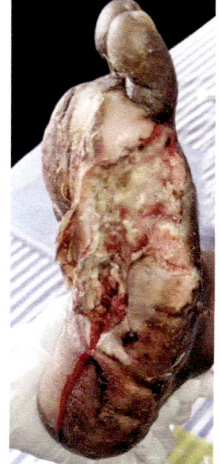

Fig. 8: Foot image shows nonhealing ulcer.

results of pDVA, revealing a promising potential for this complex group of "no option patients." A retrospective study of 32 consecutive patients (66% with type 2 diabetes mellitus) treated with pDVA using the LimFlow device. After 2 years, follow-up period showed a high technical success rate (96.9%), very satisfactory limb salvage (79.8%), and complete wound healing (72.7%).[25]

ADVANCES IN ENDOVASCULAR REVASCULARIZATION TECHNIQUES

Even though open surgery is the gold standard for lower extremity revascularization, the advent of new technologies and devices has improved the outcomes of endovascular therapy. Some of the recent technological advances available are cryoplasty balloons, drug-eluting stents, balloon expandable stents, self-expanding metallic stents, vasculomimetic stents, bioabsorbable stents, atherectomy

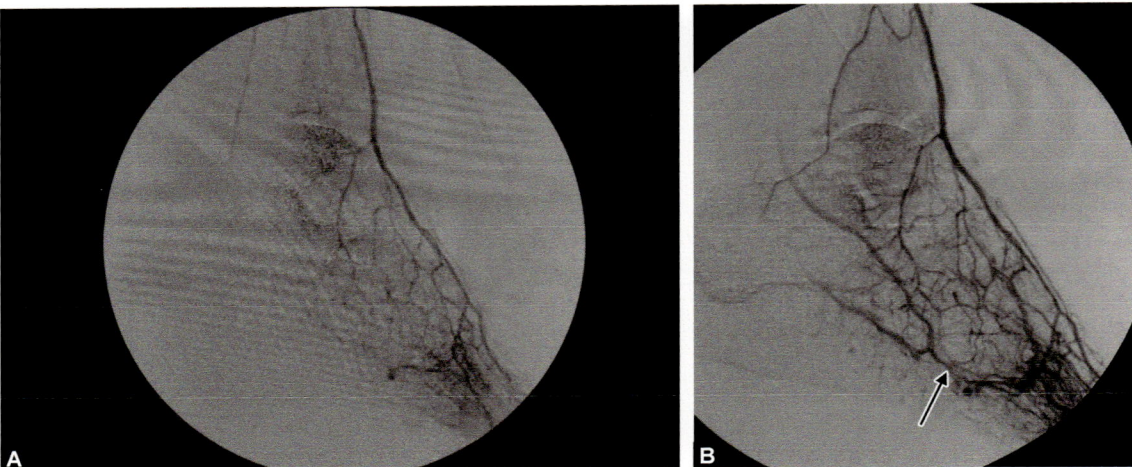

Figs. 10A and B: Arterialization of the plantar vein by creating a fistulous communication between the terminal portion of the dorsalis pedis artery and plantar vein (arrow).

devices, laser technology, intravascular lithoplasty (IVL), etc., which have been added in the armamentarium for treating PVD. Further research and development on the recently evolved technologies are required to enhance the outcomes over more standardized interventions.

POSTREVASCULARIZATION OUTCOMES

Outcomes of revascularization procedure reported limb salvage rates of 80–85% and ulcer healing in >60% at 12 months. In patients with diabetes, PAD, and end-stage renal disease, increased risk of perioperative mortality (5%), 1-year mortality (40%), and 1-year limb salvage rates (70%) were observed. There is not sufficient evidence to assess the superiority of various revascularization techniques available and it becomes imperative to make decisions based on comorbidities of the patient, autogenous vein availability as well the distribution of PAD.[8]

CONCLUSION

Diabetic foot ulcers are a challenging pathology with a broad spectrum of pathophysiological mechanisms and clinical manifestations. DM is a significant risk for PAD, resulting in increased morbidity and mortality. We need to understand that the several types of PAD may present with different clinical presentations although they share common risk factors. A comprehensive arterial assessment is thus required for early diagnosis, prompt treatment as well as rapid and appropriate wound healing. Adequate lipid-lowering, antithrombotic, and antihypertensive treatment should be available to all patients with PAD apart from strict glycemic control and lifestyle modifications.

TAKE-HOME MESSAGES

- A multidisciplinary approach is required for the management of PAD which includes adequate medical management as well as lifestyle modifications.
- Thus, diabetologists are considered predominant crusaders for the identification of at-risk individuals who can develop PAD, to provide appropriate education as well as timely referral for adequate care. With the advancements in endovascular techniques, minimally invasive endovascular procedures seem to be a good alternative for patients suffering from peripheral arterial disease.

REFERENCES

1. Soyoye DO, Abiodun OO, Ikem RT, Kolawole BA, Akintomide AO. Diabetes and peripheral artery disease: A review. World J Diabetes. 2021;12(6):827-38.
2. Hinchliffe RJ, Brownrigg JRW, Andros G, Apelqvist J, Boyko EJ, Fitridge R, et al. Effectiveness of revascularisation of the ulcerated foot in patients with diabetes and peripheral artery disease: a systematic review. Diabetes Metab Res Rev. 2016;32(Suppl 1): 136-44.
3. Premalatha G, Shanthirani S, Deepa R, Markovitz J, Mohan V. Prevalence and risk factors of peripheral vascular disease in a selected South Indian population: the Chennai Urban Population Study. Diabetes Care. 2000;23(9):1295-300.
4. Janaka HU, Standl E, Mehnert H. Peripheral vascular disease in diabetes mellitus and its relation to cardiovascular risk factors: screening with Doppler, ultrasonic technique. Diabetes Care. 1980;3(2):207-13.
5. Palumbo PJ, Melton LJ. Peripheral vascular disease and diabetes. In: Harris MI, Hamman RF (Eds). Diabetes in America. National Institutes of Health: Bethesda; 1985. pp. 1-21.
6. Krishnan MN, Geevar Z, Mohanan PP, Venugopal K, Devika S. Prevalence of peripheral artery disease and risk factors in the elderly: A community based cross-sectional study from northern Kerala, India. Indian Heart J. 2018;70(6):808-15.
7. Prathibha Divya Radha T, Arthi PS, Annamalai S. Screening for peripheral vascular disease among type 2 diabetes patients of lower socio economic status using ankle brachial index - a descriptive cross sectional study. Int J Contemp Med Res. 2020;7(6):F10-F15.

8. Hinchliffe RJ, Forsythe RO, Apelqvist J, Boyko EJ, Fitridge R, Hong JP, et al.; International Working Group on the Diabetic Foot (IWGDF). Guidelines on diagnosis, prognosis, and management of peripheral artery disease in patients with foot ulcers and diabetes (IWGDF 2019 update). Diabetes Metab Res Rev. 2020;36 Suppl 1:e3276.
9. Potier L, Abi Khalil C, Mohammedi K, Roussel R. Use and utility of ankle brachial index in patients with diabetes. Eur J Vasc Endovasc Surg. 2011;41:110-6.
10. Aboyans V, Björck M, Brodmann M, Collet JP, Czerny M, De Carlo M, et al.; ESC Scientific Document Group. Questions and answers on diagnosis and management of patients with Peripheral Arterial Diseases: a companion document of the 2017 ESC Guidelines for the Diagnosis and Treatment of Peripheral Arterial Diseases, in collaboration with the European Society for Vascular Surgery (ESVS): Endorsed by: the European Stroke Organisation (ESO) The Task Force for the Diagnosis and Treatment of Peripheral Arterial Diseases of the European Society of Cardiology (ESC) and of the European Society for Vascular Surgery (ESVS). Eur Heart J. 2018;39:e35-e41.
11. Mishra N. Use of ABI to detect peripheral arterial disease in diabetes - A recommendation for primary care physicians. J Family Med Prim Care. 2021;10(1):154-7.
12. American Diabetes Association. Peripheral arterial disease in people with diabetes. Diabetes Care. 2003;26:3333-41.
13. Sommer WH, Bamberg F, Johnson TR, Weidenhagen R, Notohamiprodjo M, Schwarz F, et al. Diagnostic accuracy of dynamic computed tomographic angiographic of the lower leg in patients with critical limb ischemia. Invest Radiol. 2012;47(6):325-31.
14. Olin JW, Kaufman JA, Bluemke DA, Bonow RO, Gerhard MD, Jaff MR, et al.; American Heart Association. Atherosclerotic Vascular Disease Conference: Writing Group IV: imaging. Circulation. 2004;109(21):2626-33.
15. Donohue CM, Adler JV, Bolton LL. Peripheral arterial disease screening and diagnostic practice: A scoping review. Int Wound J. 2020;17(1):32-44.
16. Rooke TW, Hirsch AT, Misra S, Sidawy AN, Beckman JA, Findeiss L, et al. American College of Cardiology Foundation Task Force; American Heart Association Task Force. Management of patients with peripheral artery disease (compilation of 2005 and 2011 ACCF/AHA Guideline Recommendations): a report of the American College of Cardiology Foundation/American Heart Association Task Force on Practice Guidelines. J Am CollCardiol. 2013;61:1555-70.
17. Lane R, Harwood A, Watson L, Leng GC. Exercise for intermittent claudication. Cochrane Database Syst Rev. 2017;12:CD000990.
18. Gerhard-Herman MD, Gornik HL, Barrett C, Barshes NR, Corriere MA, Drachman DE, et al. 2016 AHA/ACC guideline on the management of patients with lower extremity peripheral artery disease: executive summary: a report of the American College of Cardiology/American Heart Association task force on clinical practice guidelines. Circulation. 2017;135:e686-e725.
19. McDermott MM. Exercise Rehabilitation for Peripheral Artery Disease: A review. J Cardiopulm Rehabil Prev. 2018;38:63-9.
20. Suza DE, Hijriana I, Ariani Y, Hariati H. Effects of Lower Extremity Exercises on Ankle-Brachial Index Values among Type 2 Diabetes Mellitus Patients. Open Access Maced J Med Sci. 2020;8(E):1-6.
21. Hinchliffe RJ, Andros G, Apelqvist J, Bakker K, Friederichs S, Lammer J, et al. A systematic review of the effectiveness of revascularization of the ulcerated foot in patients with diabetes and peripheral arterial disease. Diabetes Metab Res Rev. 2012;28Suppl 1:179-217.
22. Pearce BJ, Toursarkissian B. The current role of endovascular intervention in the management of diabetic peripheral arterial disease. Diabet Foot Ankle. 2012;3.
23. Moxey PW, Chong PFS. Surgical revascularisation of the diabetic foot. In: Shearman CP (Ed). Management of Diabetic Foot Complications. Springer London; 2015. pp. 113-25.
24. Comerota AJ. Endovascular and surgical revascularization for patients with intermittent claudication. Am J Cardiol. 2001;87(12A):34D-43D.
25. Spiliopoulos S, Festas G, Paraskevopoulos I, Mariappan M, Brountzos E. Overcoming ischemia in the diabetic foot: Minimally invasive treatment options. World J Diabetes. 2021;12(12):2011-26.
26. Fusaro M, Dalla Paola L, Biondi-Zoccai G. Pedal-plantar loop technique for a challenging below-the-knee chronic total occlusion: a novel approach to percutaneous revascularization in critical lower limb ischemia. J Invasive Cardiol. 2007;19(2):E34-7.

Surgical Approach to the Management of Diabetic Foot Infections and Complex Diabetic Foot Wounds

Senthil Govindan

INTRODUCTION

Diabetic foot is the most underestimated major problem in diabetes due to the classical triad of neuropathy, angiopathy, and immunopathy, which play a significant role in the pathophysiology of diabetic foot infections (DFI). It has been projected that around 15% of people with diabetes will develop foot ulcers in their lifetime.[1] It has also been estimated that around 85% of amputations are caused by poorly treated diabetic foot ulcer infections secondary to plantar pressure ulcers, injuries, and web spaces infections.[2] This catastrophe can be averted to a great extent by timely intervention and the proper multidisciplinary approach with medical, surgical, and vascular interventions. This article discusses the surgical management of DFIs and complex wounds.

DIAGNOSIS

Diagnosis of DFI is by clinical examination. Cardinal signs of inflammation such as redness, pain, swelling warmth, and loss of function have to be observed in diabetic foot ulcers. A wound swab is not reliable; it may show bacterial colonization, not an infection.[3] Only ulcer with signs of infection needs to be tested for culture sensitivity. The wound is cleaned well with saline and a tissue specimen is obtained from the base of the ulcer either by curettage or tissue biopsy. Probe-to-bone (PTB) test can suggest an underlying bone infection. A plain X-ray may take 2 weeks to show the signs of osteomyelitis. Magnetic resonance imaging (MRI) is useful to detect bone infection early. Deep-seated soft tissue infections and Charcot foot can be diagnosed early.

Leukocytosis and raised erythrocyte sedimentation rate (ESR) or C-reactive protein (CRP) are the indicators to start systemic antibiotic therapy empirically. Palpable pedal pulses (dorsalis pedis and posterior tibial) are good signs of vascularity in the foot. However, handheld Doppler, ankle–brachial index, duplex scan, and transcutaneous oxygen pressure ($TcPO_2$) can aid in the diagnosis and assess the severity of the peripheral arterial disease. Computed tomography (CT) angiogram and digital subtraction angiogram (DSA) can detect the levels and number of lesions and will be useful for vascular intervention.

CLASSIFICATION

It is considered an important tool for decision-making which is helpful for setting meaningful goals and expectations for the patients as well as for their priorities. There are so many classification systems such as Meggitt–Wagner, the University of Texas, PEDIS, DSA, WIFI, SINBAD, and many more. There are potential merits and demerits in every method.

MANAGEMENT

Medical Management

A comprehensive examination to assess dehydration, electrolyte imbalance, anemia, glycemic control, and the evaluation of respiratory and cardiovascular systems are also considered essential for the management for DFI. Based on severity, patients are started on an empirical antibiotic regimen. Oral antibiotics such as cephalexin, amoxicillin–clavulanate, clindamycin, levofloxacin, or doxycycline are recommended for mild infections. Ceftriaxone, linezolid, and cefoperazone with sulbactam can be used for moderate infections and piperacillin with tazobactum, imipenem, meropenem, vancomycin, or tigecycline are considered for severe infections. These antibiotics can be switched to more specific culture-sensitive antibiotics after the tissue culture reports are obtained.

Surgical Management

Incision

Incision and drainage (I&D) is one of the common surgical procedures for abscesses and deep-seated infections. But, in DFIs, I&D may not suffice as the infected tissue component will be more than the pus. Wound debridement will be needed in most deep-seated DFIs. Placing the correct incision is important to access the infected compartment thoroughly. So, the incision is based on the location of the wound and its potential involvement. Grodinsky identified three major plantar spaces and published them in 1929.[4] These include medial, central (superficial and deep), and lateral spaces. The incision is also planned not to disturb the neurovascular bundle and the angiosome territory. Loeffler et al. described a plantar incision that begins posterior to the medial malleolus and extends medially and distally toward the midline, ending between the heads of the first and second metatarsals.[5] Any portion of the incision can be used depending on the location and the extent of the infection.

There are so many modifications of these techniques, which start incision distally and proceed proximally so as to trace the infection. DFI usually spreads to the ankle and leg through infected tendons. They act as "pus highways." Extrinsic muscular tendons such as flexor hallucis longus (FHL) and flexor digitorum longus (FDL) are responsible to spread the infection to the medial compartment of the leg. Peroneus longus and brevis tendons will spread the infection to the lateral compartment of the leg. Extensor tendons may carry dorsal foot infection to the anterior compartment of the leg. We have proposed a tarsal tunnel sparing incision for foot and ankle infections to safely remove the infected flexor tendons (FHL and FDL), avoiding incision over the heel and ankle. This technique stops the plantar incision distal to the heel and continues above the ankle starting just behind the medial malleolus **(Case 1—Figs. 1 to 4)**.

Debridement (Radical/Conservative)

Devitalized tissue will act as a shelter to infective microorganisms that can worsen the infection and delay the healing process. Debridement should be optimal and not necessarily radical. Conservative wound debridement can be achieved by removing the grossly contaminated, nonviable tissues en masse and leaving viable or potentially viable tissues as much as possible.

This helps in the preservation of more tissues for better reconstruction to maintain the form and function of the limbs. Bones affected by osteomyelitis can be debrided along with infective necrotic tissue. Limb salvage can be done even in extreme bony infections associated with fractures involving hind foot Charcot cases **(Case 2—Figs. 5 to 10)**. Most people are less afraid of dying than losing their limbs/toes. Our aim is to eradicate the infection and also preserve a maximum of viable or potentially viable tissues. One amputation leads to another by altering biomechanics and transferring lesions. Saving the toe means saving the limb in the best form and function **(Case 3—Figs. 11 to 16)**.

Some extensive infections may need serial debridement in order to achieve a healthy granulation wound bed for reconstruction **(Case 4: Figs. 17 to 22)**. Time is an important component of healing. There should not be any time delay in acute phase management during infection control. Optimal time should be given for the wound bed preparation for better reconstruction.

Prophylactic Surgeries

Percutaneous Achilles tendon lengthening (PAL) is used to treat nonhealing/recurrent plantar forefoot ulcers to correct equinus deformity of the diabetic foot caused by stiffness and contracture of TA due to altered collagen metabolism. Exostectomy is done by excising prominent bony bump/exostosis, thereby reducing the peak plantar pressure so as to heal/prevent ulcer recurrence. Metatarsal head resection (MTHR) surgery is performed to heal plantar ulcer over the first metatarsal head (ball of the big toe). Keller arthroplasty is used to correct hallux vagus deformity/bunion. Percutaneous needle flexor tenotomy can be done as an outpatient procedure to correct mallet/hammer toe deformities to heal the toe tip ulceration. Hypertrophic skin changes may eventually lead to callus and ulceration later.

Tenotomy procedure may be toe-saving as toe tip ulcer can result in distal phalax (Dpx) osteomyelitis and toe gangrene if untreated. Some patients with tinea pedis and intertrigo due to flexion deformity and crowded toes also can benefit from tenotomy **(Case 5—Figs. 23 and 24)**.

Treating Complex Diabetic Foot Wounds

Apart from soft tissue involvement, underlying bones and joints are also involved in neglected or poorly treated diabetic foot wounds. Infected phalanges and metatarsal bones can be managed by curettage or minor debridements, but tarsal bone and joint involvement or ankle joint involvement may need orthopedic surgical debridement and external fixators either by linear fixators/Ilizarov (ring) fixator.

Neuroischemic ulcers and ischemic ulcers may need revascularization for the healing of the ulcers. Arterial disease in patients with diabetes has three components including atherosclerosis, vasculitis, and ischemia of the vessel. Classical peripheral artery disease (PAD) in patients with diabetes is infrapopliteal involvement. This problem can be better managed by an angioplasty. However, there are numerous limitations in opening the calcified vessels during balloon angioplasty and restenosis makes it more complex.

Severely stenotic or long segment occlusive lesions in the proximal vessel like the femoral artery can be successfully managed by femoropopliteal bypass surgery. Diffuse, long-segment infrapopliteal lesions can be better managed by balloon angioplasty 3 years of patency rates of stenosis and occlusion were 61 and 48%, respectively.

Some patients present with multilevel lesions, which may require both open and endovascular procedures. Modern vascular surgeons need to master both open and endovascular techniques (hybrid procedures) and combine them in a creative fashion to the benefit of patients.

Wound Preparation

Once the acute phase management is complete, the wound needs to be prepared for the final reconstruction. Moist wound dressings are used to maintain a good environment for healing. Hydrogel, hydrofiber, alginate, and polyurethane foam dressing materials are available for clinical use. Silver-impregnated materials are also available for potentially infective wounds. Dressing material should also absorb exudate so as to avoid "strike-through" dressings.

Sucrose octa sulfate-impregnated dressings, platelet, and placenta-derived products can be used as adjuvant therapy in addition to standard care in difficult-to-heal wounds.[6] Vacuum-assisted closure can be used in post-operative wounds to facilitate healing. Systemic hyperbaric oxygen therapy can be used for nonhealing diabetic foot ulcerations.

Offloading

Diabetic neuropathy may not be reversible but diabetic feet can be protected. Educating patients to examine their feet daily, application of moisturizers, use the proper footwear, looking for corns, callus, or any ulcerations. Self-treatment with medications or bathroom surgeries should be avoided.

Customized insoles, peg-assisted insoles, molded footwear, and orthowedge footwear are used to achieve local offloading of ulcers or deformities. Total contact cast (TCC) has been used for healing of grade 1 and 2 ulcers and in acute Charcot foot for mechanical stabilization. Removable cast walker (RCW), instant total contact cast (ITCC), or Charcot restrained orthotic walker (CROW) can be used as an alternative to TCC to achieve similar results for those who are not candidates for TCC.

Follow-up

Regular follow-up is mandatory to save the foot. A healed ulcer is a potential spot for recurrent ulceration as the scar has less tensile strength with loss of protective fat cushioning and altered biomechanics make it more vulnerable to recurrent ulceration. A study shows the rate of recurrent ulcers is 50% in 2 years, 60% in 3 years, and 75% in 5 years. The usage of appropriate foot care and footwear has to be emphasized in every visit and follow-up protocol should be as per the International Working Group on the Diabetic Foot (IWGDF) guidelines.

CONCLUSION

Most diabetic foot ulcers are simple to treat initially. If neglected, diabetic wounds become complex with spreading infection and underlying bone with joint involvement. This issue is further complicated by the underlying peripheral arterial disease. So, DFI with or without PAD needs a multidisciplinary approach in order to save the limb and life of patients with diabetic foot wounds. Early referral of complex diabetic wounds to a tertiary care center can minimize the number of amputations. A better understanding of surgical management, orthopedic intervention, growing success in peripheral angioplasty, and above all the proper medical care to treat the patient as a whole has revolutionized the management of complex diabetic foot wounds for the better outcome to reduce the lower limb amputations.

TAKE-HOME MESSAGE

Diabetic foot ulcer is considered a sleeping volcano, which can erupt anytime once infected. Preventive foot care practices and early prompt treatment with a holistic approach can prevent lower extremity amputations to a greater extent.

REFERENCES

1. Reiber GE, Boyko EJ, Smith DG. Lower extremity foot ulcers and amputation in diabetics. Diabetes in America, 2nd edition. Rockeville MD: National Institute of Diabetes and Digestive and Kidney Disease, National Institute of Health; 1995. pp. 409-28.
2. Armstrong DG, Lavery LA, Harkless LB, Van Houtum WH. Amputation and reamputation of the diabetic foot. J Am Podiatr Med Assoc. 1997;87(6):255-9.
3. Pellizzer G, Strazzabosco M, Presi S, Furlan F, Lora L, Benedetti P, et al. Deep tissue biopsy vs. superficial swab culture monitoring in the microbiological assessment of limb-threatening diabetic foot infection. Diabet Med. 2001;18(10):822-7.
4. Grodinsky M. A study of the fascial spaces of the foot and their bearing on infections. Surg Gynecol Obstet. 1929;49:737-51.
5. Loeffler RD Jr, Ballard A. Plantar fascial spaces of the foot and a proposed surgical approach. Foot Ankle. 1980;1(1):11-4.
6. Rayman G, Vas P, Dhatariya K, Driver V, Hartemann A, Londahl M, et al.; International Working Group on the Diabetic Foot (IWGDF). Guidelines on use of interventions to enhance healing of chronic foot ulcers in diabetes (IWGDF 2019 update). Diabetes Metab Res Rev. 2020;36(Suppl 1):e3283.

APPENDIX: CASES

CASE 1 (FIGURES 1 TO 4)

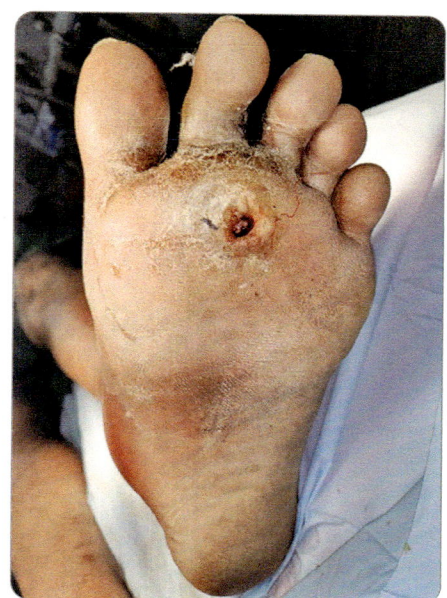

Figure 1 shows an infected diabetic foot with a nonhealing ulcer showing infection spreading to the ankle and leg via flexor tendons.

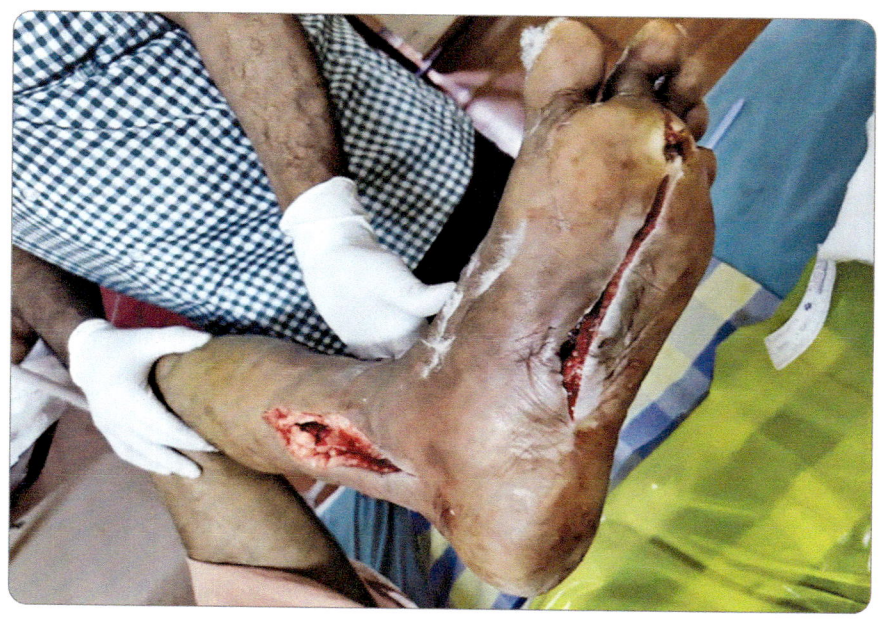

Figure 2 shows the tarsal tunnel sparing incision sparing the ankle region.

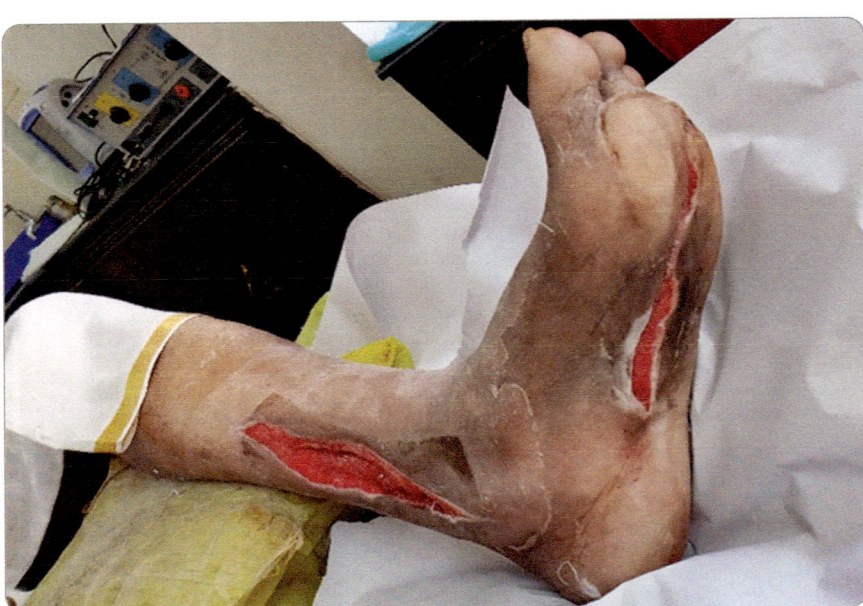

Figure 3 shows a healthy granulating wound without residual infection or cellulitis.

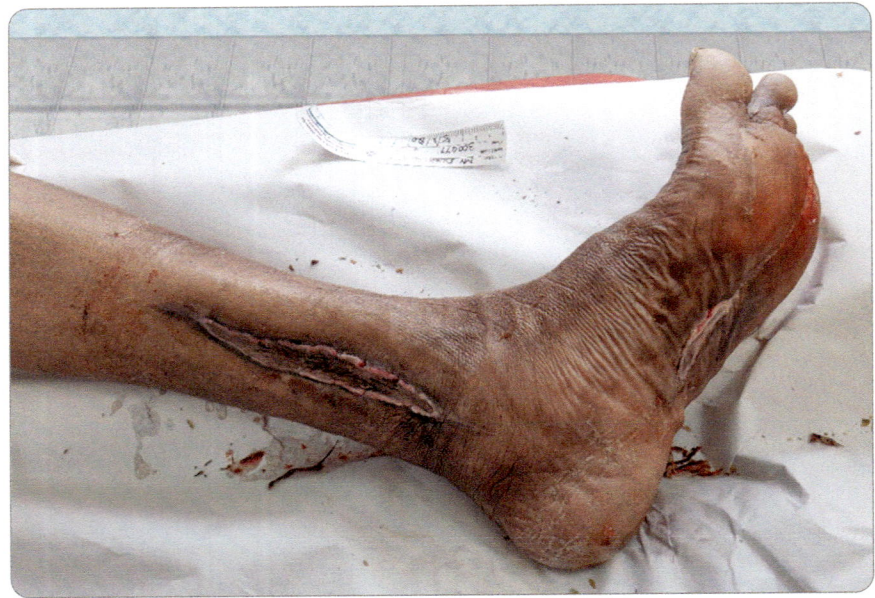

Figure 4 shows a healed wound with a skin graft.

CASE 2 (FIGURES 5 TO 10)

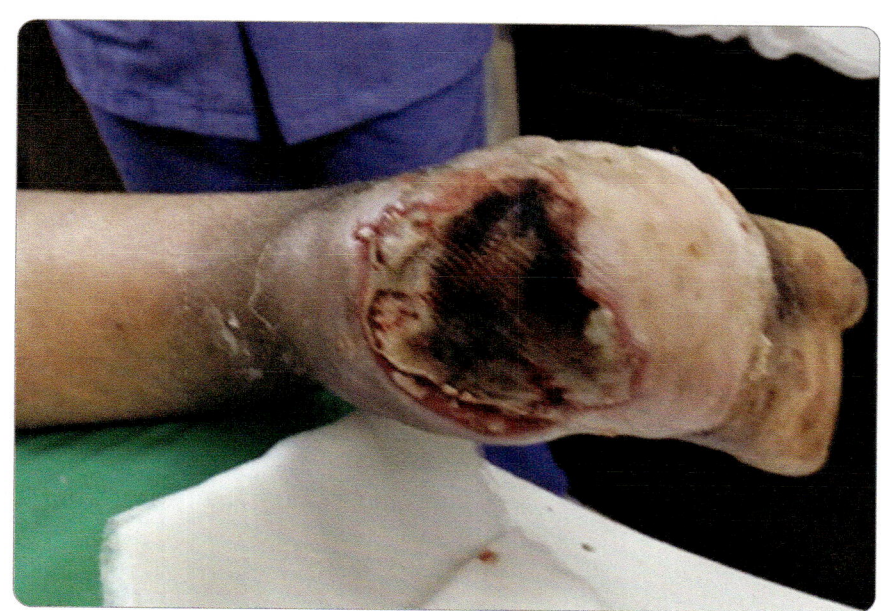

Figure 5 shows an infective necrotic wound with involvement of underlying calcaneum in Charcot foot.

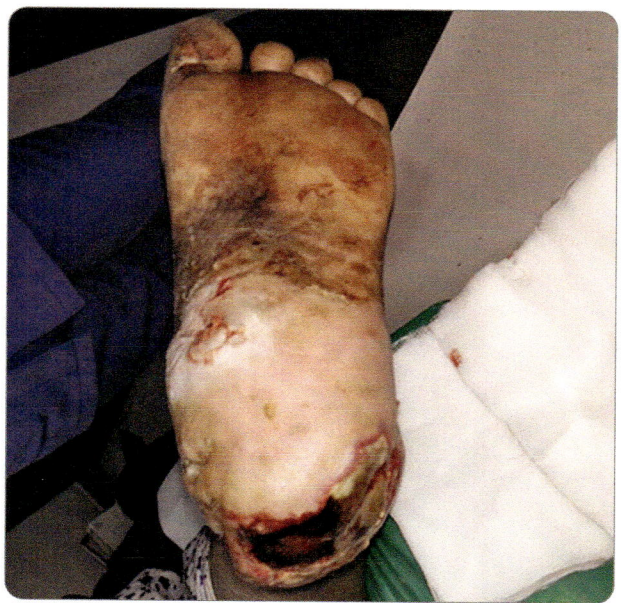

Figure 6 shows hindfoot Charcot complicated with necrotic wound infection along with underlying calcaneal bone involvement.

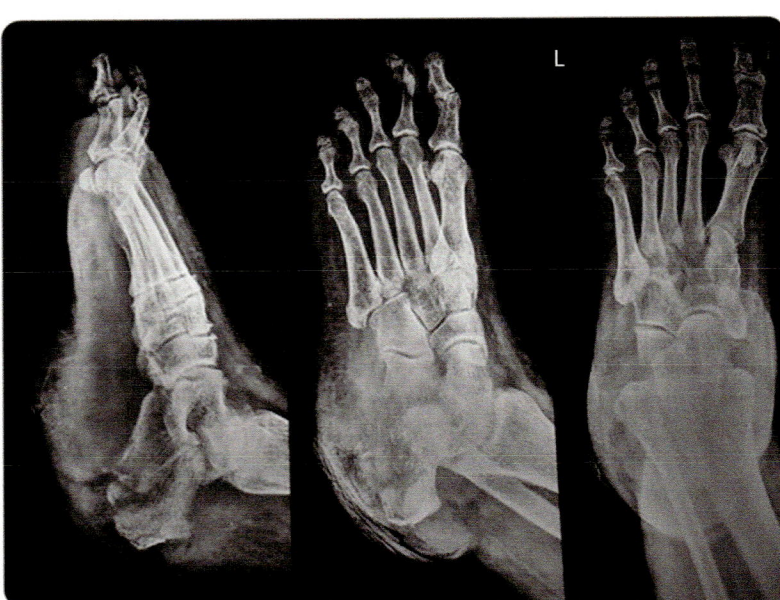

Figure 7 shows hindfoot Charcot changes associated with osteomyelitis and fractured (pathological fracture) calcaneum.

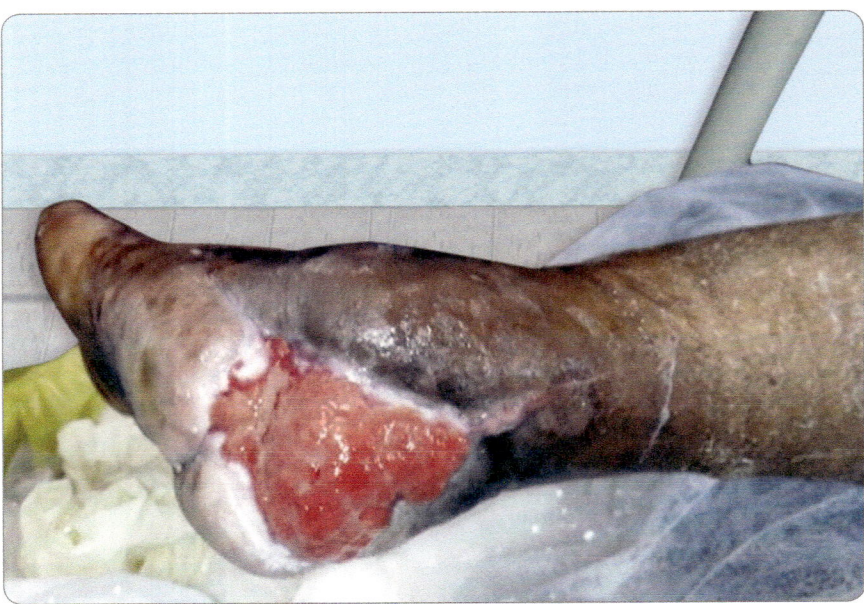

Figure 8 shows the postoperative wound with healthy granulation and no residual infection.

Surgical Approach to the Management of Diabetic Foot Infections and Complex Diabetic Foot Wounds

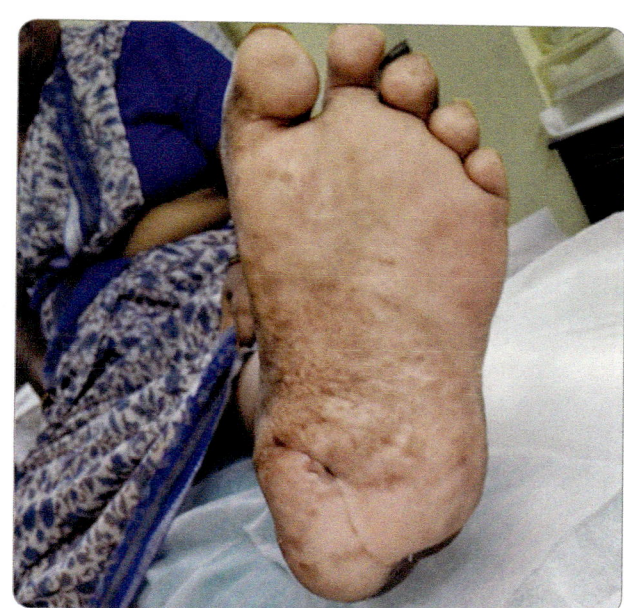

Figure 9 shows salvaged limb preserving the form and function.

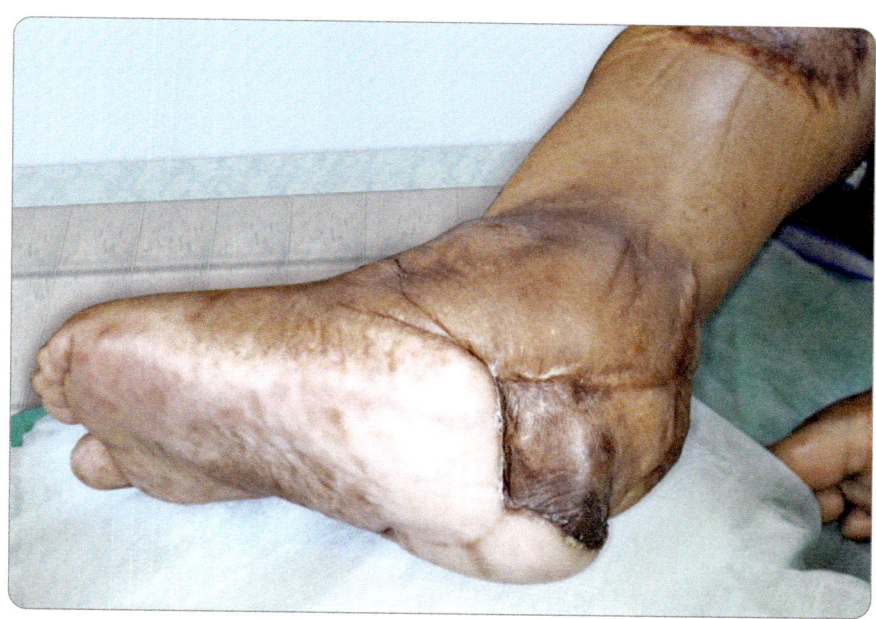

Figure 10 shows salvaged limb-healed wound with split-thickness skin grafting.

CHAPTER 6

Surgical Approach to the Management of Diabetic Foot Infections and Complex Diabetic Foot Wounds

CASE 3 (FIGURES 11 TO 16)

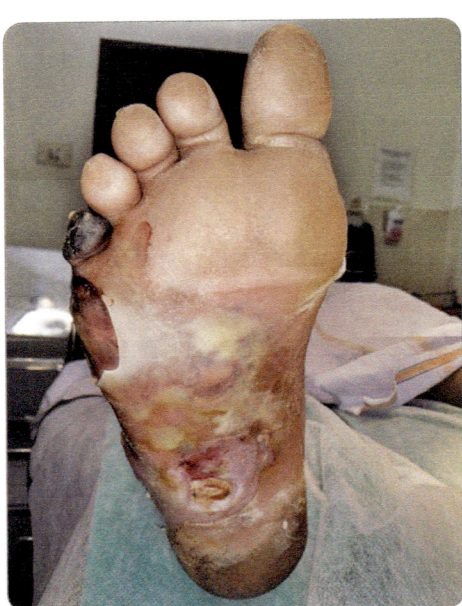

Figure 11 shows the preoperative view of a gangrenous right fifth toe with necrotic wound infection involving all three compartments of the foot.

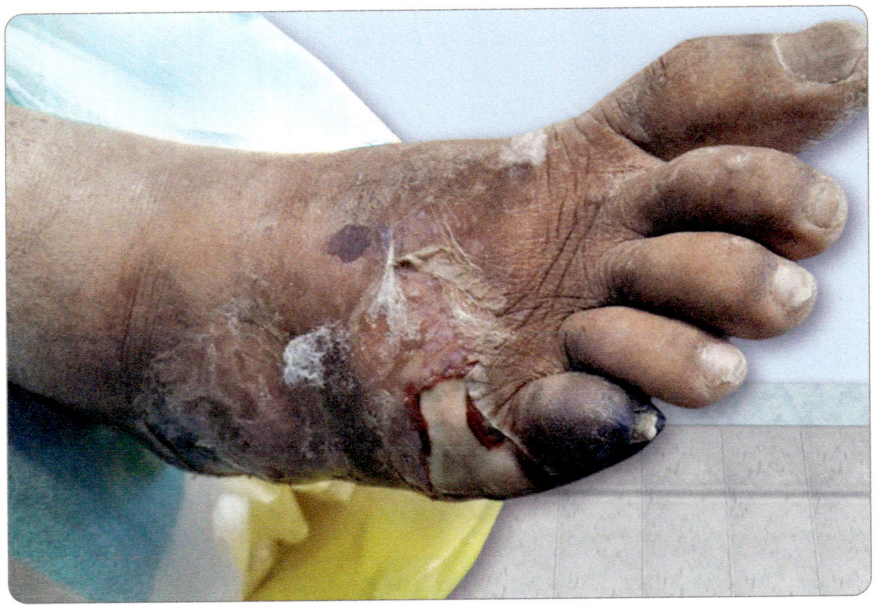

Figure 12 shows the gangrene in the fifth toe with the necrotic infection spreading to the dorsum of the foot.

Surgical Approach to the Management of Diabetic Foot Infections and Complex Diabetic Foot Wounds

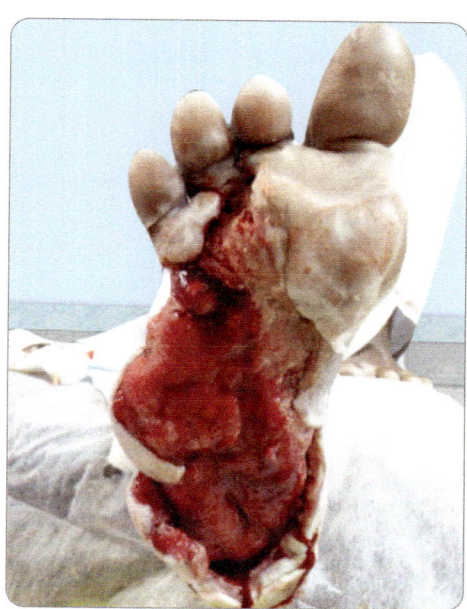

Figure 13 shows the postoperative view depicting a healthy granulating wound bed. The third and the fourth toes were saved despite marked tissue loss over the base.

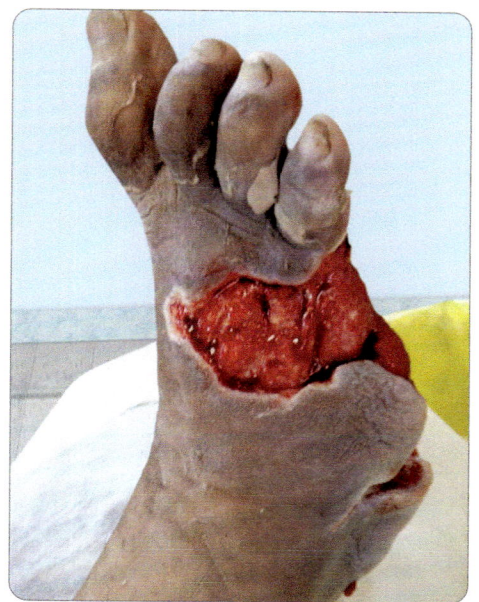

Figure 14 shows the postdebridement picture of the wound.

34 Surgical Approach to the Management of Diabetic Foot Infections and Complex Diabetic Foot Wounds

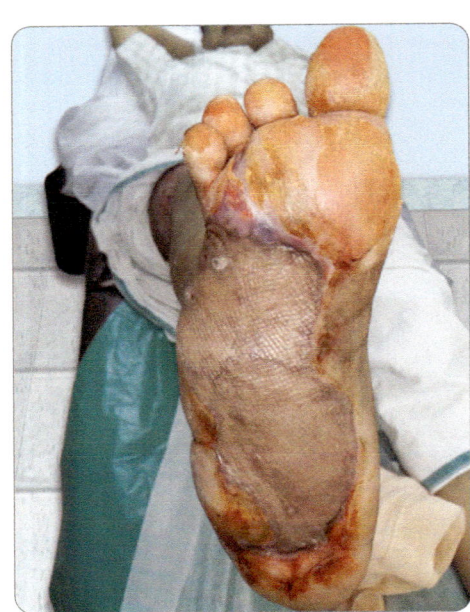

Figure 15 shows the postoperative view of the healed wound with skin graft and with good quality soft tissue bulk to withstand the pressure.

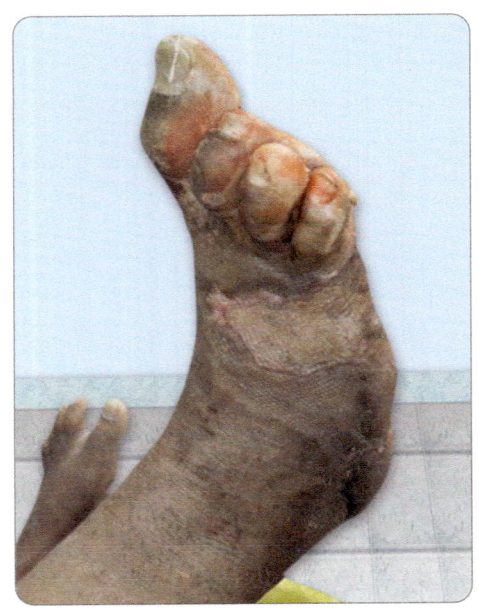

Figure 16 shows the postoperative view of the dorsum of the healed wound after split-thickness skin grafting.

Surgical Approach to the Management of Diabetic Foot Infections and Complex Diabetic Foot Wounds

CASE 4 (FIGURES 17 TO 22)

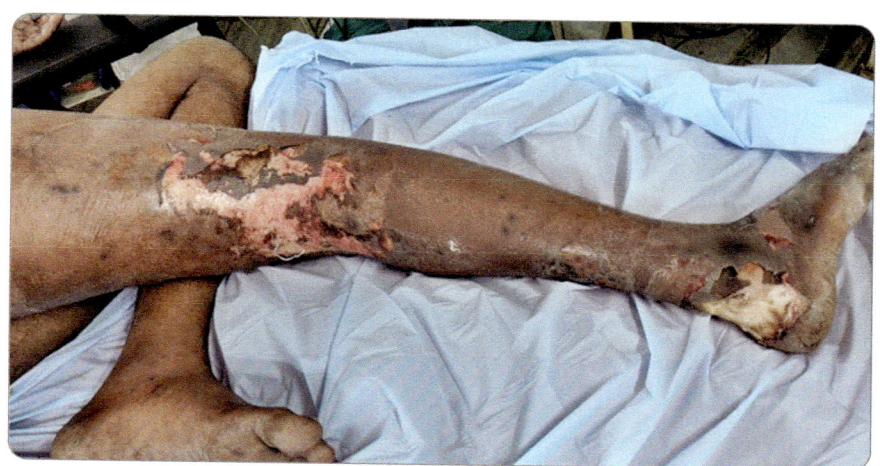

Figure 17 shows necrotizing fasciitis involving the dorsum, ankle, leg, knee, and thigh of the right foot.

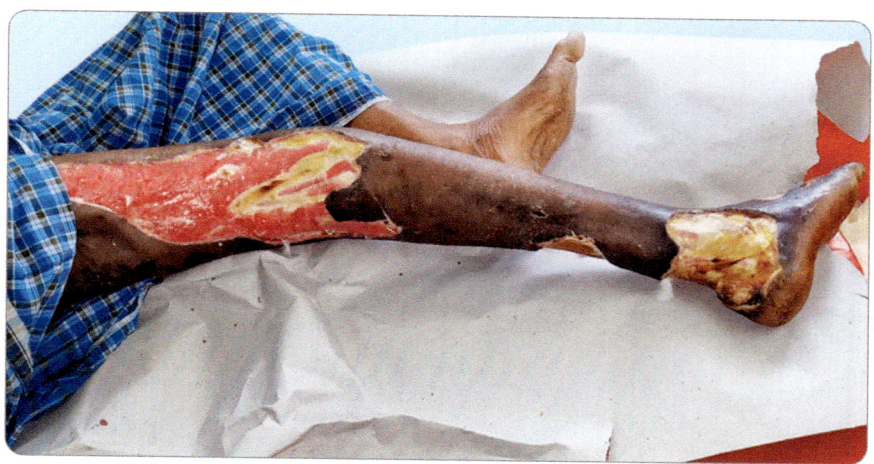

Figure 18 shows the postoperative view of a partly granulating wound. Serial debridements were done to remove the residual slough.

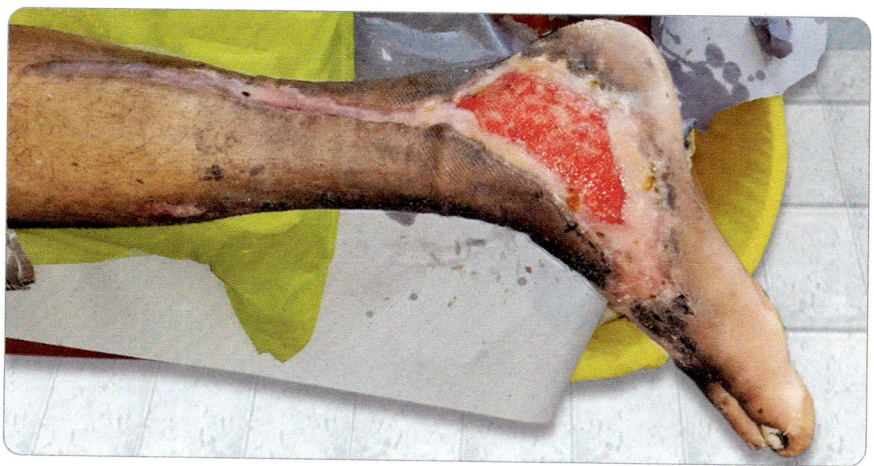

Figure 19 shows granulating healthy wound bed.

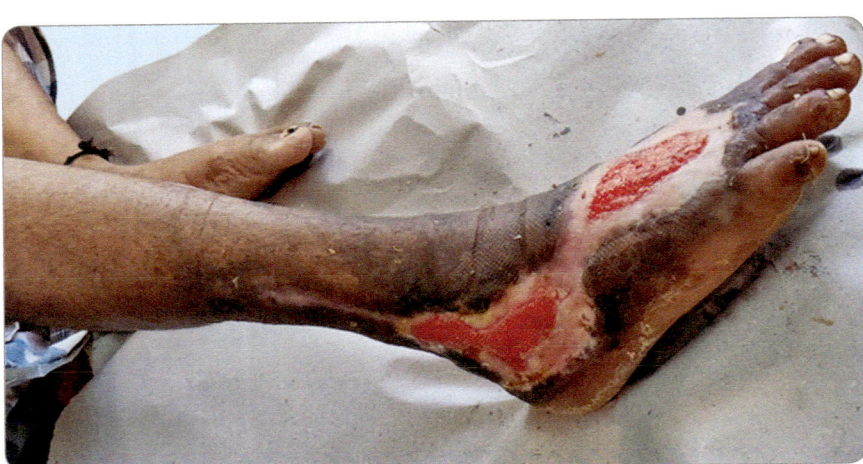

Figure 20 shows granulating healthy wound bed over the dorsum and the ankle.

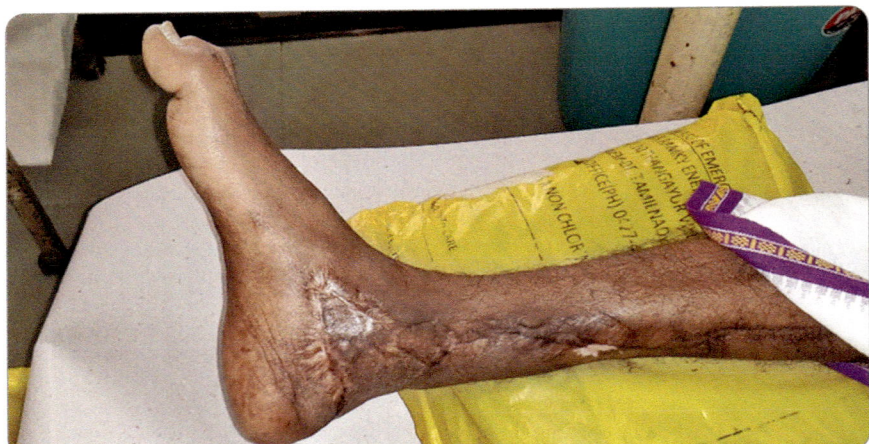

Figure 21 shows healed wound with a skin graft.

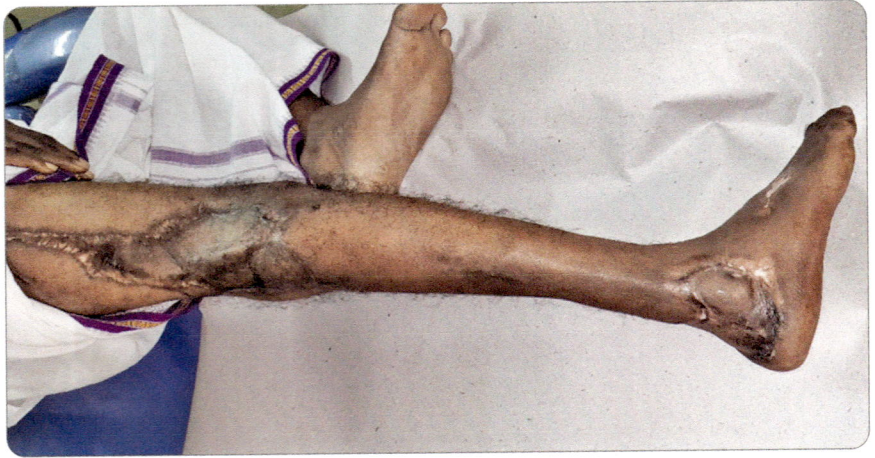

Figure 22 shows that the skin graft is maturing well without any contracture at the knee region.

Surgical Approach to the Management of Diabetic Foot Infections and Complex Diabetic Foot Wounds

CASE 5 (FIGURES 23 AND 24)

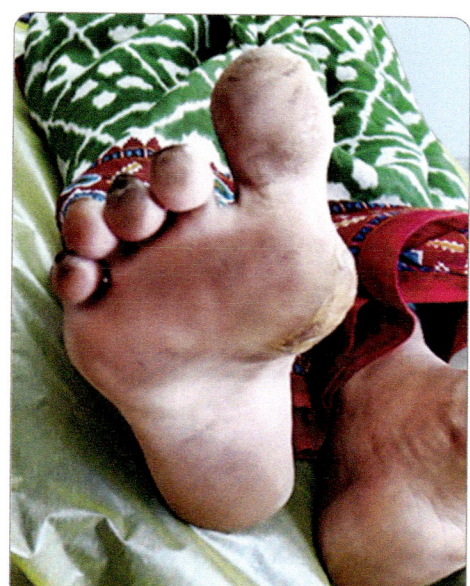

Figure 23 shows hammer toe deformity of lesser toes with skin changes.

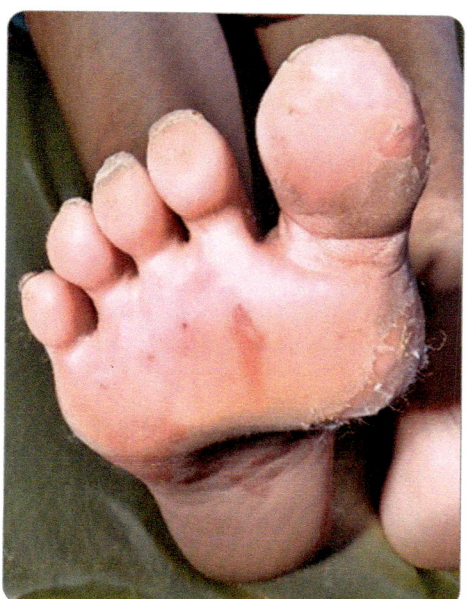

Figure 24 shows hammer toe deformity correction was done using closed needle flexor tenotomy.

Angiosome Concept: The Basics for Every Diabetic Foot Care Specialist

Sivashankari SelvaElavarasan, R Ravikumar

INTRODUCTION

Critical limb-threatening ischemia (CLTI) is considered a condition in which the arteries of the lower extremities get blocked, thereby resulting in a decrease in the blood flow. It is a significant form of peripheral arterial disease (PAD), which is caused due to atherosclerosis in which the blood vessels start narrowing due to plaque deposits causing decreased blood flow. CLTI is characterized by ischemic rest pain, which is typically felt when the person is at rest. The patient can also present with symptoms of pain or paresthesia in the feet accompanied by shiny, dry skin, toenails thickening, absence of peripheral pulses, nonhealing ulcers, or even dry gangrene.

RISK FACTORS OF CRITICAL LIMB-THREATENING ISCHEMIA

Hyperglycemia, smoking, dyslipidemia, obesity, hypertension, age, sedentary lifestyle as well as a family history of atherosclerosis are considered predominant risk factors for the development of CLTI.

DIAGNOSIS OF CRITICAL LIMB-THREATENING ISCHEMIA

Clinical and diagnostic imaging modalities for suspecting CLTI:
- *Auscultation*: A simple method used for the diagnosis of CLTI is to check for the presence of bruit in the peripheral arteries.
- *Ankle–Brachial Index (ABI)*: The ratio obtained by dividing the systolic blood pressure recorded in the arm by the systolic blood pressure in the ankle region.
- *Doppler ultrasound*: The direction and velocity of blood vessels can be accurately measured using a Doppler.
- *Computed tomography (CT) angiography*: Three-dimensional images of the foot can be developed with the help of a computer.
- *Magnetic resonance angiography*: The radiofrequency waves generated can be used to measure the energy released and can be used to develop two- or three-dimensional images.
- *Angiogram*: This remains the gold standard for the diagnosis of PAD. Contrast dyes can be used to take X-rays of the blood vessels.

The limb salvage rate has increased dramatically over the years because of the recent endovascular techniques that have been developed. In certain cases where the revascularization technique cannot be applied, the rate of major amputations was found to be >50% with a follow-up of 5 years. When the direct revascularization (DR) procedure was used, the rate of amputations was found to be between 8.2 and 21.1%.[1] The key strategy lies in the optimization of the blood flow to the ischemic regions. One of the concepts that have been focused extensively of late is the concept of angiosome.

THE CONCEPT OF ANGIOSOME

An anatomic tissue unit that is fed by a source artery and also drained by specific veins is referred to as an angiosome. Our body can be divided into 40 angiosomes, and there are six angiosomes in the foot. It becomes very important to understand the anatomy of foot angiosome to ensure better healing and also for the appropriate planning of arterial revascularization procedures. The six angiosomes in the foot are found to arise from three main below-the-knee (BTK) arteries, namely the anterior tibial artery, posterior tibial artery, and peroneal artery. There are six angiosomes that are recognized for the foot and ankle.

Angiosome Concept: The Basics for Every Diabetic Foot Care Specialist

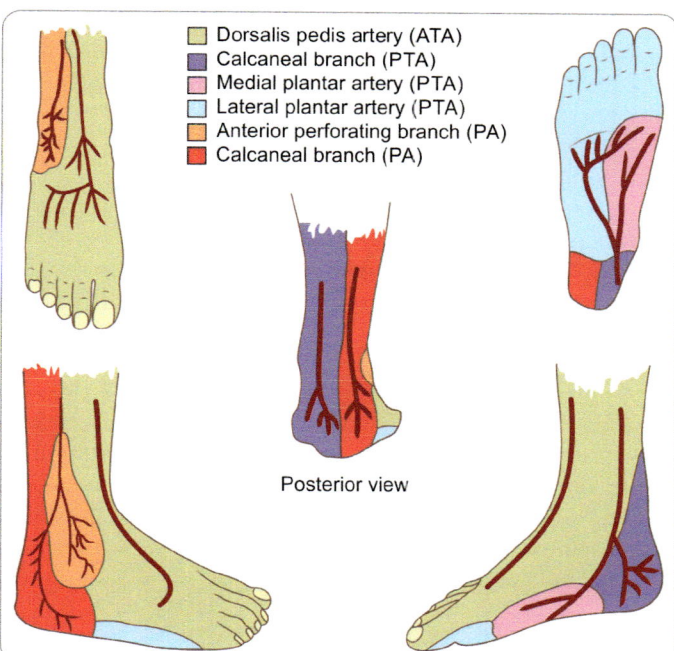

Fig. 1: It shows the six angiosomes of the foot and the ankle.[3]
(ATA: anterior tibial artery; PTA: posterior tibial artery; PA: peroneal artery)

1. *Posterior tibial artery angiosomes*:
   i. Medial calcaneal artery angiosome
   ii. Medial plantar artery angiosome
   iii. Lateral plantar artery angiosome
2. *Peroneal artery angiosomes*:
   iv. Lateral calcaneal artery angiosome
   v. Anterior perforator artery angiosome
3. *Anterior tibial artery angiosome*:
   vi. Anterior and dorsalis pedis artery angiosome

The first three angiosomes originate from the posterior tibial artery, the second two from the peroneal artery, and the last one from the anterior tibial artery **(Fig. 1)**.[2]

There are innumerable connections between the arteries called collateral arteries, which are found to feed the angiosomes. There are also small vessels called "choke vessels" that permit these angiosomes to feed the adjacent ones if any damage is found to occur to the source artery. It is imperative to understand the anatomic variants of pedal arteries to ensure optimal blood supply to the wound, especially once the direct in-line blood flow is reestablished.[4] The angiosomes of patients with PAD are distinct from the angiosomes of patients without PAD due to the occlusion of the main arteries. Hence, the identification of the correct angiosome has gained paramount importance to achieve the best possible therapeutic outcome.[5]

ANGIOSOME CONCEPT IN CLINICAL PRACTICE

In recent times, the application of the angiosome concept in revascularization has increased the rate of healing as well as the limb salvation rate. In a person living with diabetes, there can be either impairment of microcirculation due to neuropathy or sepsis as well as macroangiopathy due to atherosclerosis.[6]

In patients with CLTI, when the area of tissue loss supplied by the artery of interest is revascularized it is called DR, and in cases where the target artery is not amenable to revascularization and by revascularizing the nontarget vessel supply is reestablished to the area of tissue loss/nonhealing wound, it is called indirect revascularization (IR).

Surgical Revascularization

The concept of angiosome strategy is less relevant in bypass surgery because it is found to target the least affected artery. In a study by Rashid et al., it was found that direct angiosome revascularization through surgical bypass was practically possible in only 47% of their patients. The quality of the pedal arch was found to play a significant role in influencing both the rate of healing as well as time required for healing.[7] However, Azuma et al. stated that both direct and indirect techniques had similar healing rates, it should be kept in mind that indirect bypass revascularization had delayed healing rates.[8]

Endovascular Revascularization

There are several studies based on angiosome-guided endovascular revascularization. DR is associated with significant improvement in wound healing, major amputation as well as amputation-free survival rates when compared with IR. The similarity in outcomes between IR and DR could be attributed to the presence of collateral arteries, pedal arch, and indirect connections called "choke vessels". Patients without collaterals may benefit more from DR when it is considered a primary treatment strategy.

Points to be Considered before Planning for Revascularization (Surgery/Endovascular)

In the case of surgical revascularization, the most appropriate vessel for revascularization has to be chosen and it is not always possible to choose the artery that supplies the angiosome. However, in the case of endovascular revascularization, we have the advantage of selecting the specific angiosome that has to be targeted.[9] Endovascular revascularization also offers the benefit of treating more than one tibial vessel apart from providing the greatest advantage of treating severely affected vessels. The procedure of opening multiple vessels theoretically provides better blood flow to the foot. However, prolonged surgery and the process of trying to open multiple blood vessels at the same time can also contribute to increased perioperative complications.[10]

Severe tissue loss, the presence of arterial disease as well as infection are considered some of the limitations in angiosome guided-by-pass surgeries.[8] Medial sclerosis with diffuse calcification of the arteries makes angiosome-related arterial procedures (both surgical and endovascular) difficult, which can be overcome with the use of recent developments of novel endovascular techniques and instrumentation. It is imperative to keep in mind that in people with diabetes, the tunica media is found to be affected rather than the tunica intima, which in turn affects the collaterals as well as angiosomes anastomoses in addition to the source artery. The presence of adequate collaterals paves the way for IR to be considered.[11] Autonomic neuropathy, sepsis, and endothelial dysfunction are significant factors that can affect the outcome.[12]

ANGIOSOME REVASCULARIZATION AND WOUND HEALING

The ultimate goal of revascularization should be adequate reperfusion of tissues apart from the recanalization of vessels. Several studies have been published comparing the effects of DR and IR on wound healing, amputation-free survival, and limb salvage rates. In some cases, the rates of wound healing were similar and in clinical practice, we could use both approaches for treating patients. The procedure of using combined revascularization of both direct and indirect angiosome during angioplasty could be more beneficial and was also found to be associated with better wound healing outcomes when compared with IR.[13] In a study by Peregrin et al., it was found that patients who underwent more than one tibial artery angioplasty had increased wound healing rates and better limb salvage rates when compared to single vessel treatment. The most important variable in their cohort was identified as the number of tibial arteries opened.[14] We have discussed a few cases of angiosome-targeted angioplasty in **Appendix** for a better understanding of our readers. [Cases 1 and 2 are the examples of DR **(Figs. 2 to 8)**, whereas Cases 3 to 5 are the examples of IR **(Figs. 9 to 16)**.]

CONCLUSION

Successful revascularization and appropriate management of wound are considered as cornerstones for treatment of wounds in patients with CLTI. It becomes mandatory for the treating physician to consider the concept of angiosomes for maximum preservation of blood supply and optimum healing of wounds.

TAKE-HOME MESSAGE

A comprehensive approach which highlights the significance of achieving adequate revascularization in a diabetic foot is required to achieve good pulsatile arterial flow for the appropriate treatment of wound infection, to ensure adequate healing and most importantly to achieve better limb salvage rates.

REFERENCES

1. Faglia E, Clerici G, Clerissi J, Gabrielli L, Losa S, Mantero M, et al. Long-term prognosis of diabetic patients with critical limb ischemia: a population-based cohort study. Diabetes Care. 2009;32(5):822-7.
2. Taylor GI, Pan WR. Angiosomes of the leg: anatomic study and clinical implications. Plast Reconstr Surg. 1998;102(3):599-616.
3. Setacci C, De Donato G, Setacci F, Chisci E. Ischemic foot: Definition, etiology and angiosome concept. J Cardiovasc Sur (Torino). 2010;51(2):223-31.
4. Manzi M, Cester G, Palena LM, Alek J, Candeo A, Ferraresi R. Vascular imaging of the foot: the first step toward endovascular recanalization. Radiographics. 2011;31(5):1623-36.
5. Fujii M, Terashi H. Angiosome and Tissue Healing. Ann Vasc Dis. 2019;12(2):147-50.
6. Gibbons GW, Shaw PM. Diabetic vascular disease: characteristics of vascular disease unique to the diabetic patient. Semin Vasc Surg. 2012;25(2):89-92.
7. Rashid H, Slim H, Zayed H, Huang DY, Wilkins CJ, Evans DR, et al. The impact of arterial pedal arch quality and angiosome revascularization on foot tissue loss healing and infrapopliteal bypass outcome. J Vasc Surg. 2013;57(5):1219-26.
8. Azuma N, Uchida H, Kokubo T, Koya A, Akasaka N, Sasajima T. Factors influencing wound healing of critical ischaemic foot after bypass surgery: is the angiosome important in selecting bypass target artery? Eur J Vasc Endovasc Surg. 2012;43(3):322-8.
9. Alexandrescu V, Vincent G, Azdad K, Hubermont G, Ledent G, Ngongang C, et al. A reliable approach to diabetic neuroischemic foot wounds: below-the-knee angiosome-oriented angioplasty. J Endovasc Ther. 2011;18(3):376-87.
10. Hou X, Guo P, Cai F, Lin Y, Zhang J. Angiosome-Guided Endovascular Revascularization for Treatment of Diabetic Foot Ulcers with Peripheral Artery Disease. Ann Vasc Surg. 2022;86: 242-50.
11. Bosanquet DC, Glasbey JC, Williams IM, Twine CP. Systematic review and meta-analysis of direct versus indirect angiosomal revascularisation of infrapopliteal arteries. Eur J Vasc Endovasc Surg. 2014;48(1):88-97.
12. van den Berg JC. Angiosome perfusion of the foot: An old theory or a new issue? Semin Vasc Surg. 2018;31(2):56-65.
13. Ambler GK, Stimpson AL, Wardle BG, Bosanquet DC, Hanif UK, Germain S, et al. Infrapopliteal angioplasty using a combined angiosomal reperfusion strategy. PLoS one. 2017;12(2):e0172023.
14. Peregrin JH, Smírová S, Koznar B, Novotný J, Kovác J, Lastovicková J, et al. Self-expandable stent placement in infrapopliteal arteries after unsuccessful angioplasty failure: one-year follow-up. Cardiovasc Intervent Radiol. 2008;31(5):860-4.

Angiosome Concept: The Basics for Every Diabetic Foot Care Specialist 41

APPENDIX: CASES

Cases 1 and 2: Direct Revascularization

CASE 1 (FIGURES 2 TO 5)

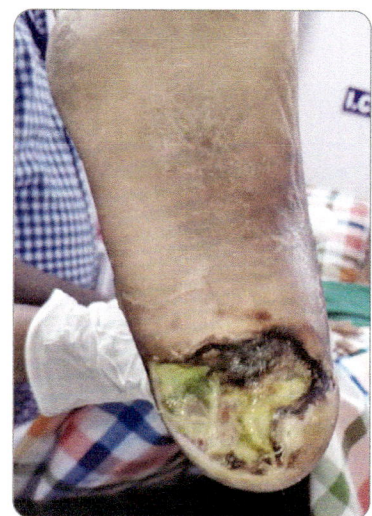

Figure 2 shows that the wound is on the plantar aspect of the calcaneum, which is supplied from both the medial calcaneal artery, which is a branch of the posterior tibial artery and the lateral calcaneal artery, which is a branch of the peroneal artery.

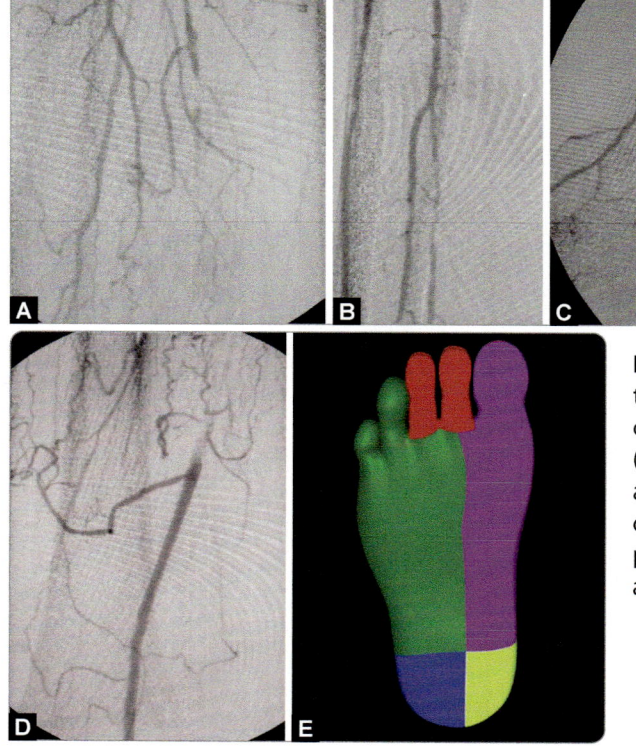

Figures 3A to E show the angiogram pictures, which depict the long segment mid superficial femoral artery (SFA) complete occlusion with infrapopliteal disease affecting all three vessels (preangioplasty pictures). **Figure 3E** shows the different angiosomes of the plantar aspect of foot. Yellow: medial calcaneal artery; Blue: lateral calcaneal artery; Violet: medial plantar artery; Green: lateral plantar artery; Red: anterior tibial artery.

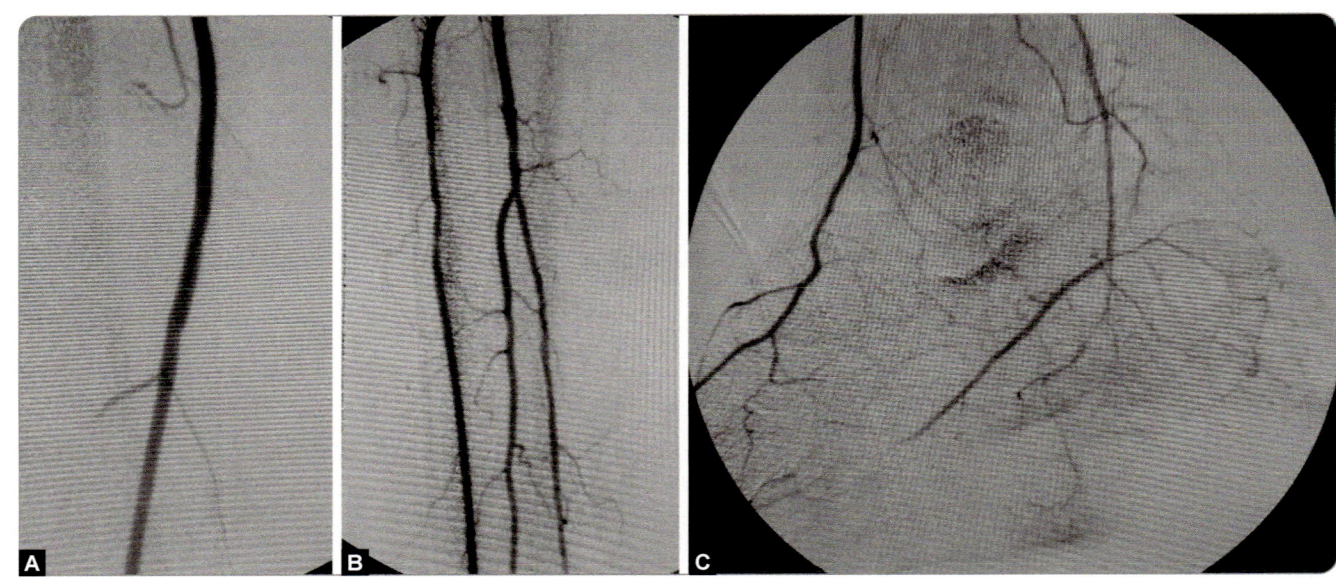

Figures 4A to C show postangioplasty pictures. Angioplasty was performed for SFA and all three infrapopliteal arteries with wound blush noted within the ulcer area.

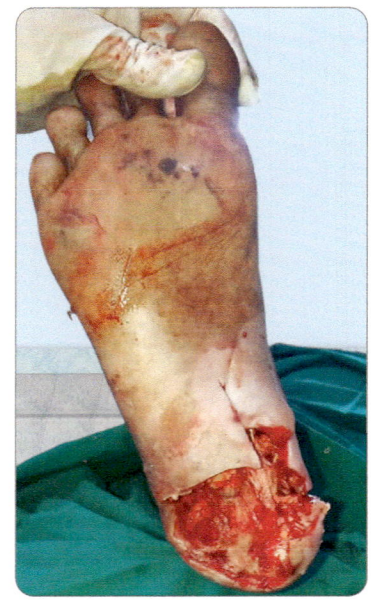

Figure 5 depicts a postdebridement foot picture showing red granulation tissue sign of healing.

Angiosome Concept: The Basics for Every Diabetic Foot Care Specialist 43

CASE 2 (FIGURES 6 TO 8)

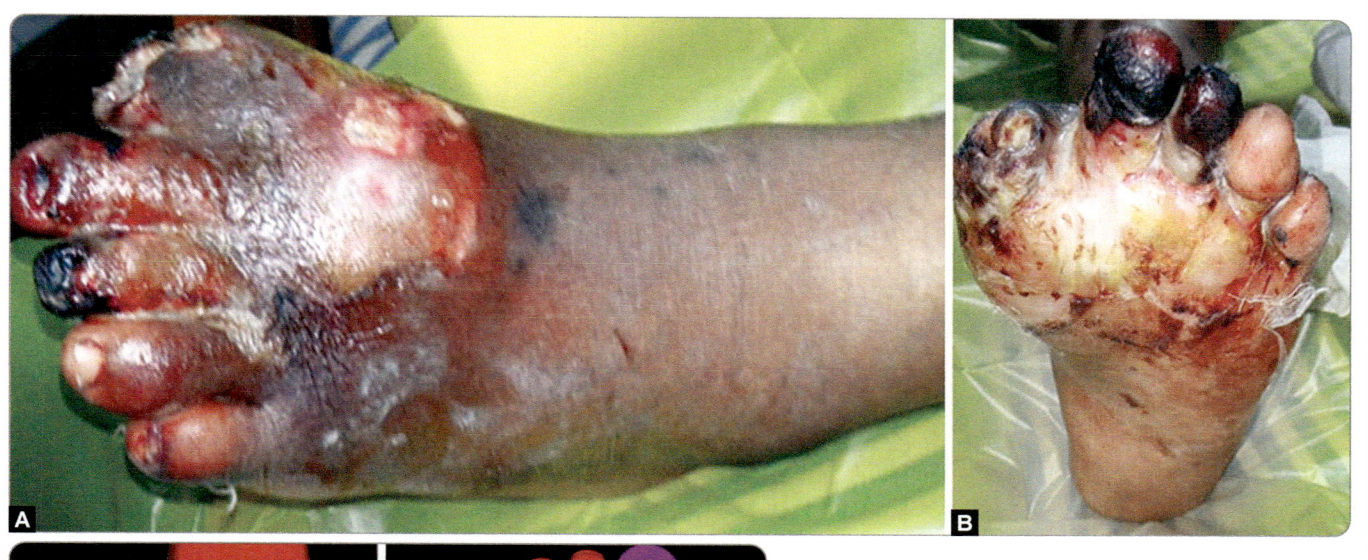
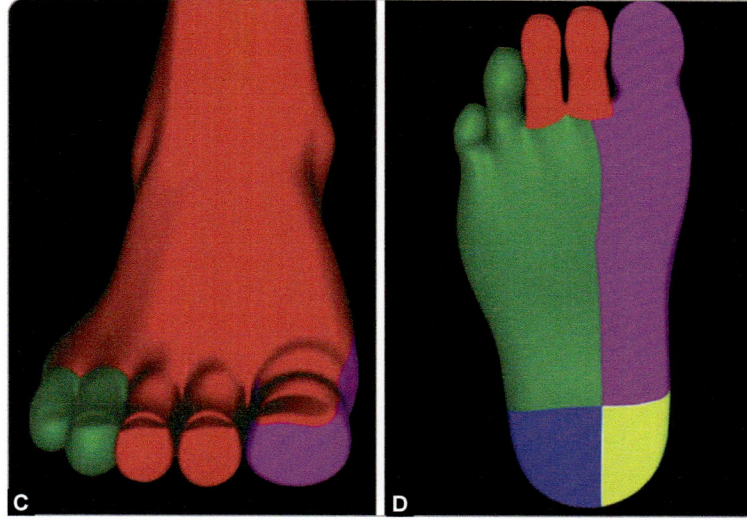

Figures 6A to D show the clinical and preangioplasty images of a nonhealing wound over the dorsal and plantar aspect of the foot. **Figures 6C and D** show the angiosome territory. The dorsum of the foot is supplied by the anterior tibial artery, and the plantar aspect is supplied by branches of the posterior tibial artery.

44 Angiosome Concept: The Basics for Every Diabetic Foot Care Specialist

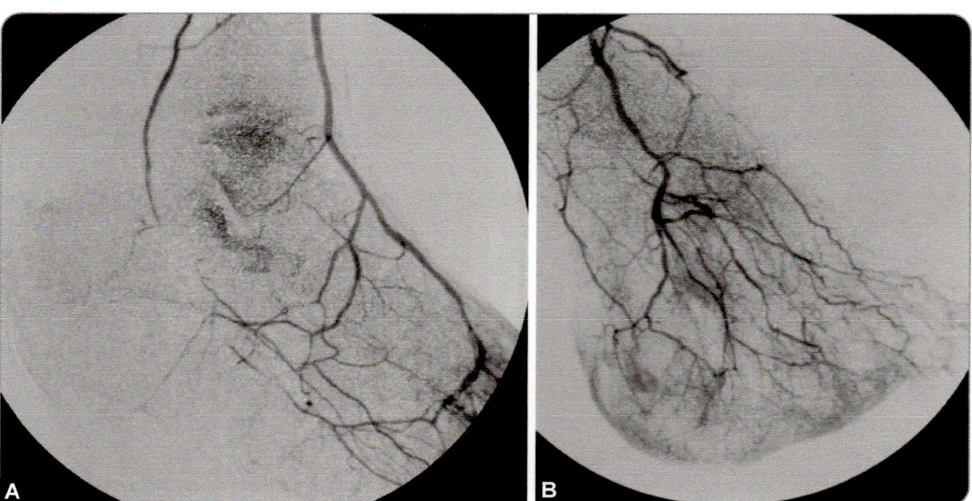

Figures 7A and B show the postangioplasty pictures in which the patient underwent both anterior tibial artery and posterior tibial artery revascularization forming the plantar arch with good wound blush.

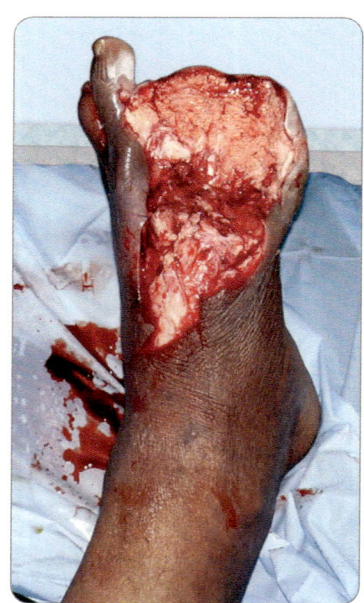

Figure 8 depicts the clinical picture of post-transplant amputation showing the stump with healthy granulation tissue.

Cases 3 to 5: Indirect Revascularization

CASE 3 (FIGURES 9A TO E)

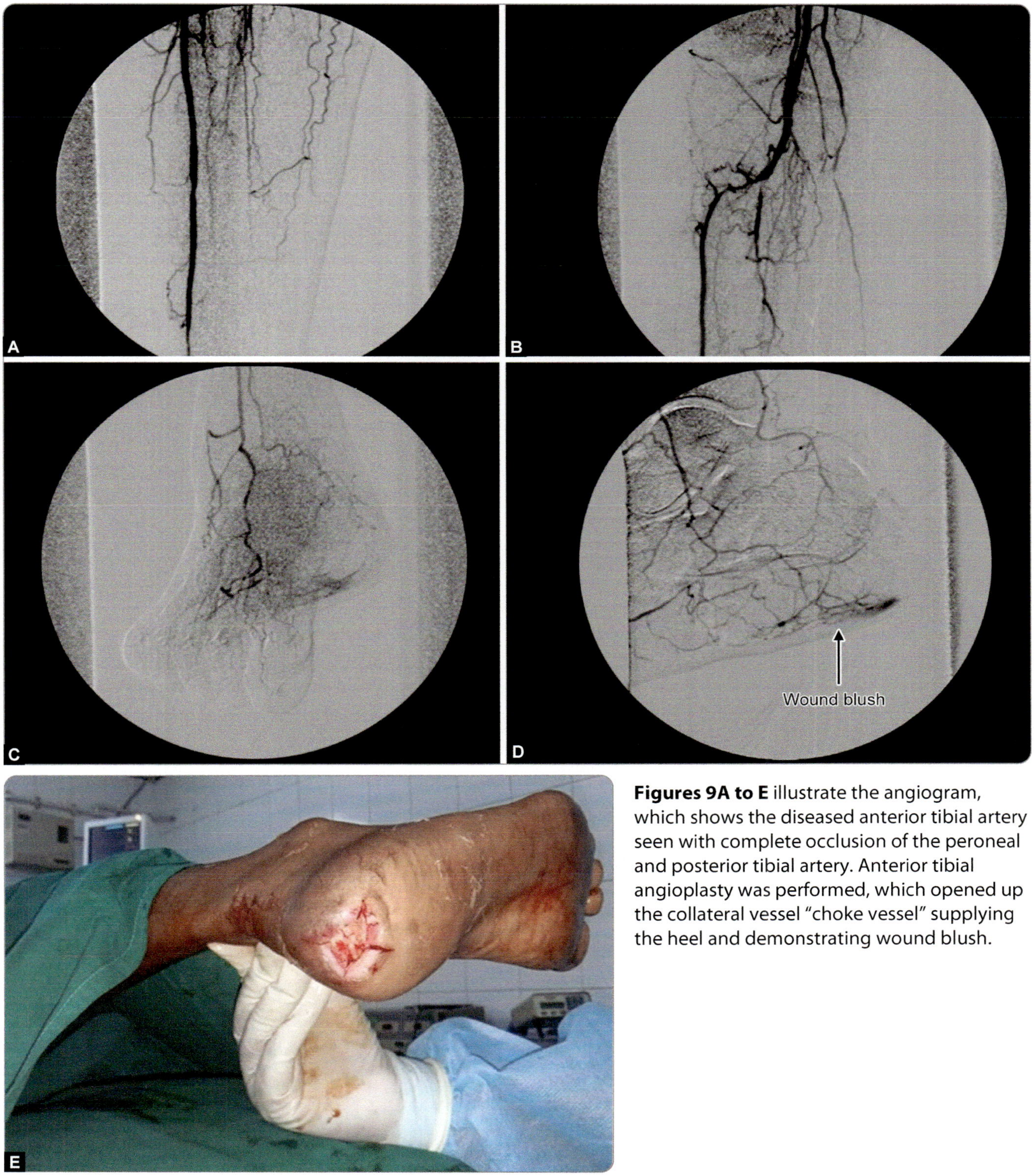

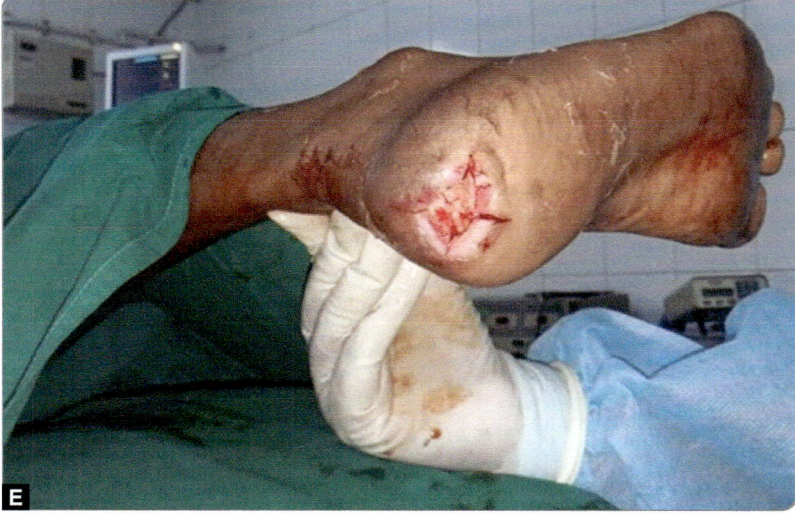

Figures 9A to E illustrate the angiogram, which shows the diseased anterior tibial artery seen with complete occlusion of the peroneal and posterior tibial artery. Anterior tibial angioplasty was performed, which opened up the collateral vessel "choke vessel" supplying the heel and demonstrating wound blush.

CASE 4 (FIGURES 10 TO 12)

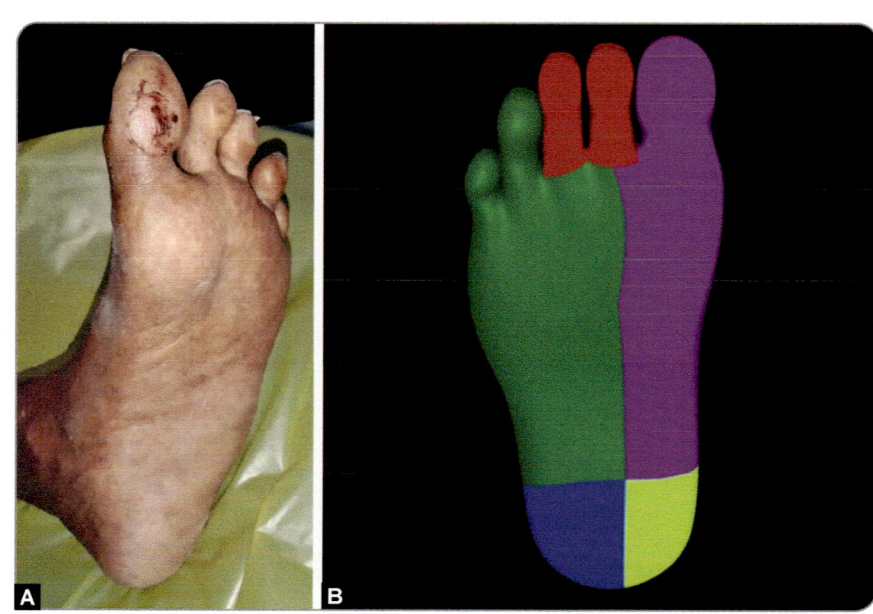

Figures 10A and B show the plantar surface of the great toe with a nonhealing ulcer. **Figure 10B** shows that this area is supplied by the medial plantar artery branch of the posterior tibial artery.

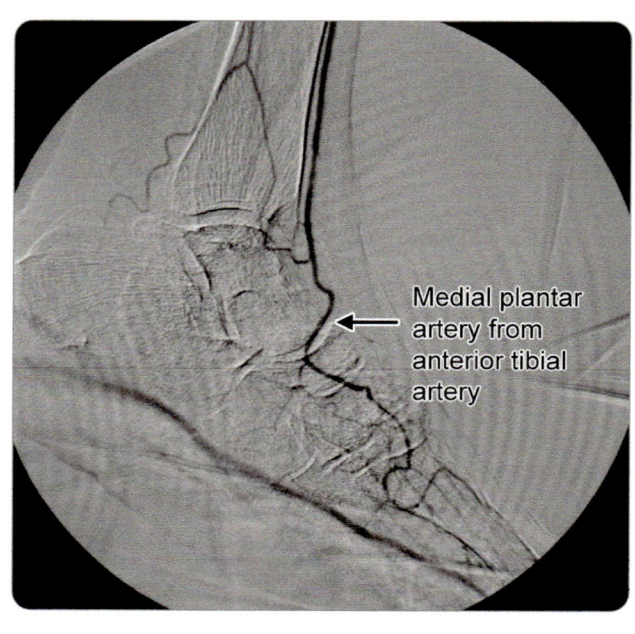

Figure 11 depicts the angiogram illustrating the diseased anterior tibial artery with the occluded posterior tibial artery. The anterior tibial artery is seen to continue as the medial plantar artery with an absent dorsalis pedis artery (variant anatomy).

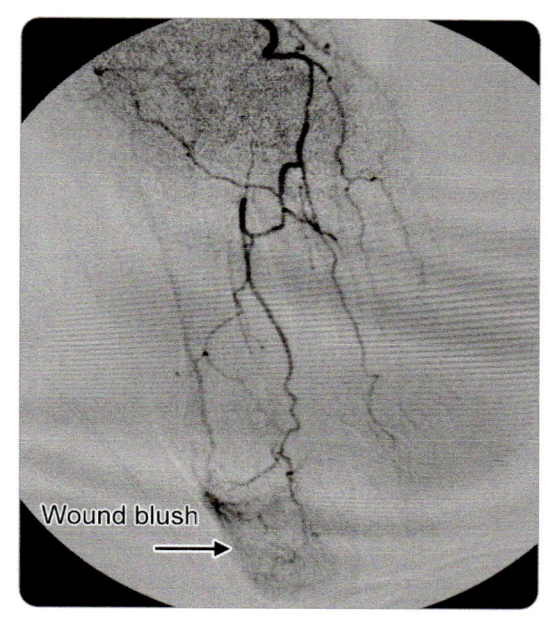

Figure 12 shows post anterior tibial angioplasty picture depicting a wound blush to the great toe.

CASE 5 (FIGURES 13 TO 16)

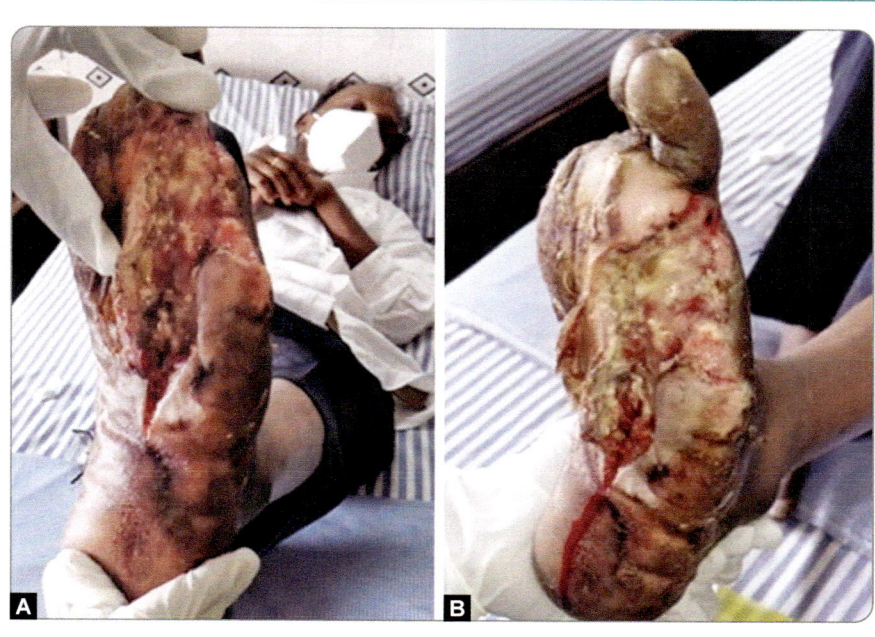

Figures 13A and B exhibit the foot images depicting a nonhealing ischemic wound over the entire plantar aspect of the foot. This area is supplied by the posterior tibial artery.

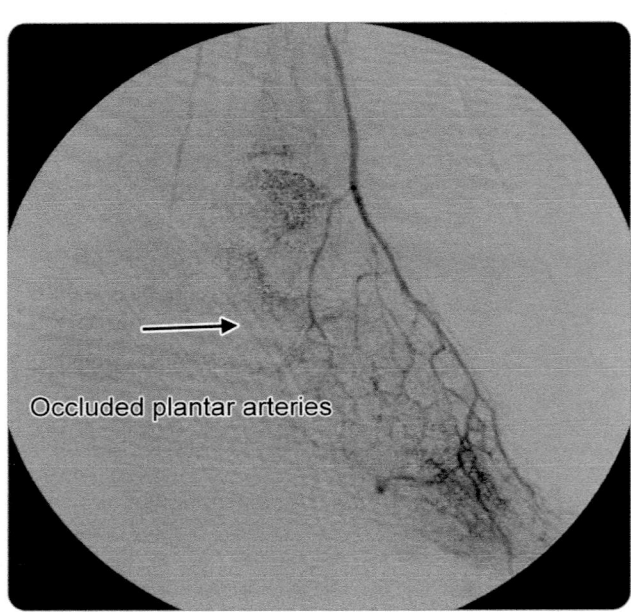

Figure 14 shows the angiogram, which revealed only flow within the anterior tibial artery with occlusion of the posterior tibial artery.

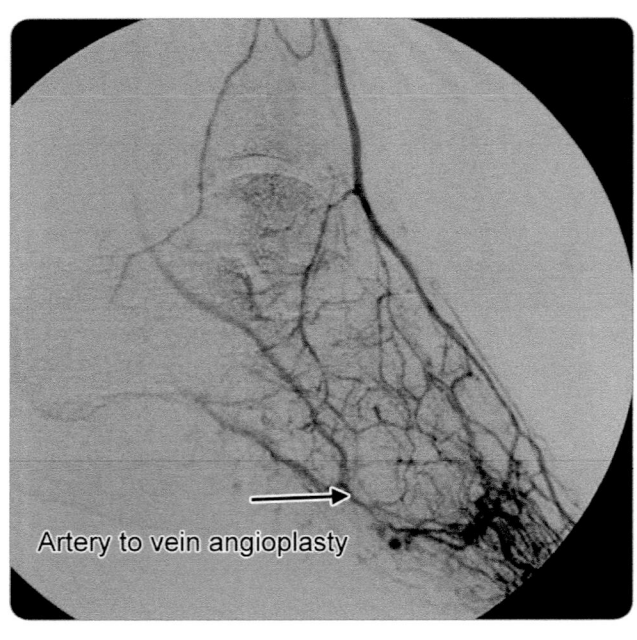

Figure 15 shows the distal venous arterialization, which was performed by connecting the plantar branch of the anterior tibial artery with the medial and plantar veins.

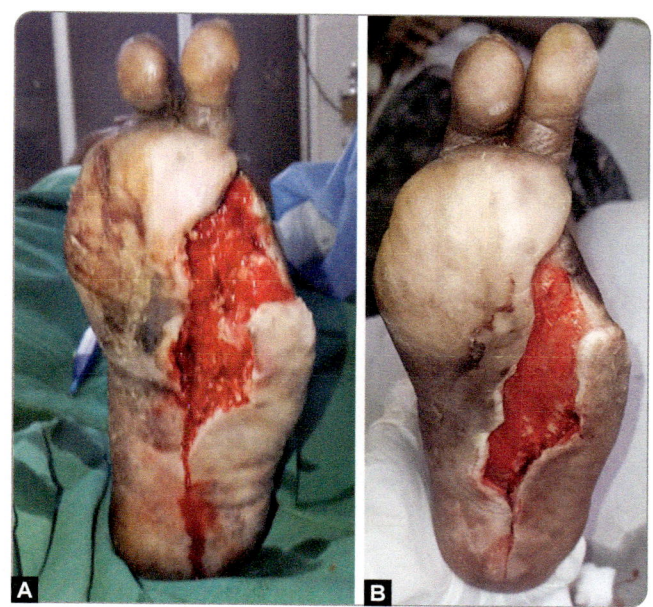

Figures 16A and B show red granulation tissue and healing in the postoperative clinical picture.

An Insight into the Radio Imaging of Diabetic Foot Infection

Senthil Govindan, Sivashankari SelvaElavarasan, Vijay Viswanathan

INTRODUCTION

Diabetic foot infection (DFI) is one of the most common and serious complications of long-standing diabetes, which can result in significant complications such as lower extremity amputations and mortality. Neuropathy remains a predominant risk factor responsible for DFI responsible for loss of protective sensation (LOPS) and is considered the principal reason for imperception of pain among neuropathic patients with skin ulcers, which can ultimately lead to soft tissue infections (STIs). If unidentified, these STIs can spread to the underlying bone resulting in osteomyelitis (OM). Thus, early identification and diagnosis of OM are considered very important to assess the prognosis and to treat patients most appropriately.

DIAGNOSIS OF DIABETIC FOOT INFECTION

A comprehensive history and clinical examination remain the fundamental principles for a good diagnosis. Imaging provides a noninvasive approach to arrive at a diagnosis compared to bone biopsy or probe-to-bone test (PTB) and is also considered complementary to the various clinical, microbiological, or laboratory assessments.[1] The various imaging modalities that can be used for the diagnosis of DFI are radiography, computed tomography (CT), and magnetic resonance imaging (MRI). Apart from this, various nuclear imaging modalities that use radiolabeled WBC (white blood cell), scintigraphy, and ^{18}F-fluorodeoxyglucose (^{18}F-FDG) positron emission tomography (PET) can help us in the evaluation of bone marrow and also achieve an accurate diagnosis of OM.

Imaging Modalities

A plain radiograph is always considered the simplest, cheapest, easily available, and first-line imaging in patients with DFI. It can help us to evaluate the alignment of the foot, analyze bony prominences, which can lead to ulcers, and assess fractures as well as dislocations of joints. It is well ascertained that it is very difficult to detect the early stages of OM using only plain radiographs.[2] It takes almost 4 weeks for radiographic changes to appear, and hence the use of serial radiographs can be considered to detect bone resorption as well as cortical destruction. Radiographs are of little paramount importance in the diagnosis of soft tissue pathologies such as ulcers, callus, cellulitis, or abscess. However, it can be used to assess any defect or swelling of the soft tissue. Although a clinical diagnosis is sufficient for cellulitis, it must be kept in mind that imaging is required to rule out OM.

Sonography is another imaging diagnostic modality that can be used to diagnose soft tissue abscesses or cellulitis. Accumulation of edema in the connective tissue can lead to the formation of striation or cobble-stone appearance.[3] The detection of foreign bodies as well as the diagnosis of necrotizing fasciitis requires the support of an ultrasound (USG).

Three-dimensional images and contrast enhancement have enabled the usage of CT for the detection of pathologies such as angiopathy or abscess. It has greater sensitivity and specificity when compared to radiographs in the identification of erosions of cortical bone, sequestra, soft tissue gas, and for the detection of foreign bodies as well as calcifications. However, the inability to differentiate between healthy and infected tissues, and ionizing radiation are some of the limitations to be considered while using CT. However, MRI remains the gold standard to diagnose soft tissue pathologies.

PREVALENCE OF RADIOGRAPHIC ABNORMALITIES IN INDIA

The prevalence of radiographic abnormalities in people with neuropathy and foot ulcers in India was studied by Viswanathan et al., which can help us in the early detection of such abnormalities and comprehensive management of DFI. People with diabetes have reduced cortical mass when compared to normal people and the presence of risk factors such as peripheral neuropathy makes them prone to bone fractures, which can in turn cause these bone and joint abnormalities (Table 1).[4] Table 1 illustrates the prevalence of various radiographic abnormalities in different study groups.

Normal Bone

The dorsoplantar, lateral, and anteroposterior views are the three important X-ray views usually considered in the radiographic imaging of a normal foot. The dorsoplantar view can be used to ascertain the metatarsal bones (heads and shafts), deformities of the forefoot as well as the phalanges. The first metatarsal bone, calcaneus, medial tarsus, and the profile of the ankle can be studied with the help of a lateral view. The various disorders of the foot related to biomechanics can be assessed using these views. The talocrural structures can be evaluated using the anteroposterior or frontal view. Lateral oblique and axial sesamoid views are some of the supplementary views, which are found useful.[5] The lateral weight bearing X-rays are useful in the diagnosis of Charcot foot (CF) deformities.

Osteomyelitis

Osteomyelitis is characterized by the classic radiologic triad of periosteal reaction, osteolysis, and destruction of bone. These radiographic changes become evident only 10–20 days after the development of clinical symptoms.[6] Small ill-defined radiolucencies seen in the medullary bone as well as the cortex are referred to as osteolysis. In some cases, destruction of the cortex might be seen. In the later stages, sequestrum or dead/sclerotic bone is evident. We have discussed five cases of OM for better comprehension of our readers (Cases 1 to 5: Figs. 1 to 5). Plain radiography for OM is expected to have a sensitivity of 60% and a specificity of 80%.[7] If an accurate diagnosis of OM cannot be achieved with the help of clinical examination and radiographs, MRI is usually recommended. However, radiographs alone can be used to exclude a diagnosis of fracture.

Charcot Foot

Charcot foot is characterized by an inflammation of the foot due to polyneuropathy. The natural course of the disease has four different phases, namely (i) inflammation, (ii) fragmentation, (iii) coalescence, and (iv) consolidation. The active phase of the disease is marked by a red, hot, and swollen foot without pain due to neuropathy. At this stage, the bone is fragile and is liable to get fractured and destruction of joints. It is imperative to diagnose an acute CF in its early stages, because it can prevent the development of deformities. During the inactive phase, there is no redness, but there is clinical evidence of soft tissue as well as bone marrow edema. There may be prominent osteophytes, palpable loose bodies, and proliferation of the bone, which may ultimately result in characteristic rocker-bottom deformity. Conventional radiographs remain the standard imaging technique to arrive at an accurate diagnosis of CF. However, MRI remains the best imaging modality to diagnose early active CF.[8]

Focal demineralization along with flattening of the metatarsal head seems to be the earliest finding in a conventional radiograph of acute CF. Few cases might present with periarticular or subchondral changes in the midfoot region.[9] Case 6 is a description of both clinical and radiographic changes seen in a case of CF (Case 6: Fig. 6). However, plain radiography is found to have very low sensitivity as well as specificity (<50%) for the detection of CF in its early stages.[10] MRI is considered an imaging modality with high sensitivity to diagnose an acute case of CF. MRI

Details	Group I (DM)	Group II (DM + neuropathy)	Group III (DM + neuropathy + ulcer)
Bone abnormalities, n (%)			
Traumatic fracture	–	3 (6)	6 (12)
Periosteal reaction	–	5 (10)	23 (46)*
Osteopenia	3 (6)	14 (28)	30 (60)*
Exostoses	–	1 (2)	1 (2)
Infection	1 (2)	7 (14)	27 (54)*
Erosion	–	4 (8)	14 (28)*
Atrophy of metatarsal	1 (2)	1 (2)	8 (16)*
Penciling	–	–	1 (2)
Amputation	1 (2)	1 (2)	16 (32)*
Joint abnormalities, n (%)			
Charcot changes	–	7 (14)	27 (54)*
Subchondral sclerosis	1 (2)	1 (2)	2 (4)
Osteophytes	1 (2)	1 (2)	9 (18)*
Fragmentation	–	–	9 (18)
Destruction	–	4 (8)	14 (28)*
Dislocation	–	2 (4)	4 (8)

TABLE 1: Prevalence of radiographic abnormalities in different study groups.[4]

*$p < 0.05$ versus group II

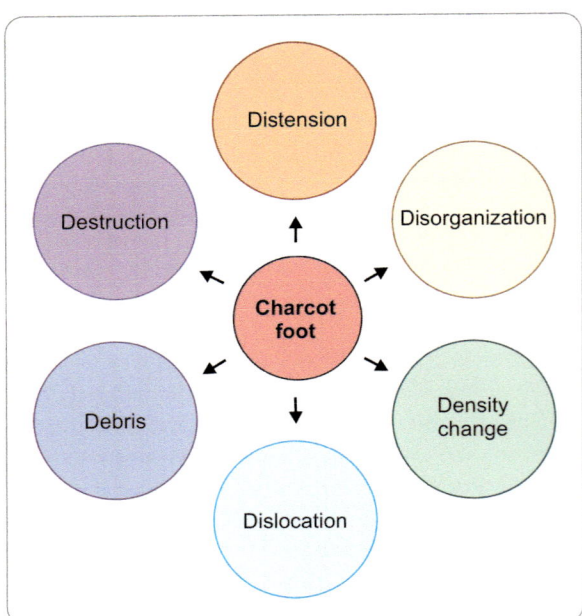

Fig. 7: Radiographic features of Charcot foot.

TABLE 2: Radiographic findings of OM and CF.		
Radiographic features	OM	CF
Location	Metatarsal head and toes, forefoot	Midfoot
Cortical destruction	Distinct	Absent
Proximity to soft tissue	In close proximity to STI or ulcer	Distant from STI or ulcer

(CF: Charcot foot; OM: osteomyelitis; STI: soft tissue infection)

of active CF can show subchondral bone marrow edema, effusion of the joints as well as edema of the soft tissue.[11]

In chronically stable cases of CF, the use of conventional radiographs is considered highly beneficial in the follow-up of patients.[12] The radiographic features of a CF are characterized by 6 Ds as depicted in **Figure 7**.[13] Figure 7 summarizes the radiographic changes in a CF.

Any subchondral osteopenia or sclerosis may contribute to changes in the density of the bone, osseous fragmentation, and bone resorption, which may lead to destruction; the presence of interarticular loose bodies is considered responsible for the debris; joint effusion may lead to distension, and the malalignment of the joints due to ligamentous laxity is the predominant reason for disorganization as well as dislocation. The forefoot can also present with a "pencil and cup appearance", which may develop secondary to metatarsophalangeal involvement. Sometimes, it can present with the involvement of the tarsometatarsal joint, which can result in the collapse of the longitudinal arch, and can ultimately result in a rocker-bottom deformity. The hind foot can also present with calcaneal fractures, collapse of the talus bone, or dislocation of the talocalcaneal joint.[14] Sometimes, there can be a deadly combination of both OM and CF. Case 7 is an example of CF with OM in distal phalanx (DPX) **(Case 7: Fig. 8)**.

Osteomyelitis versus Charcot Foot

Sometimes, it can be very difficult to distinguish between OM and CF. **Table 2** illustrates the radiographic findings of both conditions, which will enable us to easily differentiate between the two substantiating the importance of understanding both their imaging characteristics **(Table 2)**.[15]

ROLE OF MAGNETIC RESONANCE IMAGING IN THE DIAGNOSIS OF OSTEOMYELITIS AND CHARCOT FOOT

Magnetic resonance imaging has a very high sensitivity (77–100%) and high specificity (80–100%) in the precise diagnosis of OM.[16] An early and accurate diagnosis of CF has become possible with the advent of MRIs. They are also highly beneficial in monitoring the activity of the disease as well as in detecting complications in advanced stages of CF, STI, or OM. Conventional radiographs sometimes appear very normal in the very early stages of CF. In such cases, MRI remains the best imaging modality for an accurate diagnosis of early active CF. Edema of the bone marrow and soft tissues, subchondral microfractures, and joint effusions are some of the early signs of CF in MRI. In advanced stages, cortical fractures, dislocations, and destructions of joints may be seen. In cases where MRI is contraindicated, CT and PET-CT are alternative imaging modalities that can be considered.

FOOT DEFORMITIES

The predominant risk factors for DFI are high plantar pressure and structural foot deformities. Prominent metatarsal heads, CF, hammertoes, hallux limitus, or any history of previous amputations are some of the predisposing factors, which can lead to high pressures and can ultimately result in inflammation as well as the formation of ulcers. Removal of bony prominences or structural realignment remains the mainstay of treatment of these patients. Sometimes, the treatment may further get complicated due to the presence of infections, OM, or cellulitis.[1] Thus radiographs play a very significant role in the early identification of these deformities and their subsequent treatment.

CONCLUSION

Radiographs are always considered a good, noninvasive diagnostic aid to detect various bone and joint abnormalities, especially in resource-constrained settings. It also substantially reduces the morbidity and complications associated with deformities as well as ulcerations. It also becomes mandatory to use other imaging modalities like MRI in recommended cases to arrive at a more accurate diagnosis. Thus, an integrated and systematic approach is required to correlate clinical, laboratory as well as imaging findings for the most appropriate therapeutic management.

> **TAKE-HOME MESSAGE**
>
> Radiographs are recommended in patients with nonhealing ulcers with a duration of more than 4 weeks and when the PTB test becomes positive. They are also considered highly beneficial in the early diagnosis of acute CF and various foot deformities. Thus, diagnosis and management of DFI require a multidisciplinary approach, which includes the pertinent usage of multimodality imaging techniques to assess the involvement of underlying bone and the magnitude of infection, to differentiate STI from OM, and to identify the bony abnormalities associated with CF, which can help us to understand the pathology behind DFI, which in turn is found beneficial for its appropriate management.

REFERENCES

1. Lauri C, Leone A, Cavallini M, Signore A, Giurato L, Uccioli L. Diabetic Foot Infections: The Diagnostic Challenges. J Clin Med. 20208;9(6):1779.
2. Wang CL, Cohan RH, Ellis JH, Caoili EM, Wang G, Francis IR. Frequency, outcome, and appropriateness of treatment of nonionic iodinated contrast media reactions. AJR Am J Roentgenol. 2008;191(2):409-15.
3. Adhikari S, Blaivas M. Sonography first for subcutaneous abscess and cellulitis evaluation. J Ultrasound Med. 2012;31(10):1509-12.
4. Viswanathan V, Kumpatla S, Rao VN. Radiographic Abnormalities in the Feet of Diabetic Patients with Neuropathy and Foot Ulceration. J Assoc Physicians India. 2014;62(11):30-3.
5. Bouysset M, Tavernier T. Radiography of the foot. In: Bouysset M (Ed). Bone and Joint Disorders of the Foot and Ankle: A Rheumatological Approach. Berlin, Heidelberg: Springer; 1998.
6. Crim JR, Seeger LL. Imaging evaluation of osteomyelitis. Crit Rev Diagn Imaging. 1994;35(3):201-56.
7. Donovan A, Schweitzer ME. Current concepts in imaging diabetic pedal osteomyelitis, Radiol Clin North Am. 2008;46(6):1105-24.
8. Rosskopf AB, Loupatatzis C, Pfirrmann CWA, Böni T, Berli MC. The Charcot foot: a pictorial review. Insights Imaging. 2019;10(1):77.
9. Toledano TR, Fatone EA, Weis A, Cotten A, Beltran J. MRI evaluation of bone marrow changes in the diabetic foot: a practical approach. Semin Musculoskelet Radiol. 2011;15(3):257-68.
10. Chantelau E, Poll LW. Evaluation of the diabetic charcot foot by MR imaging or plain radiography—an observational study. Ex Clin Endocrinol Diabetes. 2006;114(8):428-31.
11. Morrison WB, Ledermann HP. Work-up of the diabetic foot. Radiol Clin North Am. 2002;40(5):1171-92.
12. Ergen FB, Sanverdi SE, Oznur A. Charcot foot in diabetes and an update on imaging. Diabet Foot Ankle. 2013;20:4.
13. Radswiki T, Lokhandwala D, Knipe H. Radiographic features of a Charcot joint (mnemonic). [online] Available from https://radiopaedia.org/articles/radiographic-features-of-a-charcot-joint-mnemonic#:~:text=The%20radiographic%20features%20of%20a,Ds%20(separating%20disorganization%20and%20dislocation) [Last accessed August, 2023].
14. Rajbhandari SM, Jenkins RC, Davies C, Tesfaye S. Charcot, neuroarthropathy in diabetes mellitus. Diabetologia. 2002;45(8): 1085-96.
15. Hochman MG, Cheung Y, Brophy DP, Parker JA. Imaging of the diabetic foot. In: Veves A, Giurini JM, Logerfo FW (Eds). The Diabetic: Foot Contemporary Diabetes. Totowa, NJ: Humana Press; 2006.
16. Mautone M, Naidoo P. What the radiologist needs to know about Charcot foot. J Med Imaging Radiat Oncol. 2015;59(4):395-402.

APPENDIX: CASES

CASE 1 (FIGURES 1A TO C)

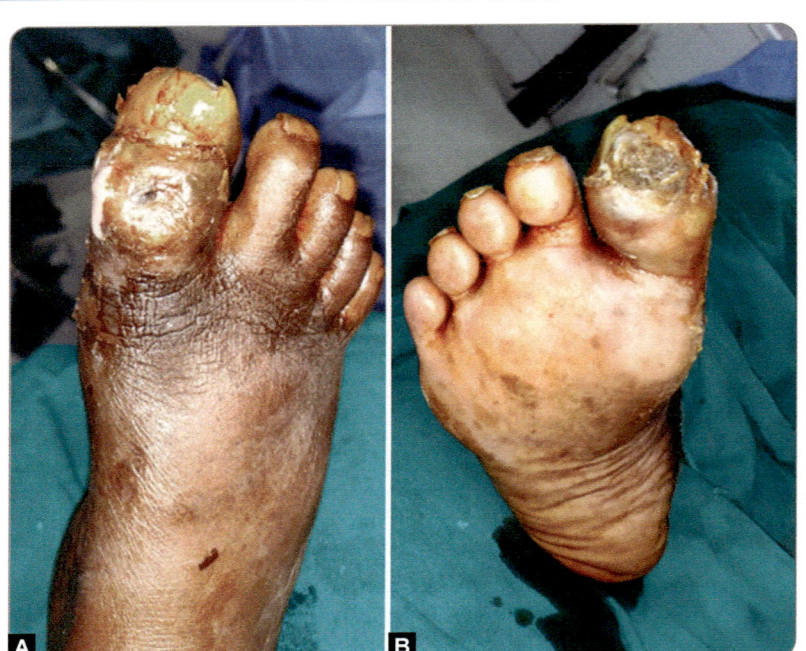

Figures 1A and B show a case of necrotic wound infection of the right great toe (dorsal and plantar aspect).

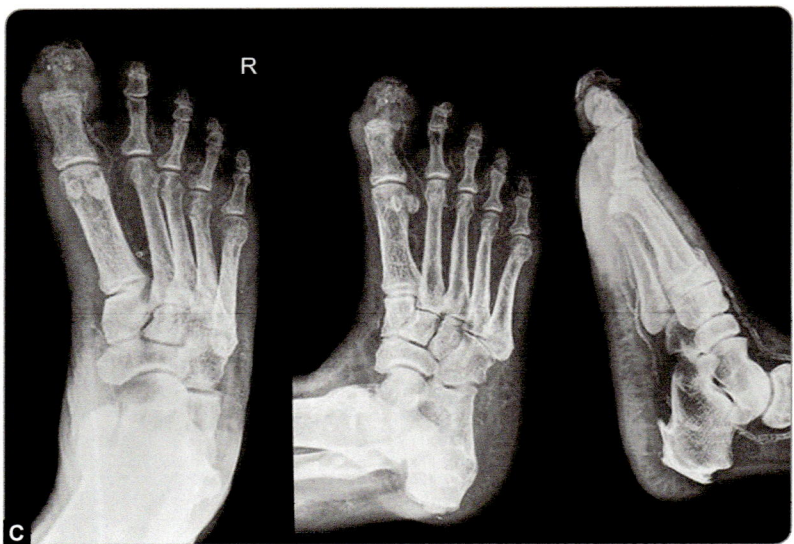

Figure 1C depicts X-ray showing OM with destruction of DPX.

CASE 2 (FIGURES 2A AND B)

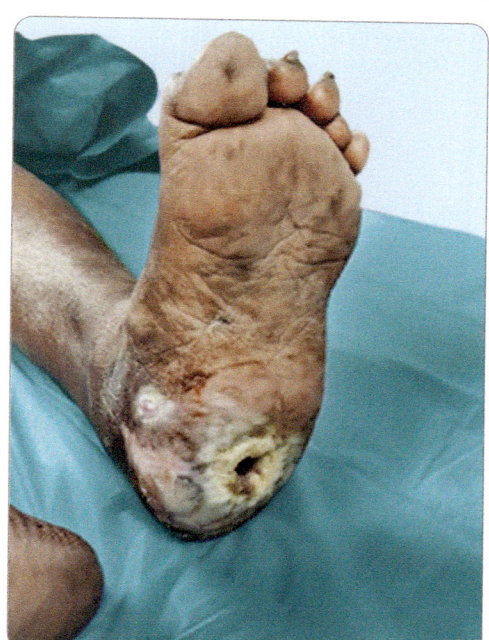

Figure 2A shows a nonhealing ulcer over the left heel.

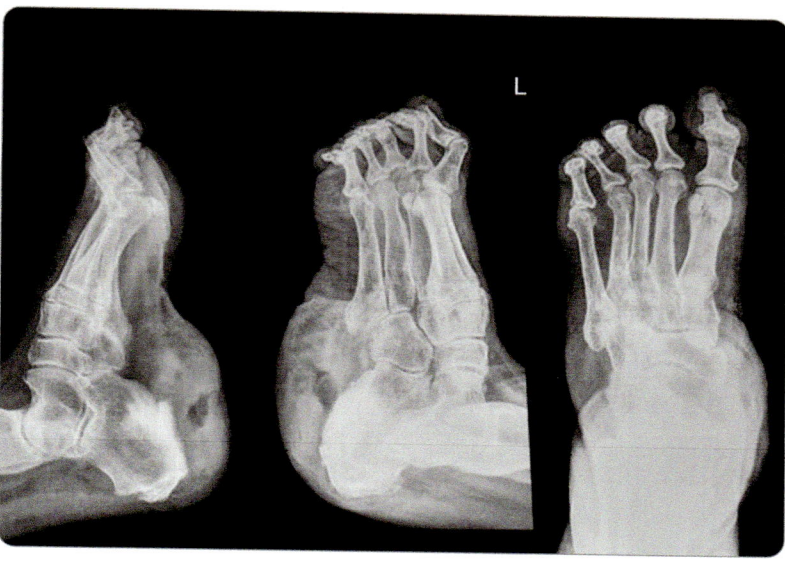

Figure 2B shows portion of calcaneal sequestrum with soft tissue defect.

CASE 3 (FIGURES 3A TO C)

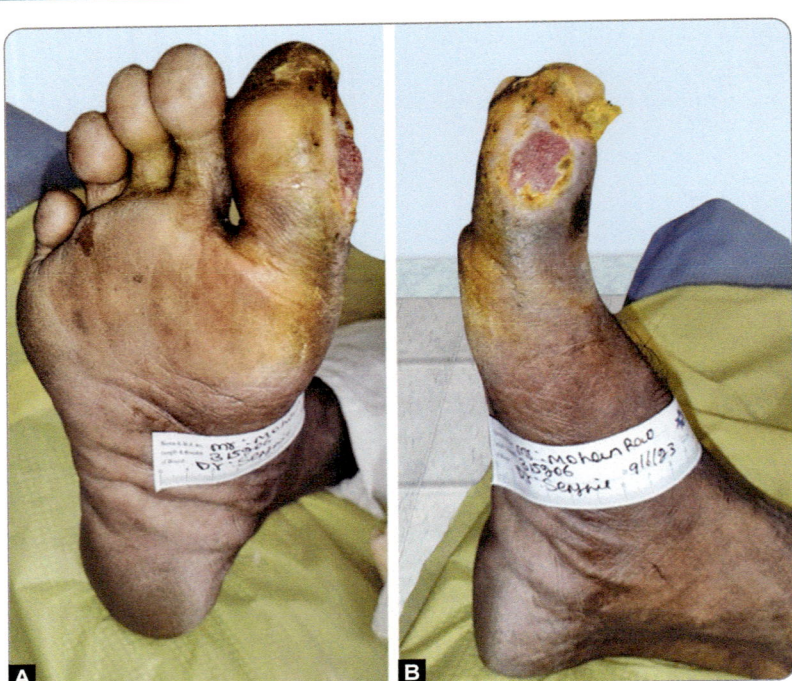

Figures 3A and B show a clinical picture of a nonhealing wound over the right great toe.

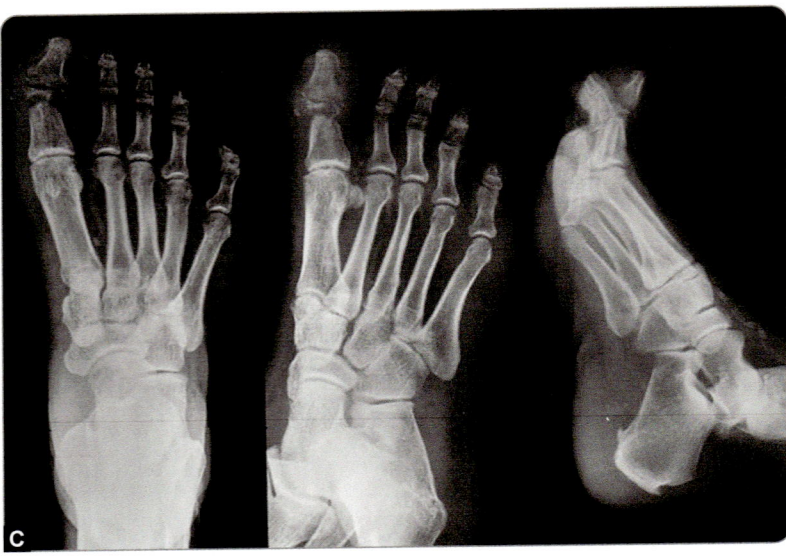

Figure 3C shows a radiograph showing areas of osteomyelitic changes in DPX and PPX (proximal phalanx) with sequestrum at the interphalangeal (IP) joint.

An Insight into the Radio Imaging of Diabetic Foot Infection

CASE 4 (FIGURES 4A TO C)

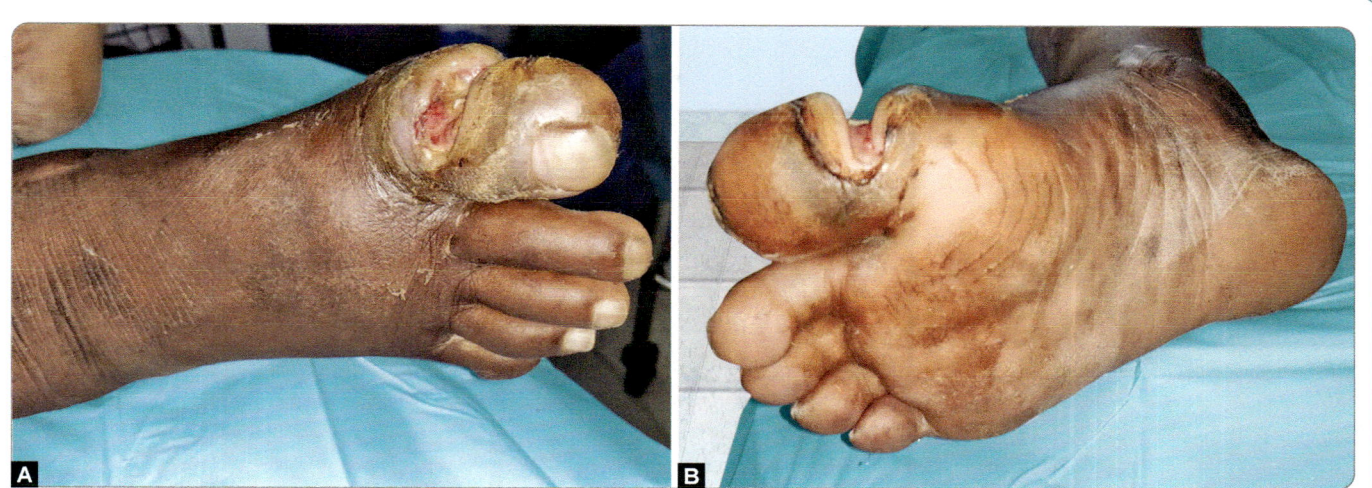

Figures 4A and B show clinical pictures of an infected wound in the right great toe with a positive PTB test.

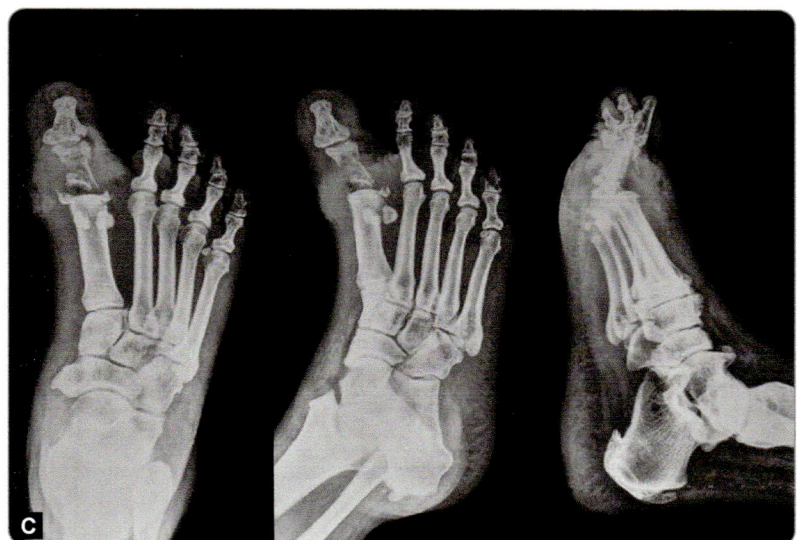

Figure 4C shows osteomyelitic changes seen in PPX.

CASE 5 (FIGURES 5A TO C)

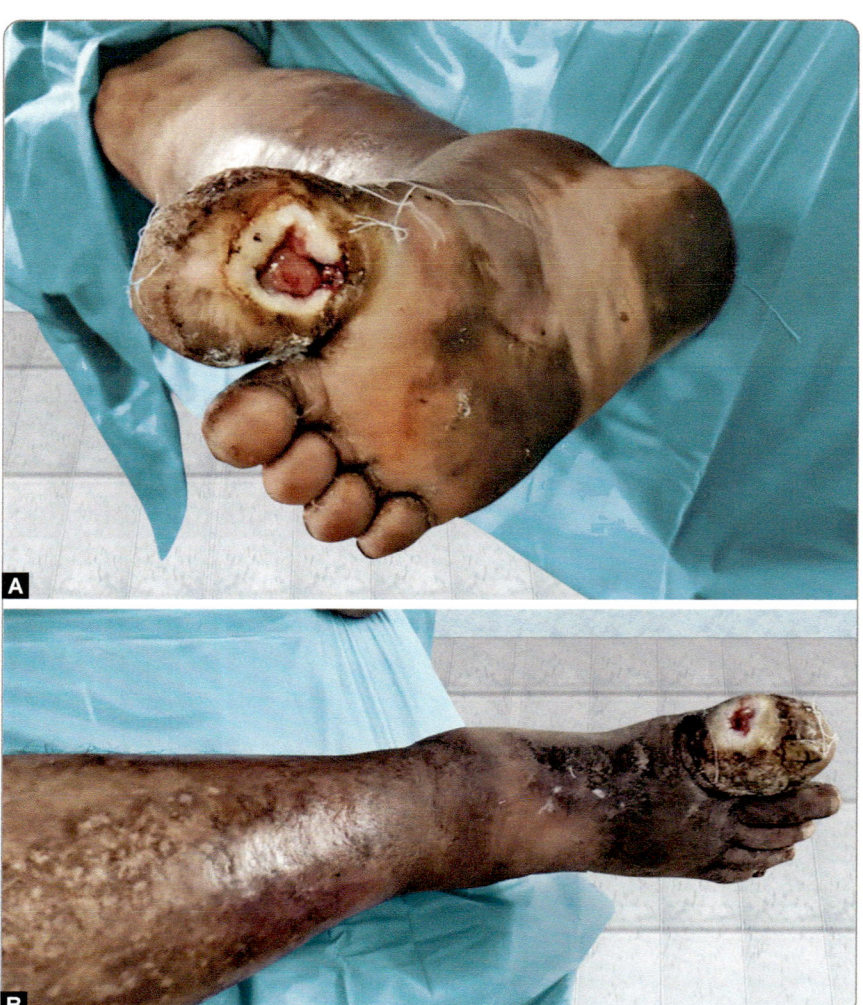

Figures 5A and B show a clinical picture of a wound infection in the right great toe.

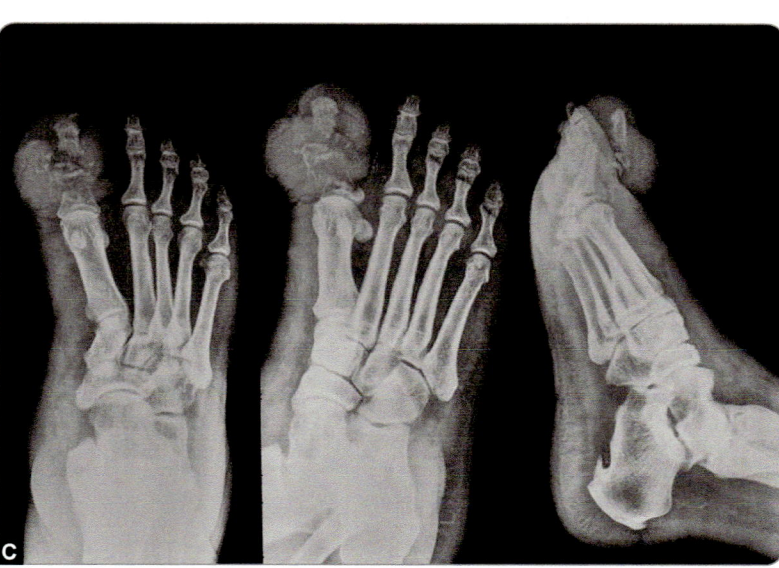

Figure 5C shows an X-ray showing OM involving DPX and PPX of the great toe.

CASE 6 (FIGURES 6A TO C)

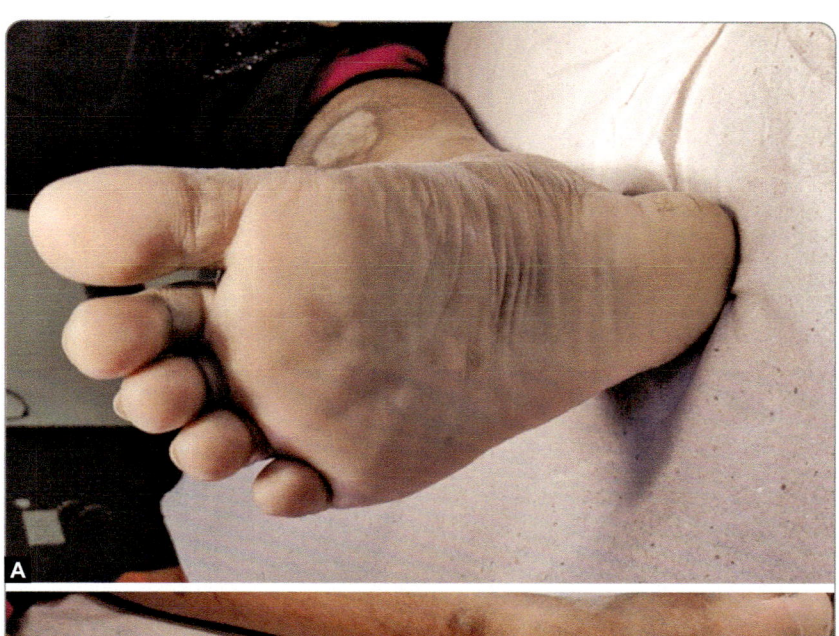

Figures 6A and B show a red, hot, and swollen CF (plantar and dorsal aspect).

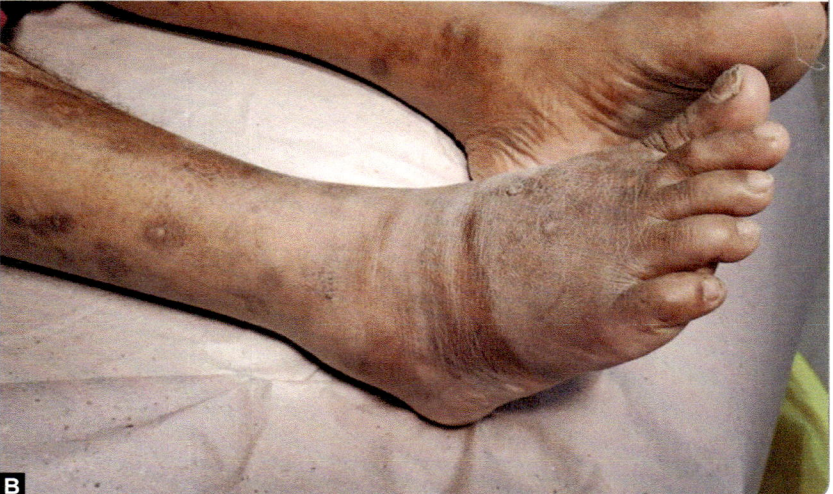

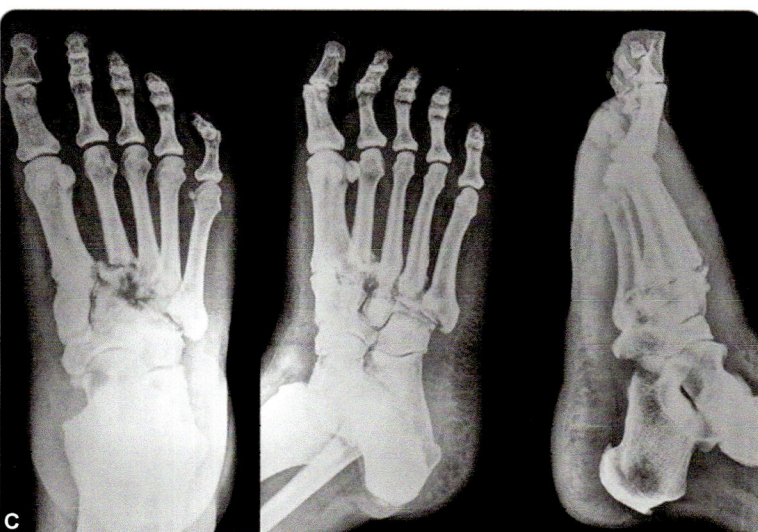

Figure 6C shows the widening of I and II metatarsal base, tarsometatarsal joint dislocation, and destruction of II and III metatarsal base, and intermediate cuneiform bone. High-arched foot and claw toe deformity are seen. Flat foot deformity and flexion deformity of the lesser toes are evident. Bone resorption and osteophytes are also noted.

CASE 7 (FIGURES 8A TO C)

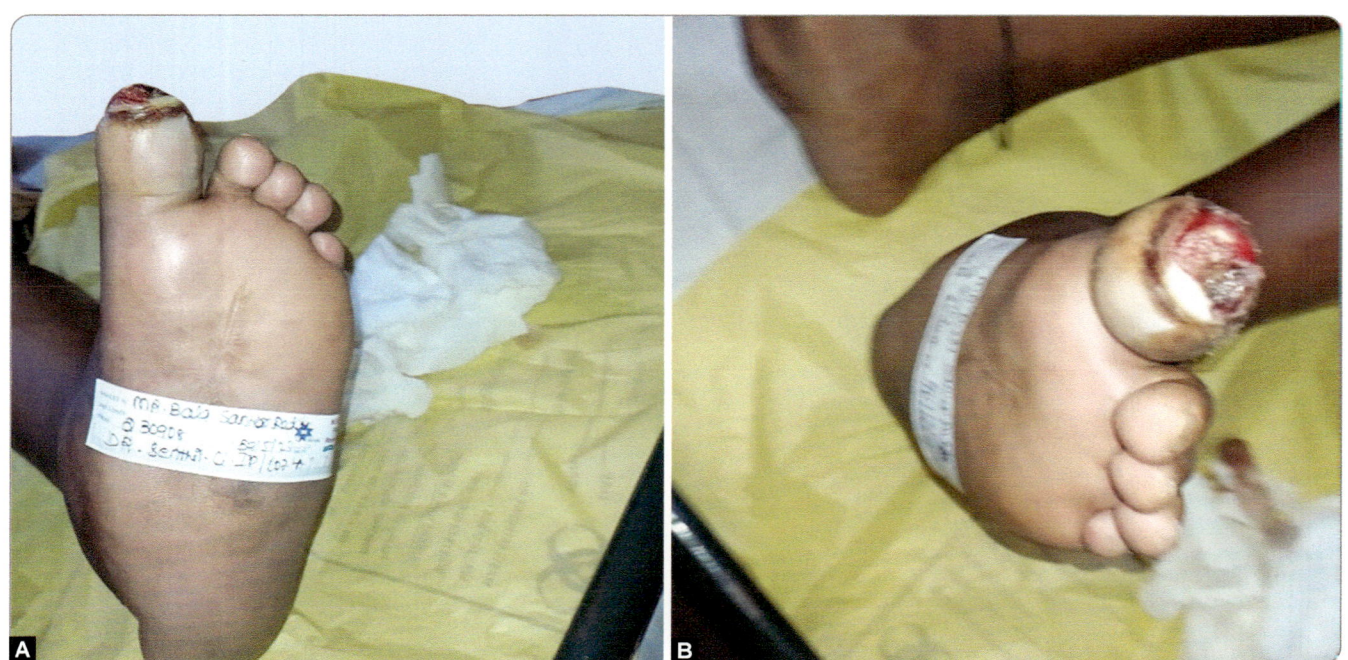

Figures 8A and B show an infected wound in the left great toe.

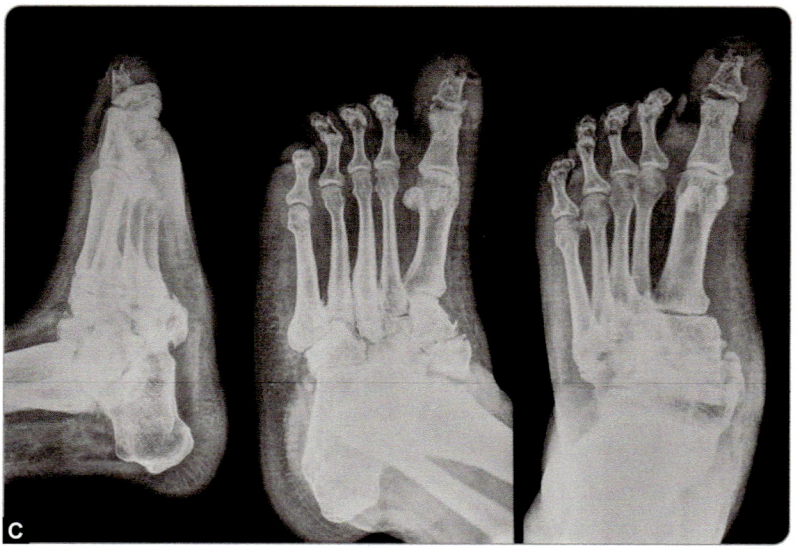

Figure 8C shows X-ray showing CF with DPX OM.

CHAPTER 9

The Indispensable Role of Orthotics in the Prevention and Management of Diabetic Foot

Sivashankari SelvaElavarasan, Bamila Selvaraj, Seena Rajsekar, Vijay Viswanathan

INTRODUCTION

Diabetic foot ulcer (DFU) is a serious emerging global health problem, affecting nearly 34% of people living with diabetes in their lifetime.[1] According to the American Diabetes Association, it has been projected that nearly 20% of people with diabetes are being hospitalized due to foot-related complications.[2] Any repetitive trauma due to weight-bearing or inappropriate use of footwear may result in DFU, which when left untreated can result in dreadful consequences like amputation. Shoe modifications and orthoses are highly recommended to maintain stability, reduce pressure, and protect the feet from ulcers or any other external stimuli.

PATHOPHYSIOLOGY BEHIND THE DEVELOPMENT OF DIABETIC FOOT ULCERS AND THE USE OF ORTHOTICS

Peripheral neuropathy and ischemia are two predominant factors responsible for DFUs. Apart from this, altered biomechanics, improper weight-bearing, and ill-fitting shoes are other reasons for their occurrence and if not treated appropriately can also be considered responsible for their recurrence. The two important determinants of DFUs are limited joint mobility and increased plantar pressure. Similarly, in the case of Charcot arthropathy, the bone becomes weak and liable to fracture, and the ligaments may also get weakened causing either subluxation or dislocation. Patients with Charcot foot are unable to perceive the pain and continuous application of pain could even result in permanent bone deformities. Thus, orthotic devices play a very significant role in minimizing stress, distributing the pressure evenly, stabilizing the joint as well as in reducing edema. They are also considered highly useful in limiting joint mobility and controlling foot deformity.[3]

IDEAL CHARACTERISTICS OF APPROPRIATE FOOTWEAR

Appropriate footwear must essentially contain the following characteristics as depicted in **Figure 1**.

EXAMINATION OF THE DIABETIC FOOT

The examination of the diabetic foot plays a predominant role in prescribing the appropriate footwear for a person with diabetes. It becomes mandatory to inspect the foot

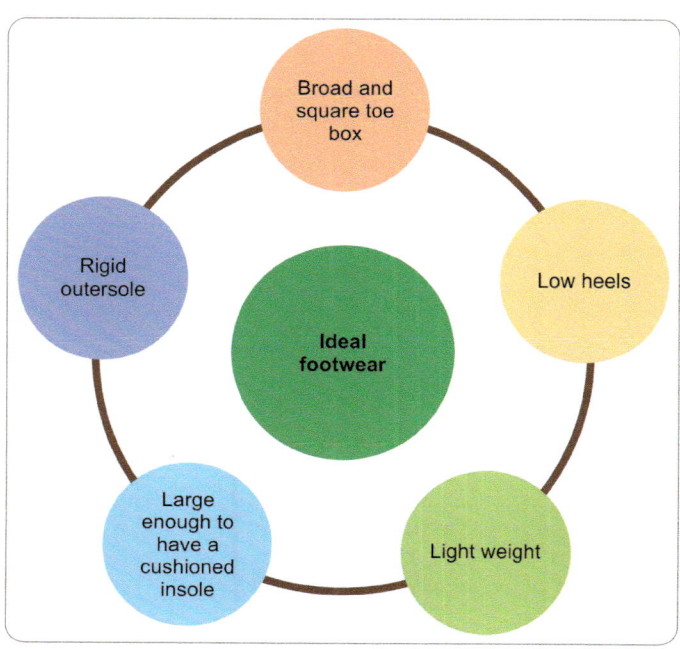

Fig. 1: The ideal characteristics of an appropriate footwear.

for sensation, foot abnormalities, disorders of muscle, or any changes in temperature before prescribing the footwear. A general assessment of skin for ulceration, areas of inflammation, or any other changes related to vascular disease, the evaluation of protective sensation, or identification of muscle paralysis which in turn is recognized as a key factor for the formation of claw toe deformity are recognized as important factors in the comprehensive examination of diabetic feet. The two important classic indicators that also act as surrogate markers for the identification of at-risk feet are the magnitude of deformity as well as the presence of callus, which are found to be extremely useful for prescribing the proper footwear.[4]

CLASSIFICATION BASED ON RISK CATEGORIES

The modified American Diabetes Association classification was given for the holistic examination of feet as well as for the assessment of risk, which is found beneficial for the prescription of footwear and the appropriate management of diabetic foot infection (DFI) **(Table 1)**.[4,5]

PRESCRIBING THE PROPER FOOTWEAR BASED ON RISK CATEGORIES

Risk Category 0

All people with diabetes with no loss of protective sensation (LOPS) or peripheral artery disease (PAD) are categorized under the low-risk category. It is very important to educate these patients on appropriate footwear and proper foot care practices, because they are liable to lose sensation or vascular supply at any stage. Therapeutic footwear can be fabricated for people with heel pain and cracked heels as well as obese people. This footwear is intended to relieve the high plantar pressure in the forefoot region and distribute the plantar pressure, thereby preventing callus formation. They are also designed to re-equilibrate the foot for patients at risk, increase stability, and reduce the sheer stress.

Risk Category 1

The Semmes-Weinstein monofilament test can be used to test LOPS. People placed under risk category 1 exhibit LOPS, and they are unable to perceive the pain due to burns or small cuts. They should avoid the practice of walking barefoot and also follow regular hygienic foot care measures. Sports shoes are usually recommended because they reduce the plantar pressure as well as the formation of callus. However, these shoes cannot be used for people with foot deformities. In such cases, customization of the insole might be required. Customized footwear with low heels and soft insoles is preferred for people under the risk category.

Figures 2A to C are the examples of footwear prescribed for risk category 0 and 1.

Ideally, the shoes should be neither loose nor tight. An ideal toe box should be either round, high, or oblique, which provides the most appropriate fit when compared to a narrow, tapered toe box. The internal width of the shoe must be equal to the foot width, especially in the regions of metatarsophalangeal joints, and the height should be spacious enough to accommodate the toes **(Fig. 3)**.

Risk Category 2

An electronic baropodogram can be used to prepare customized therapeutic molded insole for people under risk category 2 **(Fig. 4A)**. It can be used to evaluate the

TABLE 1: The modified American Diabetes Association (ADA) classification given for risk assessment in a diabetic foot.			
Risk category/priority	**Indications**	**Referral**	**Management and Follow-up**
Very low (Risk category 0)	No LOPS/PAD	1–3 months	• Annual foot examination • Education of the patient on the appropriate selection of footwear
Low (Risk category 1)	LOPS ± Deformity	Within 1 month	• Foot examination every 6 months • The footwear worn by the patient should be reviewed and soft insoles have to be added
Moderate (Risk category 2)	• PAD ± LOPS • Peripheral pulses diminished • Swelling, edema present	1–3 weeks	• Foot examination every 3–4 months • The use of custom-molded orthotic devices as well as prescription footwear are considered necessary
High (Risk category 3)	• Diabetes with a previous history of ulcer or LEA • Chronic venous insufficiency	Immediate	Customized orthotic devices and prescription footwear are required
Urgent	• Active Charcot foot • New neuropathic pain or pain at rest • Open wound or ulceration • Absent peripheral pulses	Immediate	As determined by the specialist

(LEA: lower extremity amputation; LOPS: loss of protective sensation; PAD: peripheral artery disease)

The Indispensable Role of Orthotics in the Prevention and Management of Diabetic Foot

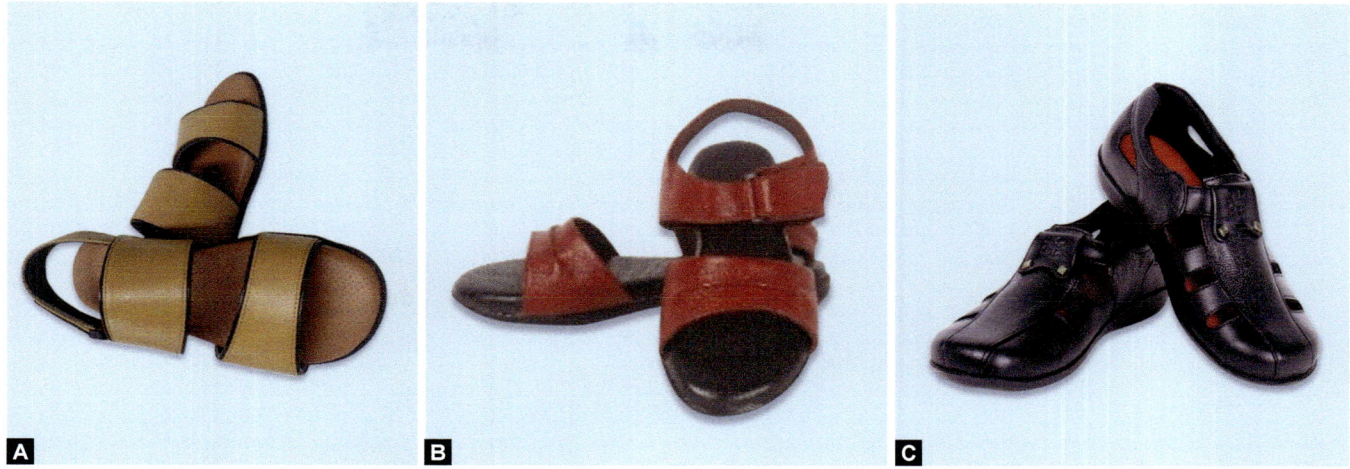

Figs. 2A to C: Footwears prescribed for risk category 0 and 1.

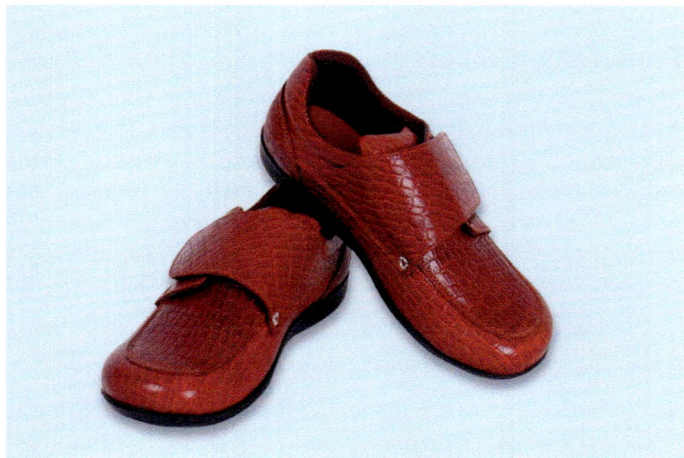

Fig. 3: A special diabetic shoe prescribed for risk categories 0 and 1.

stability, and pressure distribution in both the orthostatic and dynamic positions, and is capable of individualization of certain areas of the at-risk feet. The customized insoles are usually prescribed to offload high pressures from the metatarsal heads and other predominant areas and thereby help in the reduction of the risk of plantar ulcerations **(Fig. 4B)**. Therapeutic footwear designed using a baropodometry platform reduces the plantar pressure by 31 and 21% in dynamic and static analysis, respectively.[6]

Peg Insoles

The peg-assisted insoles are prepared by removing the pegs from specific regions to promote granulation and healing. They also assist in reducing pressures, especially in wounded areas **(Figs. 5A and B)**.

In a follow-up study to assess the effectiveness of different types of footwear insole by Vijay et al., it was concluded that

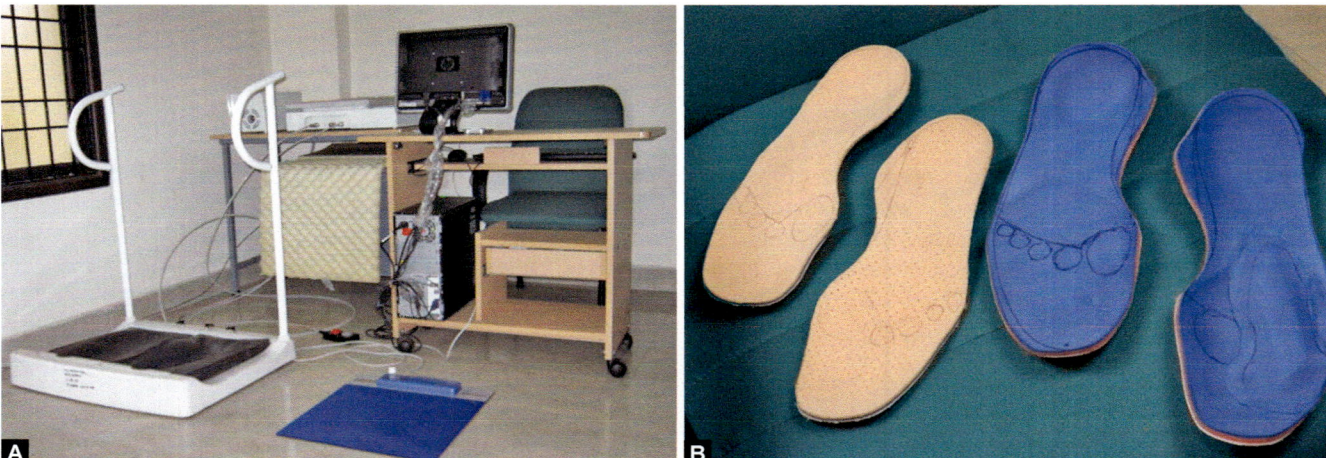

Figs. 4A and B: (A) The image of an electronic baropodogram (BPG). (B) BPG insoles prepared and inserted into BPG sandals.

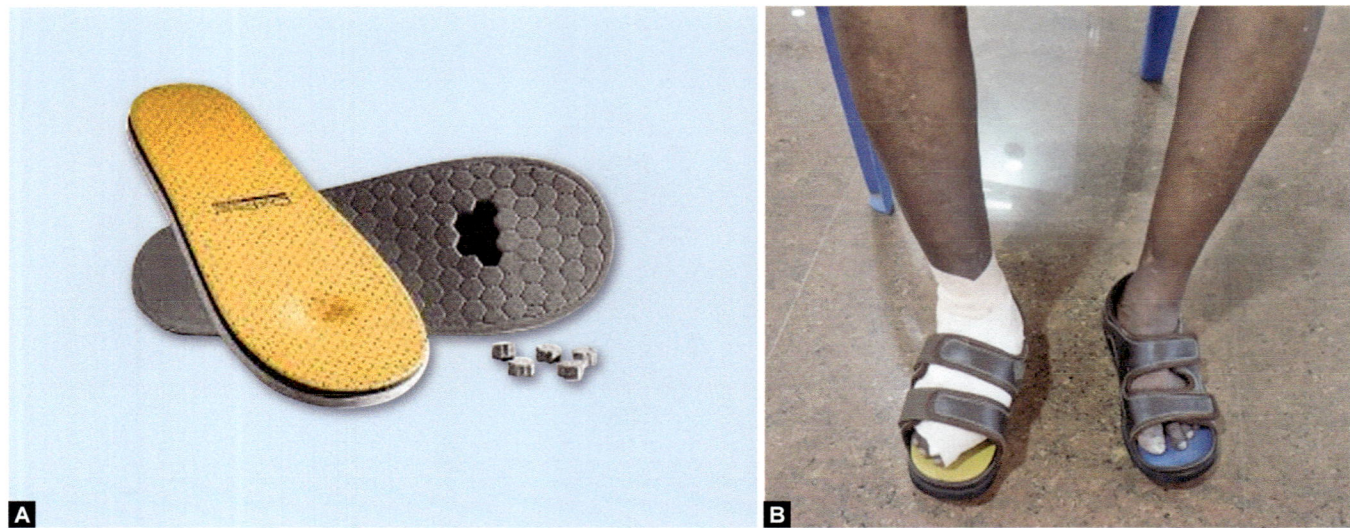

Figs. 5A and B: The use of peg-assisted insoles, which help to promote healing of the wound.

a reduction of plantar pressure by 10–19% was observed with the use of therapeutic footwear when compared to the hard leather board insole in the control group.[7]

Similarly, Uccioli et al. suggested that customized footwear was found to be highly useful for people with a previous history of ulceration. Reulceration was found to occur in 58% of people who continued to wear their own footwear when compared to 28% of people who wore customized footwear.[8]

Risk Category 3

Offloading is a principal component of integrated and holistic wound care, which requires the pressure and sheer to be minimized, especially in areas of wound. An ideal offloading device should have the following features **(Box 1)**.[7]

There are several forefoot and hindfoot offloading footwear available. A forefoot offloading footwear is designed to reduce the pressure in metatarsal heads and phalanges, whereas the hindfoot offloading footwear is customized to reduce the pressure in the calcaneal region.[9] Stabil D, Tera heel, Pneumatic walkers, and Charcot Restraint Orthotic Walker (CROW) are removable offloading devices considered for people placed under risk category 3 with both high and urgent priorities. It is very important to provide good therapeutic footwear to allow consolidation of the new tissue in the healing phase and prevent the recurrence of ulceration as well as amputation.

> **BOX 1: The characteristics of an ideal offloading device.**
>
> - Promote wound healing effectively
> - Affordable
> - Easy to use and patient compliant
> - Appropriate for ambulation

Pneumatic Walkers

A pneumatic walker is used to offload acute Charcot foot with rocker bottom deformity and plantar ulcers. It facilitates easy inspection of the wound and regular dressing as it is removable offloading footwear. It has inflatable sections that hold the ankle as well as the feet in proper position and also limit mobility **(Figs. 6A and B)**. They help to establish total contact with the plantar surface of the feet, redistribute the forces, reduce the edema, and prevent callus formation.[10]

Charcot Restraint Orthotic Walker

A customized orthotic device designed for the treatment of Charcot neuroarthropathy and foot ulcers is capable of establishing total contact with the plantar aspect of the ankle and the foot. It is recommended for a wide range of ankle and foot deformities and is responsible for causing triphasic motion restriction to enable better offloading. A rocker sole is usually required to move the foot forward, because it otherwise makes the foot immobile. It is considered an effective offloading footwear similar to total contact cast (TCC), which lasts for a longer period but it is removable.[10] However, CROW has limited patient compliance, because it is bulky and the patient experiences both lumbar and knee pain due to lower extremity immobility.[11]

Total Contact Casting

Total contact casting is always considered the gold standard method for offloading. It is capable of relieving the pressure by redistributing the force across the entire sole and also minimizes mobility of foot and ankle joints to prevent the risk of injury to the tibia and malleolus. However, it is time-consuming and quite expensive.[12] TCCs can be given to a patient either with a nonhealing ulcer **(Figs. 7A and B)** or with acute Charcot foot **(Figs. 8A and B)**.

The Indispensable Role of Orthotics in the Prevention and Management of Diabetic Foot

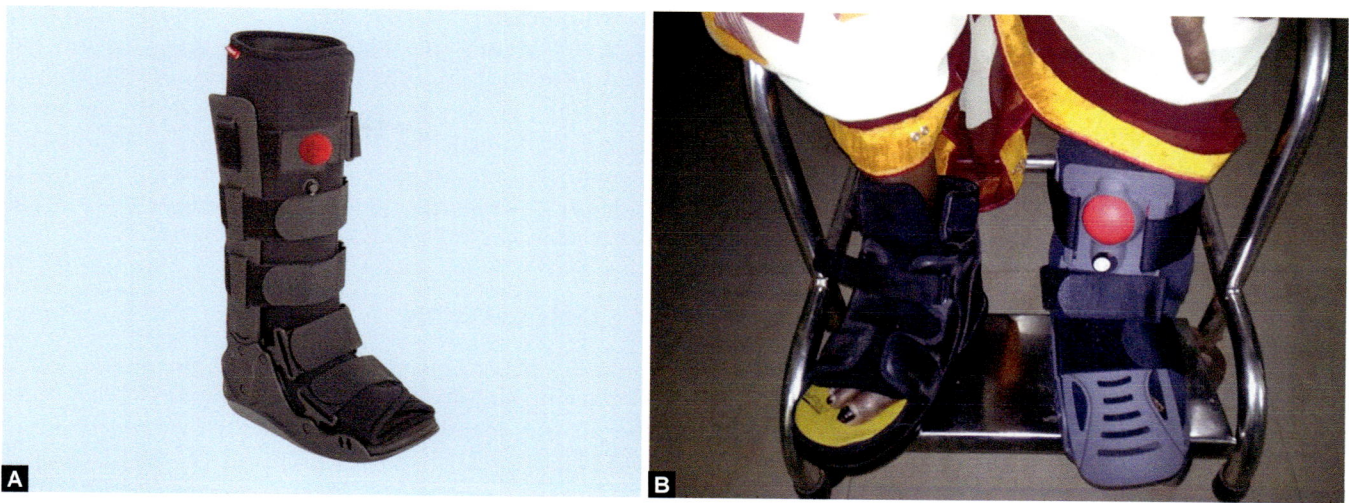

Figs. 6A and B: Pictures of a pneumatic walker.

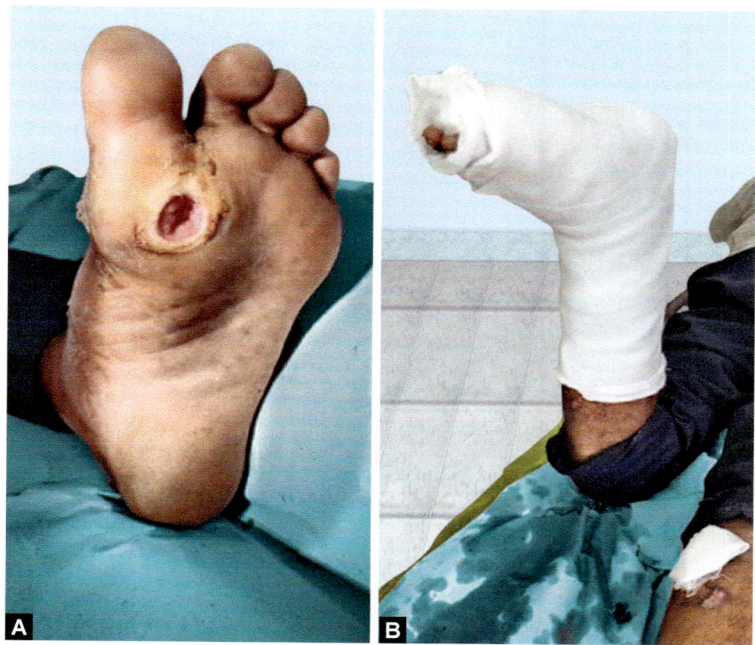

Figs. 7A and B: Total contact casting (TCC) given to a patient with nonhealing diabetic foot ulcer.

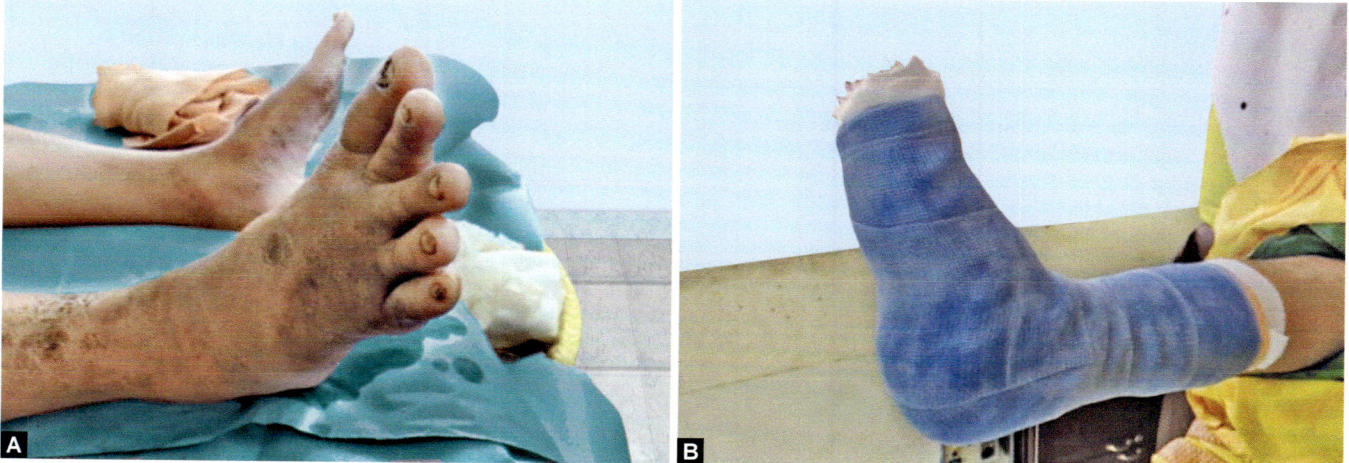

Figs. 8A and B: Total contact casting (TCC) given for a case of acute Charcot foot.

IWGDF Offloading Guidelines 2023

The IWGDF guidelines 2023 recommend the usage of a nonremovable knee-high offloading device like TCC for the treatment of neuropathic ulcers in the plantar aspect of the forefoot, midfoot, or heel regions. In certain cases where nonremovable offloading devices are contraindicated, removable offloading devices can be considered to promote healing of the wound. In cases where a knee-high offloading device cannot be used, a removable ankle-high offloading device is recommended as the third choice of offloading treatment. It recommends the use of therapeutic footwear only when the either the patient is not willing or when none of the offloading devices are available. Felted foam in combination with therapeutic footwear is recommended as the fourth choice of offloading treatment. When there is a failure of non-surgical offloading treatment in case of a plantar ulcer in the metatarsal head, Achilles Tendon Lengthening, metatarsal head resection, and joint arthroplasty are all recommended. Similarly, in the case of a digital ulcer in the plantar aspect, Digital flexor tenotomy can be considered. The choice of the offloading device is based on the ambulatory and functioning status of the patient as well as their level of activity to promote the healing of the ulcer. In the case of non-plantar foot ulcers, a removable ankle-high offloading device, modifications of footwear, and the use of toe spacers or orthoses can also be considered to encourage the healing of the ulcers.[13]

In recent times, instant TCCs and removable cast walkers can be used, because they are less time-consuming. Lack of motivation to use these devices and patients' misconception that these offloading devices should be used only outside their homes are the reasons responsible for them to perform strain-bearing activities at home without proper offloading.[14]

Hence, it is imperative to comprehend these challenges and overcome them by providing proper education on foot care and the use of offloading devices.[15] In a study by Vijay et al., it was estimated that around 65% of the study population did not practice regular foot care procedures, which ultimately was considered the major reason for the high prevalence of DFIs.[16] A comprehensive, intensive management and appropriate foot care education are considered key cornerstones for the prevention of complications of diabetic foot. In another study by Vijay et al., it was concluded that patients who did not follow strict foot care advice developed new complications when compared to the ones who followed the advice provided.[17]

CONCLUSION

Orthotics play a very significant role in the prevention and management of diabetic foot. They provide stability, reduce the plantar pressures, aid in effective wound healing of foot ulcers, and control symptoms of Charcot arthropathy and thereby avert potential consequences like amputation. Customized or therapeutic footwear is more effective than normal footwear, especially for people identified to be at risk for developing foot ulcers. The choice of the effective offloading device must unquestionably depend on the patient's compliance also because unless it is patient-centered the optimum result would be very difficult to achieve. Prescribing appropriate footwear and orthoses is an integral component of the prevention of foot infections and thus requires a collaborative approach among healthcare providers to provide intensive education about the various foot care practices.

TAKE-HOME MESSAGE

A multidisciplinary podiatric team should essentially consist of podiatrists and orthotists who are capable of assessing the diabetic feet in their earliest stages, providing the appropriate offloading devices and thereby preventing serious consequences like amputation. It is imperative to provide and promote adequate knowledge both among the patients as well as clinicians about the invaluable role of orthotic devices in reducing the global burden of the disease.

REFERENCES

1. Armstrong DG, Boulton AJ, Bus SA. Diabetic foot ulcers and their recurrence. N Engl J Med. 2017;376:2367.
2. Skrepnek GH, Mills JL Sr, Lavery LA, Armstrong DG. Health Care Service and Outcomes Among an Estimated 6.7 Million Ambulatory Care Diabetic Foot Cases in the U.S. Diabetes Care. 2017;40:936-42.
3. Chang MC, Choo YJ, Park IS, Park MW, Kim DH. Orthotic approach to prevention and management of diabetic foot: A narrative review. World J Diabetes. 2022;13(11):912-20.
4. Prescribing footwear. In: Vijay V (Ed). Contemporary Management of the Diabetic foot. New Delhi: Jaypee Brothers Medical Publishers; 2014. pp. 176-84.
5. Boulton AJM, Armstrong DG, Kirsner RS, Attinger AC, Lavery LA, Lipsky BA, et al. (Eds). Diagnosis and Management of Diabetic Foot Complications. Arlington (VA): American Diabetes Association; 2018. [online] Available from https://www.ncbi.nlm.nih.gov/books/NBK538977/ [Last accessed September, 2023].
6. Faraco de Oliveira A, Bertoletti De Marchi AC, Leguisamo CP. Diabetic footwear: is it an assistive technology capable of reducing peak plantar pressures in elderly patients with neuropathy? Fisioter Mov. 2016;29(3):469-76.
7. Viswanathan V, Madhavan S, Gnanasundaram S, Gopalakrishna G, Das BN, Rajasekar S, et al. Effectiveness of Different Types of Footwear Insoles for the Diabetic Neuropathic Foot: A follow-up study. Diabetes Care. 2004;27(2):474-7.
8. Uccioli L, Faglia E, Monticone G, Favales F, Durola L, Aldeghi A, et al. Manufactured shoes in the prevention of diabetic foot ulcers. Diabetes Care. 1995;18(10):1376-8.
9. Robinson C, Major MJ, Kuffel C, Hines K, Cole P. Orthotic management of the neuropathic foot: an interdisciplinary care perspective. Prosthet Orthot Int. 2015;39(1):73-81.
10. Caroline M, Greg H. Offloading Strategies for the Diabetic Foot. Wounds Essential. 2009;4:117-21.

11. Oh-Park M, Kim DD, Lee JM. Footwear and insole. In: Ko YJ, Kang SY (Ed). Physical Medicine and Rehabilitation, 1st edition. Seoul: Jungmunkag; 2009. pp. 286-9.
12. Faglia E, Caravaggi C, Clerici G, Sganzaroli A, Curci V, Vailati W, et al. Effectiveness of removable walker cast versus nonremovable fiberglass off-bearing cast in the healing of diabetic plantar foot ulcer: a randomized controlled trial. Diabetes Care. 2010;33: 1419-23.
13. Bus SA, Armstrong DG, Crews RT, Gooday C, Jarl G, Kirketerp-Moller K, et al. Guidelines on offloading foot ulcers in persons with diabetes (IWGDF 2023 update). Diabetes Metab Res Rev. 2023:e3647.
14. van Netten JJ, Seng L, Lazzarini PA, Warnock J, Ploderer B. Reasons for (non-) adherence to self-care in people with a diabetic foot ulcer. Wound Repair Regen. 2019;27:530-9.
15. Lazzarini PA, Jarl G, Gooday C, Viswanathan V, Caravaggi CF, Armstrong DG, et al. Effectiveness of offloading interventions to heal foot ulcers in persons with diabetes: a systematic review. Diabetes Metab Res Rev. 2020;36 Suppl 1:e3275.
16. Viswanathan V, Thomas N, Tandon N, Asirvatham A, Rajasekar S, Ramachandran A, et al. Profile of diabetic foot complications and its associated complications--a multicentric study from India. J Assoc Physicians India. 2005;53:933-6.
17. Viswanathan V, Sivagami M, Seena R, Snehalatha C, Ramachandran A. Amputation Prevention Initiative in South India: Positive impact of foot care education. Diabetes Care. 2005;28:1019-21.

CHAPTER 10

Wound Dressings in the Management of Diabetic Foot Infections

Senthil Govindan, Vijay Viswanathan

INTRODUCTION

The management of diabetic foot infections (DFIs) is quite challenging and currently requires a multidisciplinary approach for its effective management. Dr Frederick Treves discovered three main principles in the management of DFI, namely debridement, offloading, and education about foot care.[1] The key principles of management of DFI include effective wound care along with surgical debridement, use of dressing materials to provide an adequate moist environment for good healing, offloading of wounds, appropriate treatment of active infection, vascular assessment as well as optimum glycemic control.[2]

PRINCIPLES OF OPTIMUM WOUND CARE

Figure 1 summarizes the essential key principles involved in establishing optimum wound care.

Surgical debridement involves the removal of necrotic tissue to promote granulation tissue formation and re-epithelialization. The removal of devitalized tissue is considered important, because it can enhance bacterial proliferation, act as a barrier to the penetration of antibiotics, and decrease immunity. Sharp debridement is preferred over the application of topical chemical or biological debridement techniques by the Infectious Disease Society of America (IDSA).[3] An ideal dressing material should be able to provide a moist environment to enhance the formation of granulation tissue, promote angiogenesis, and effectively manage the exudates. Wound offloading plays a crucial role in the management of DFI. The two important factors are reduction in the sheer stress and redistribution of plantar pressure. Offloading involves modifications of shoes, orthotic walkers, total contact casting (TCC), and nonremovable high knee devices, which are highly beneficial in promoting healing and preventing the recurrence of DFIs. Peripheral arterial disease (PAD) can be evaluated by palpating the pedal pulses or by using ankle-brachial index (ABI). IDSA recommends the treatment of active infection using antibiotics when two or more signs of inflammation are present. The five cardinal signs of inflammation are Rubor (redness), Calor (warmth), Dolor (pain), Tumor (swelling), and Loss of function. A tissue culture must be ideally obtained before initiating an empirical antibiotic regimen. Culture-sensitive antibiotics can be initiated once the culture reports are available. Optimum glycemic control is always considered quintessential to achieve improvement in wound healing.

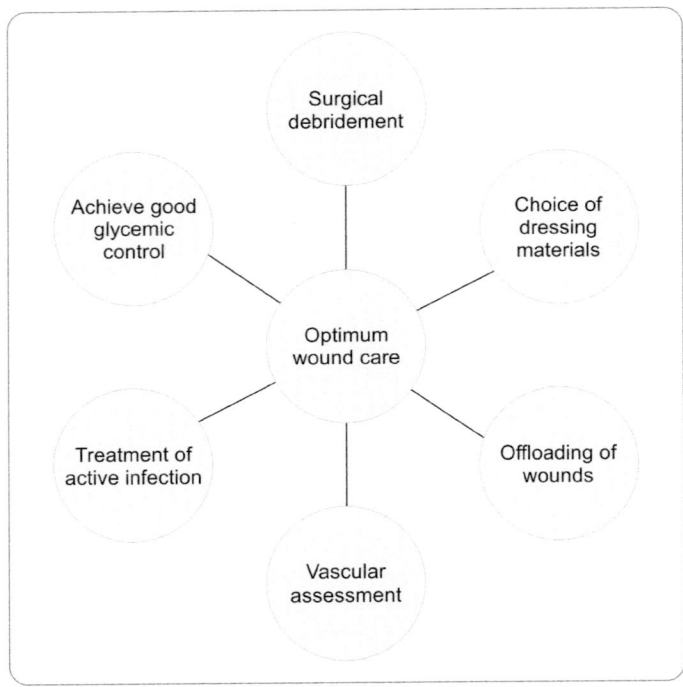

Fig. 1: Essential principles of optimum wound care.

The ultimate aim of the treatment should be to initiate the appropriate preparation of the wound bed for the removal of biofilm. A biofilm comprises a complex microbial composition that develops over the surface of the wounds, is not visible to the naked eye, and is undetectable even in routine cultures.[4] The two ideal treatment strategies are to cause disruption of the biofilm through proper debridement and prevention of attachment of the biofilm with the help of appropriate dressing materials.[5]

We will be discussing the role of dressing materials in the management of DFI in this chapter.

Traditionally, saline was used and is known to have a good debridement action and also helps in the preparation of wound beds. It is one of the cheapest, easily available, and considered to be a good adherent. However, it has certain disadvantages as it requires frequent change of dressings, removal of dressings can be painful, the granulation tissue may be damaged, or sometimes the cotton fiber that sticks on the wound may cause foreign body reaction. It must always be kept in mind that dressings must be moistened before their removal in order to prevent any bleeding.[6]

CHARACTERISTICS OF AN IDEAL DRESSING MATERIAL

An ideal dressing material should be able to:
- Create a moist environment to promote healing of the wound.
- Provide mechanical protection of the wound.
- Control the microbial growth and reduce the symptoms.
- Comfortable, acceptable, and affordable for the patient.[7]

The advantages of using wound dressing materials are that it prevents the wound from getting desiccated, and helps to remove granulation tissue. Most importantly, it can be done by the patient himself. At times, even home dressing is possible. Apart from this, it also helps to reduce the pain, preserves the wound from the environment, and enhances wound healing.

THE CONCEPT OF TIME

The European Wound Management Association (EWMA) recommends four distinct components for the preparation of wound beds and thereby suggests the *TIME* framework for the management of DFUs:[8]
- *T*issue debridement
- *I*nfection and inflammation control
- *M*oisture balance
- *E*pithelial edge advancement

The emphasis should be laid on frequent debridement, regular inspection of the wound, and control of moisture and infection to prevent any risk of maceration, thereby optimizing wound care.

The various modern dressing materials that are currently available are:
- Hydrogels
- Hydrocolloid
- Poly urethane foam ± ionic silver
- Polyester mesh ± ionic silver
- Vacuum-assisted closure (VAC)
- Biocomposite material
- Hydrofiber
- Alginate
- Medical grade honey

The different types of dressing materials available with their indications and contraindications are shown in **Table 1**.[4]

The clinical implication of the various dressing materials used can be explained with the help of different cases of DFUs (Cases 1 to 3).

Case 1 **(Figs. 2A to C)** is a clinical picture of the patient using a dressing material made up of polyester mesh impregnated with nanosilver, which is found to be effective against methicillin-resistant *Staphylococcus aureus* and *Pseudomonas aeruginosa*. It is a soft and flexible material, less adherent, absorbs minimal exudate, and provides an antibacterial environment that constitutes the primary dressing. Secondary dressing is required to cover this primary dressing.

Figures 2A to C depict the clinical pictures of a patient in which a combination of polyester mesh and nanosilver was used.

Case 2 **(Figs. 3A to D)** is a clinical picture of a patient using hydrogel dressing material along with topical administration of mupirocin, collagen granules, and metronidazole.

A secondary dressing is done to cover the wound.

Case 3 **(Figs. 4A and B)** is an example of a shoe-bite ulcer where a dressing made up of polyurethane foam incorporated with healing accelerators is used to achieve better healing, stimulate the proliferation of fibroblasts, and also minimize pain during change of dressing.

Similarly, in the case of medium or high exuding heel ulcers, certain foam dressings can be used to absorb and retain the exudates, maintain moisture, and prevent the risk of maceration and strike-through effects. Case 4 **(Figs. 5A to C)** depicts clinical pictures of the management of a heel wound using a five-layered nonadherent foam material with an adhesive silicon border. The exudate is absorbed by the absorbent foam pad, protects the periwound area, and also helps to reduce the development of blisters in the postoperative region. Heel ulcers are protected with foam dressing to confirm the contour of the heel wound. Various foam dressings are now available, which can be contoured to fit specific areas like the heel.

Wound Dressings in the Management of Diabetic Foot Infections

TABLE 1: Various dressing materials available.[4]

Type of dressing material	Mechanism of action	Indications	Contraindications/Precautions
Hydrogel	Rehydrates the wound bed, good moisture control, and also promotes autolytic debridement	• Low-moderate exuding wounds • Can be combined with silver for their antimicrobial activity	• High exuding wounds or in cases of anaerobic infection • Capable of causing maceration
Hydrocolloids	• Waterproof adhesive • Exudates produced by the wound can be absorbed into the dressing and can form a gel	• Low-moderate exuding wounds • Can be combined with silver for their antimicrobial property	• Dry, necrotic/high exuding wounds • Can cause overgranulation or maceration of tissue
Foams	Provides semipermeable membrane for adequate moisture, loosens the slough and promotes healing	• Moderate-high exuding wounds • Low adherent versions for fragile tissue are available	Minimal exudate, dry/necrotic wounds
Polyurethane film	Transparent and allows easy monitoring of the wound without removal of the dressing, the permeable barrier maintains a moist environment to promote healing	• Low exuding wounds • Secondary dressing over hydrogel or alginate to promote rehydration of the wound	• Moderate/high exuding wounds • Fragile skin
Silver	Antimicrobial action	• Low-high exuding wounds • Infected or colonized wounds	Discoloration/known sensitivity
Alginates	Controls moisture, absorbs fluid, and also enhances autolytic debridement	Moderate-high exuding wounds	• Dry/necrotic wounds • Weak/friable tissue
Honey	Rehydrates the wound bed, antimicrobial and anti-inflammatory properties	• Low-moderate exuding wounds • Wounds with clinical signs of infection or critically colonized wounds	Drawing pain due to osmotic effect and known sensitivity

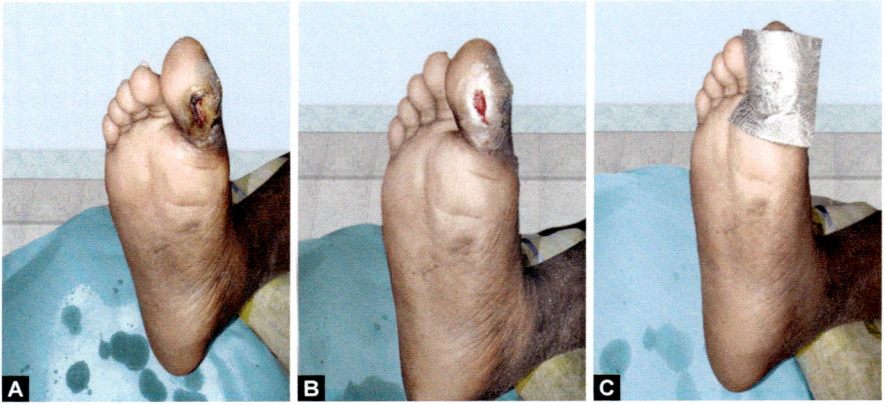

Figs. 2A to C: (A) A nonhealing ulcer with callus; (B) The callus was excised and saline irrigation was done; (C) The dressing material made of polyester mesh and nanosilver applied over the wound.

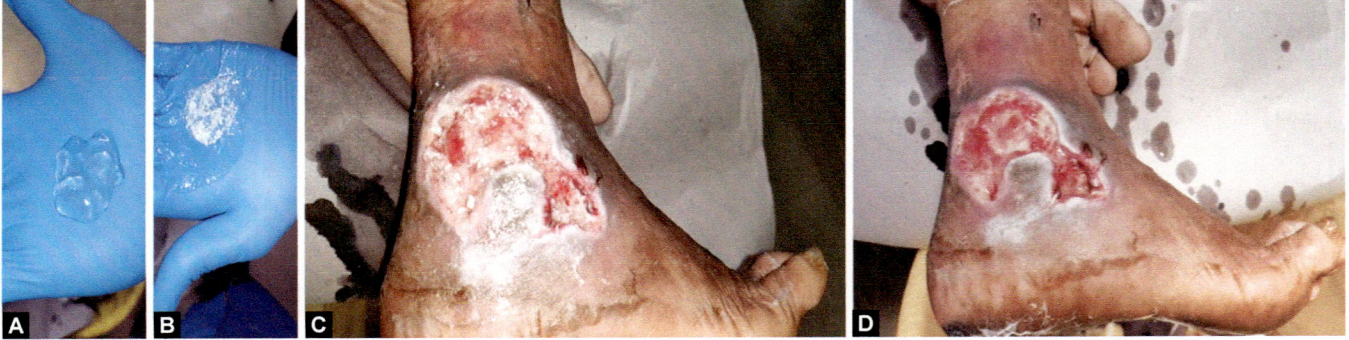

Figs. 3A to D: (A and B) The mixing of hydrogel dressing material with mupirocin, collagen, and metronidazole; (C) The application of the mixed dressing material over the wound; (D) A clean wound after the application of the mixed dressing material.

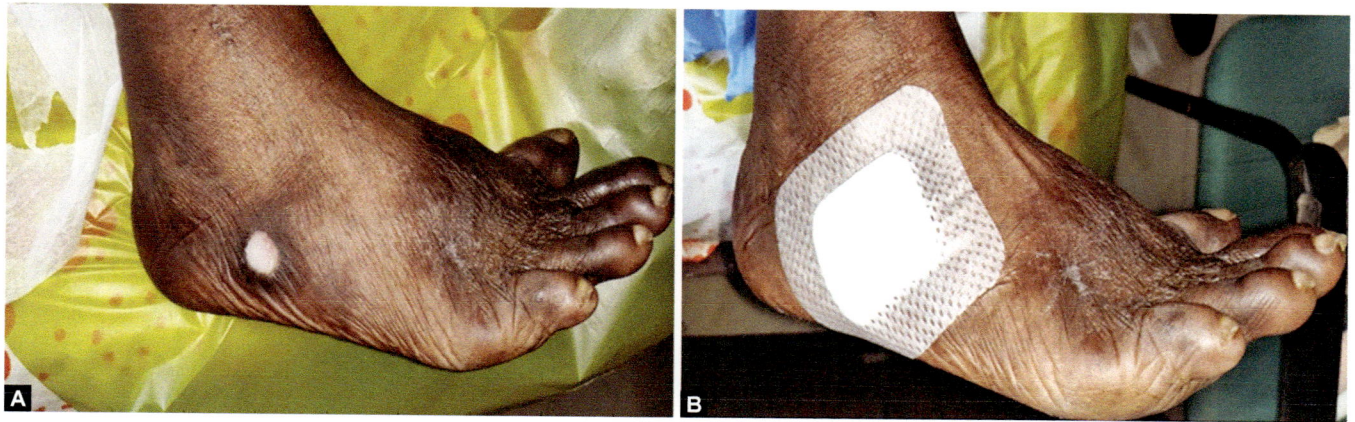

Figs. 4A and B: (A) A clinical picture of a shoe-bite ulcer; (B) Combined primary and secondary dressings made of five-layered polyurethane foam with silicon adhesive border.

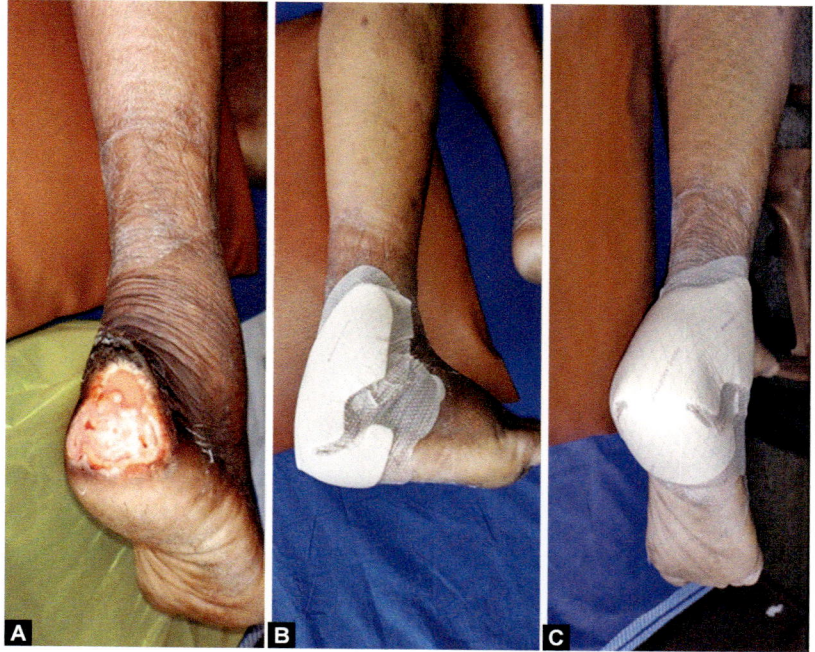

Figs. 5A to C: (A) The clinical picture of a heel ulcer; (B and C) Clinical pictures of foam dressing, which has been adapted to contour the wound in the heel region.

IMPORTANCE OF CLEANSING THE WOUND IN THE REMOVAL OF BIOFILM

It is very important to clean the wounds properly at every dressing change, because it can help us to reduce the exudate, remove the devitalized tissue, maintain an equilibrium of the bioburden and thereby help promote healing of the wound.[9] A biofilm is a microbial complex produced by the colonizing bacteria, which are considered responsible for the progression of infection. It is therefore very important to eradicate the biofilm to ensure appropriate healing. Thus, regular and adequate removal of infected tissue known as debridement either using surgical instruments or through irrigation is considered a quintessential strategy for the removal of biofilm.[10] This, in turn, helps in the preparation of the wound bed, which remains the gold standard procedure for the removal of biofilm.[11]

The presence of biofilms, microbes, slough, and other wound debris as well as increased exudate are all considered predominant factors involved in the formation of a vicious cycle that can cause damage to the tissues as well as delayed wound healing. An effective antimicrobial therapy and complete cleaning of the wound are essential to fight infection and thereby break the vicious cycle.[12] Case 5 **(Figs. 6A and B)** are the clinical pictures showing the complete cleaning action and the use of polyacrylate fibers and silver ions for efficient debriding action on invisible biofilms and visible slough along with antibacterial activity to prevent the reattachment of biofilms.

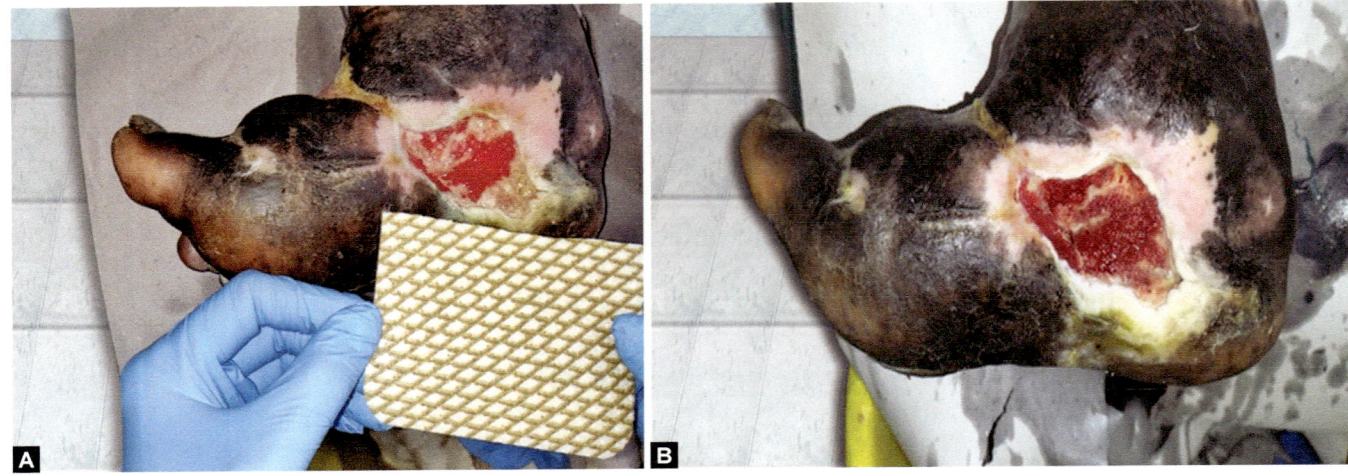

Figs. 6A and B: (A) An invisible biofilm and visible slough covering the wound; (B) A post-treatment picture where the slough has been removed after treatment with polyacrylate material and nanosilver.

ADVANCEMENTS IN WOUND DRESSING

Sustained Local Delivery of Antibiotics

It is well known that systemic antibiotics are given for the treatment of DFI. Some soft tissue infections and deep-seated bone and joint infections may require long-term use of antibiotics. However, there are certain limitations to their long-term usage. This can be overcome by delivering antibiotics to the site of infection directly. In this system, culture-sensitive antibiotics are impregnated with calcium sulfate powder (Biocomposites) to form small beads or pellets and applied over the wound[13] [**Fig. 7**; Case 6 (**Figs. 8A and B**)].

Figure 7 shows a case of nonhealing ulcer after debridement. A bioabsorbable material made up of antibiotics mixed with calcium sulfate is used in which the effect of antibiotics is expected to last for even 2 months when applied

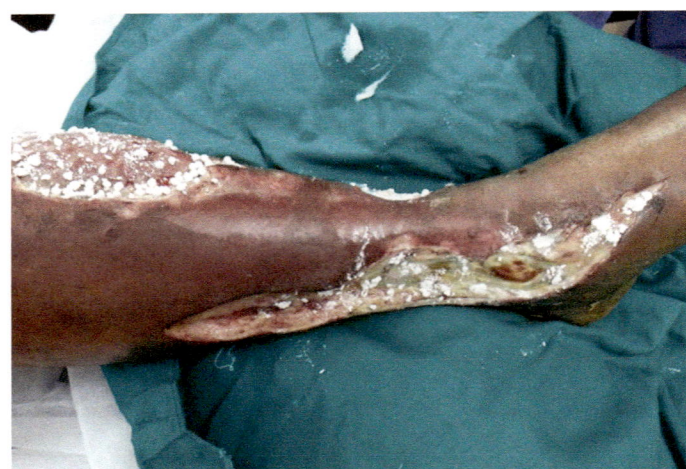

Fig. 7: A case of nonhealing ulcer treated using Biocomposites.

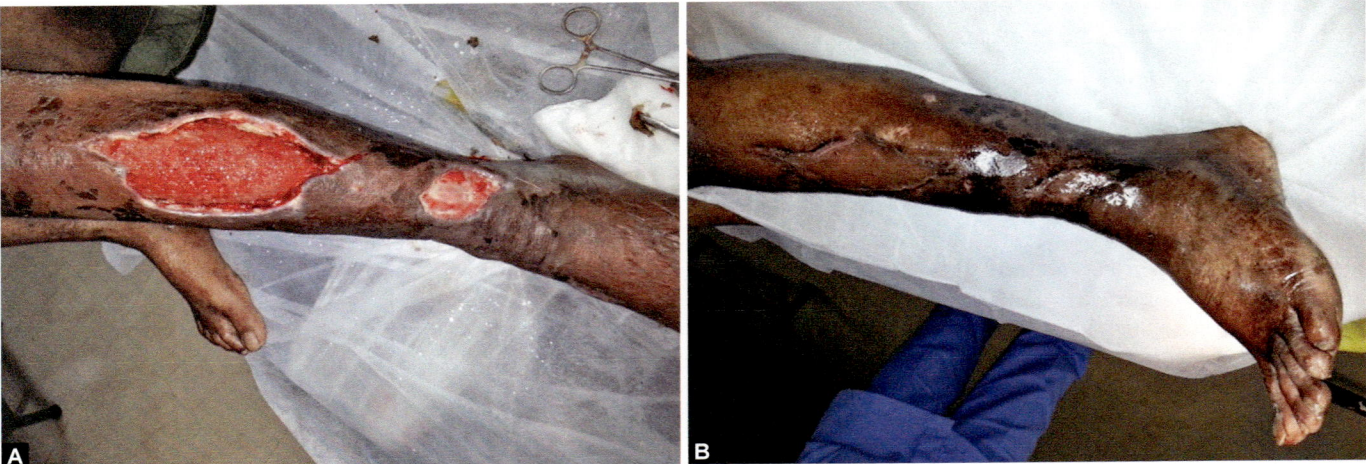

Figs. 8A and B: (A) A nonhealing foot ulcer after clean granulation; (B) A Biocomposite treated wound after skin grafting.

over the wound region. The whole material will dissolve after a month. Residual infection is present over the leg and ankle-joint regions exposing the skin under the fascia. Further debridement may pose the risk of exposing the ankle joint. Conservative management paved the way for skin grafting.

Growth Factors

There are several growth factors like transforming growth factor [TGF (α and β)], insulin-like growth factor (IGF), platelet-derived growth factor (PDGF), and epidermal growth factor (EGF) that aid in wound healing and also promote angiogenesis and cellular proliferation.[14] In a study by Vijay et al., it was found that recombinant human (rh) EGF was found to play a significant role in accelerating the healing of wounds and thereby preventing complications like amputation.[15]

Nanofibers

Electrospun nanofibers have evolved as one of the most recent advanced wound dressings in the treatment of diabetic foot ulcers. Its structural similarity to the extracellular matrix (ECM), high porosity, excellent ability to absorb moisture, and increased rate of oxygen exchange in addition to its antibacterial properties are some of the major advantages of using this recent dressing material.[16] Their outstanding potential to encapsulate and deliver the necessary active substances is considered significant in the process of wound healing.[17]

Negative Pressure Wound Therapy or Vacuum-assisted Closure

This is a mechanical method that uses subatmospheric pressure for the removal of exudate, reduction of edema, and promotion of granulation tissue. VAC is indicated for the management of both chronic as well as acute wounds. A negative pressure of 125 mm is generated over the wound bed which facilitates wound healing. It also helps in the restoring the dermal integrity of complex wounds and is recognized as a cornerstone in advanced wound care therapy.[18] It is contraindicated in untreated osteomyelitis, necrotic wounds, malignancy, avascular wounds, or exposed tendons, bones, organs, or blood vessels.[19] In a comparative study on various dressing materials in DFUs, it was reported that VAC was the best option available to promote early recovery as it shortens the healing time and also decreases the duration of hospitalization.[20] A case of necrotizing fasciitis for which VAC therapy was given which shortens the healing time and thereby promotes early recovery has been discussed for further understanding [Case 7 (**Figs. 9A to F**)].

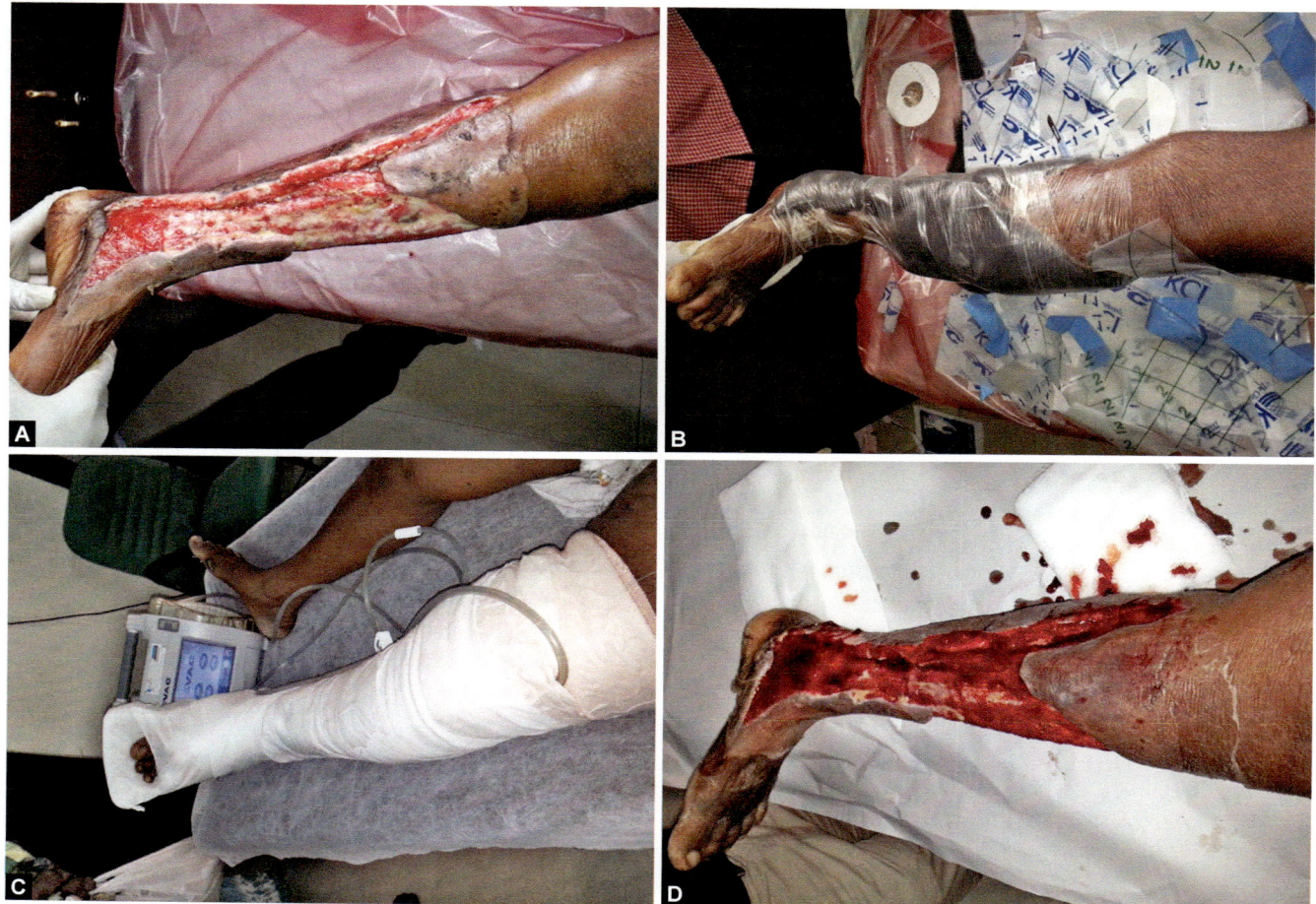

Figs. 9A to F: *Continued*

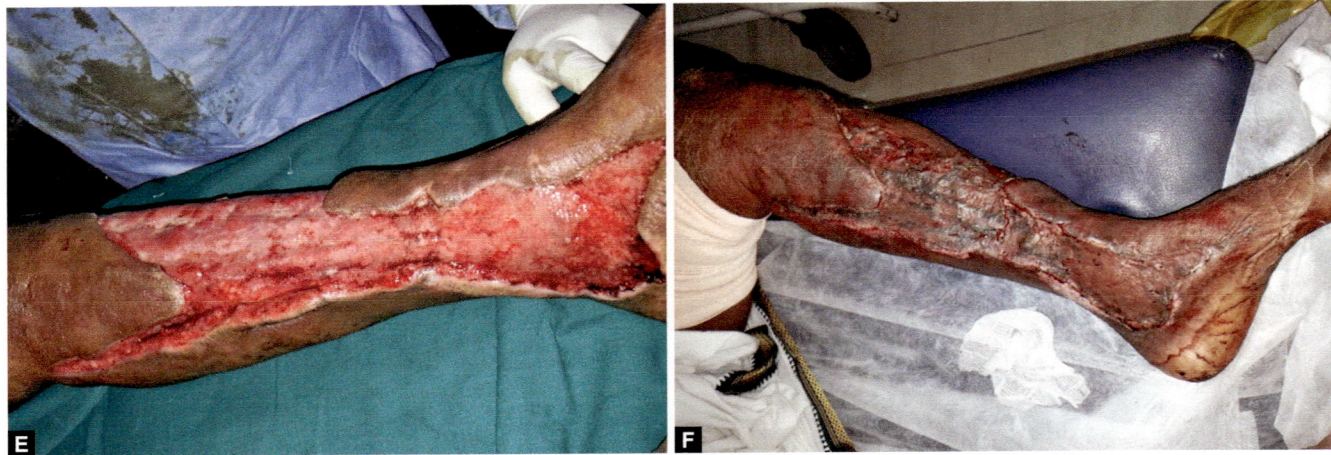

Figs. 9A to F: (A) A case of necrotizing fasciitis after debridement; (B) The application of vacuum-assisted closure (VAC); (C) VAC in situ. (D) The clinical picture at the first sitting; (E) A clinical picture of a granulating wound after two sittings of VAC; (F) The postoperative clinical picture after skin grafting.

IWGDF WOUND HEALING GUIDELINES 2023

The International Working Group on the Diabetic Foot (IWGDF) guidelines (2023) on intervention to enhance wound healing in people with DFUs do not recommend the use of topical antibiotics, collagen, alginate dressings, herbal remedies, or growth factors for the healing of wounds related to diabetic foot. However, the use of hyperbaric oxygen can be considered as a supplemental therapy for treating neuroischemic or ischemic foot ulcers. In cases where the standard of care for treatment of DFU has failed, topical oxygen and placental-derived products are to be considered. Negative pressure wound therapy (NPWT) has also been recommended for the healing of postsurgical wounds related to DFUs.[21]

CONCLUSION

Dressing materials are an integral part of optimum wound care and management of DFUs. It becomes imperative to choose the most appropriate dressing material that is capable of protecting the wound as well as accelerating the wound closure. Apart from this, adequate debridement and offloading of the wound, establishment of good glycemic control, and selection of the most appropriate choice of antibiotics are considered important pillars of standard of care practices. Thus, a comprehensive approach is required to reduce the healing time required for DFUs and also reduce the incidence of potential consequences like amputation.

TAKE-HOME MESSAGE

Successful management of DFUs requires the correct choice of dressing materials suitable for a particular wound from a wide array of various dressing modalities currently available. An ideal dressing material should be able to alleviate pain, provide a moist environment, achieve good control of exudate, and also be patient-compliant. Regular inspection of the wound and frequent dressing changes are considered quintessential to promote good healing. Advanced thin dressing materials serve this purpose and also help accommodate offloading footwear.

REFERENCES

1. Naves CCLM. The Diabetic Foot: A Historical Overview and Gaps in Current Treatment. Adv Wound Care. 2016;5(5):191-7.
2. Lavery LA, Davis KE, Berriman SJ, Braun L, Nichols A, Kim PJ, et al. WHS guidelines update: Diabetic foot ulcer treatment guidelines. Wound Repair Regen. 2016;24(1):112-26.
3. Lipsky BA, Berendt AR, Cornia PB, Pile JC, Peters EJ, Armstrong DG, et al. 2012 Infectious Diseases Society of America Clinical Practice Guideline for the Diagnosis and Treatment of Diabetic Foot Infections. Clin Infect Dis. 2012;54(12):132-73.
4. Wound International. (2013). Best Practice Guidelines: Wound Management in Diabetic Foot Ulcers. [online] Available from https://woundsinternational.com/best-practice-statements/best-practice-guidelines-wound-management-diabetic-foot-ulcers/ [Last accessed September, 2023].
5. Phillips PL, Fletcher J, Shultz G S. Biofilms Made Easy. Wounds International. 2010;1(3):1-6.
6. Kavitha KV, Tiwari S, Purandare VB, Khedkar S, Bhosale SS, Unnikrishnan AG. Choice of wound care in diabetic foot ulcer: A practical approach. World J Diabetes. 2014;5(4):546-56.
7. Hilton JR, Williams DT, Beuker B, Miller DR, Harding KG. Wound Dressings in Diabetic Foot Disease. Clin Infect Dis. 2004;39:S100-3.
8. Wound International. (2004). EWMA Position document: Wound bed preparation in practice. London: MEP Ltd, 2004. [online] Available from https://woundsinternational.com/best-practice-statements/wound-bed-preparation-practice-ewma-position-document/#:~:text=This%20document%20arose%20out%20of,the%20highest%20standards%20of%20care. [Last accessed September, 2023].

9. Wolcott RD, Kennedy JP, Dowd SE. Regular debridement is the main tool for maintaining a healthy wound bed in most chronic wounds. J Wound Care. 2009;18(2):54-6.
10. Pouget C, Dunyach-Remy C, Pantel A, Schuldiner S, Sotto A, Lavigne JP. Biofilms in Diabetic Foot Ulcers: Significance and Clinical Relevance. Microorganisms. 2020;8(10):1580.
11. Kim S, Rahman M, Seol SY, Yoon SS, Kim J. Pseudomonas aeruginosa bacteriophage PA1Ø requires type-IV pili for infection and shows broad bacterial and biofilm-removal activity. Appl Environ Microbiol. 2012;78(17):6380-85.
12. International Wound Infection Institute (IWII). (2022). Wound Infection in Clinical Practice: Principles of best practice, 3rd edition. [online] Available from https://woundsinternational.com/consensus-documents/wound-infection-in-clinical-practice-principles-of-best-practice/ [Last accessed September, 2023].
13. Chadwick P, Ahmad N, Dunn G, Elston D, Fisher N, Haycocks S, et al. Local antibiotic delivery: early intervention in infection management strategy. The Diabetic Foot Journal. 2022;25(2):44-52.
14. Fitton AR, Drew P, Dickson WA. The use of a bilaminate artificial skin substitute (Integra) in acute resurfacing of burns: an early experience. Br J Plast Surg. 2001;54:208-12.
15. Vijay V, Sharad P, Sekar N, Murthy GSR. A phase III study to evaluate the safety and efficacy of recombinant human epidermal growth factor (REGEN-DTM 150) in healing diabetic foot ulcers. Wounds. 2006;18:186-96.
16. Yan L, Shiya Z, Yanlin G, Yinglei Z. Electrospun nanofibers as a wound dressing for treating diabetic foot ulcer. Asian J Pharm Sci. 2019;14(2):130-43.
17. Jang EJ, Patel R, Patel M. Electrospinning Nanofibers as a Dressing to Treat Diabetic Wounds. Pharmaceutics. 2023;15(4):1144.
18. Zaver V, Kankanalu P. Negative Pressure Wound Therapy. In: StatPearls [Internet]. Treasure Island (FL): StatPearls Publishing; 2023 [online] Available from https://www.ncbi.nlm.nih.gov/books/NBK576388 [Last accessed September, 2023].
19. Andros G, Armstrong DG, Attinger CE, Boulton AJ, Frykberg RG, Joseph WS, et al. Consensus statement on negative pressure wound therapy (V.A.C. Therapy) for the management of diabetic foot wounds. Ostomy Wound Manage. 2006;Suppl:1-32.
20. Yadav AK, Mishra S, Khanna V, Panchal S, Modi N, Amin S. Comparative study of various dressing techniques in diabetic foot ulcers in the Indian population: a single-center experience. Int J Diabetes Dev Ctries. 2023:1-7.
21. Chen P, Vilorio NC, Dhatariya K, Jeffcoate W, Lobmann R, McIntosh C, et al. Guidelines on interventions to enhance healing of foot ulcers in people with diabetes (IWGDF 2023 update). Diabetes Metab Res Rev. 2023;e3644.

CHAPTER 11

Peripheral Arterial Disease and Diabetic Foot: Clinical Cases and Management Strategies

Vibhakar R Vachhrajani, Ashu Rastogi

CASE 1

A female patient aged 72 years had left great toe blackening of 15 days duration without any history of injury. She had rest pain. Pedal pulsations were absent with palpable popliteal pulsations. Ankle–Brachial index (ABI) was 0.4 with diminished skin temperature up to ankle. She had loss of hair in foot and leg.

This patient had a history of diabetes and hypertension (HTN) of 22 years duration with ischemic heart disease (IHD). Her left ventricular ejection fraction (LVEF) was 50% with hemoglobin (Hb) of 8.8 g/dL. Her serum creatinine was 1.02 mg/dL. Her color Doppler report was showing multiple blocks in posterior tibial and anterior tibial vessels. There was a past history of operation of coronary artery bypass graft (CABG) before 3 years. She was operated for angiography and balloon angioplasty for below-knee vessels on March 20, 2023.

After balloon angioplasty, she did not turn up for 2 months. When she came, there was gangrene on her forefoot. Her diabetes was poorly controlled with glycated hemoglobin (HbA1c) 10.8%. Her lipid profile was normal and serum potassium was 6.7 mEq/L. Her vitals were normal respiration rate/cardiovascular system at the time of admission.

We did below-knee amputation. Perioperative course was uneventful, and the wound healed well in 30 days.

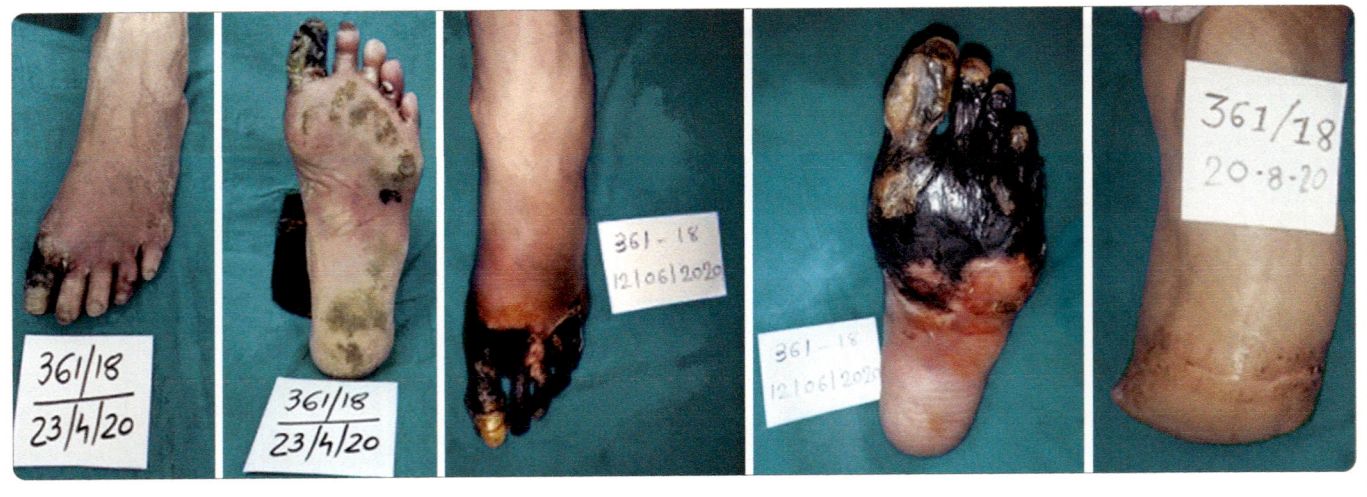

CASE 2

A 67-year-old male patient came with left great toe blackening of 4 months duration with infection. There was a history of barefoot walking and stone injury. He was a chronic smoker with tobacco chewing with a history of diabetes of 7 years duration and IHD of 5 years duration. He had claudication pain on 100 feet walk with breathlessness on exertion. He had a loss of hair on foot and leg with palpable popliteal artery and feeble posterior tibial and dorsalis pedis arteries (DPA). His ABI was 0.5.

He was anemic (Hb 9 g/dL) and had uncontrolled diabetes (HbA1c 10.6%). His lipid profile was normal with serum creatinine 0.9 mg/dL and serum potassium 6.2 mEq/L. Color Doppler was suggestive of below-knee disease. In his angiography, there was total occlusion up to distal one-thirds of anterior tibial artery (ATA) and total occlusion of proximal and middle third posterior tibial artery (PTA), and stenosis of peroneal artery. He underwent balloon angioplasty in August 2020. For angioplasty, popliteal artery was cannulated with H1 catheter. Lesion was dilated with 4 × 100-mm Rival balloon and stented. DPA and PTA were punctured at the level of ankle and cannulated retrogradely and lesion crossed with Command ES wire. Angioplasty with 2.5 × 80 mm ballooning was done. Satisfactory angiographic result was achieved.

He had diabetic cardiomyopathy with LVEF 40%. After angioplasty, he came after 2 months for the surgery of foot in October 2020. We did disarticulation at first metatarsophalangeal (MTP) joint. The wound healed nicely, and the patient was completely ambulatory with specialized footwear with toe filler. He expired on May 21 due to a cardiac problem.

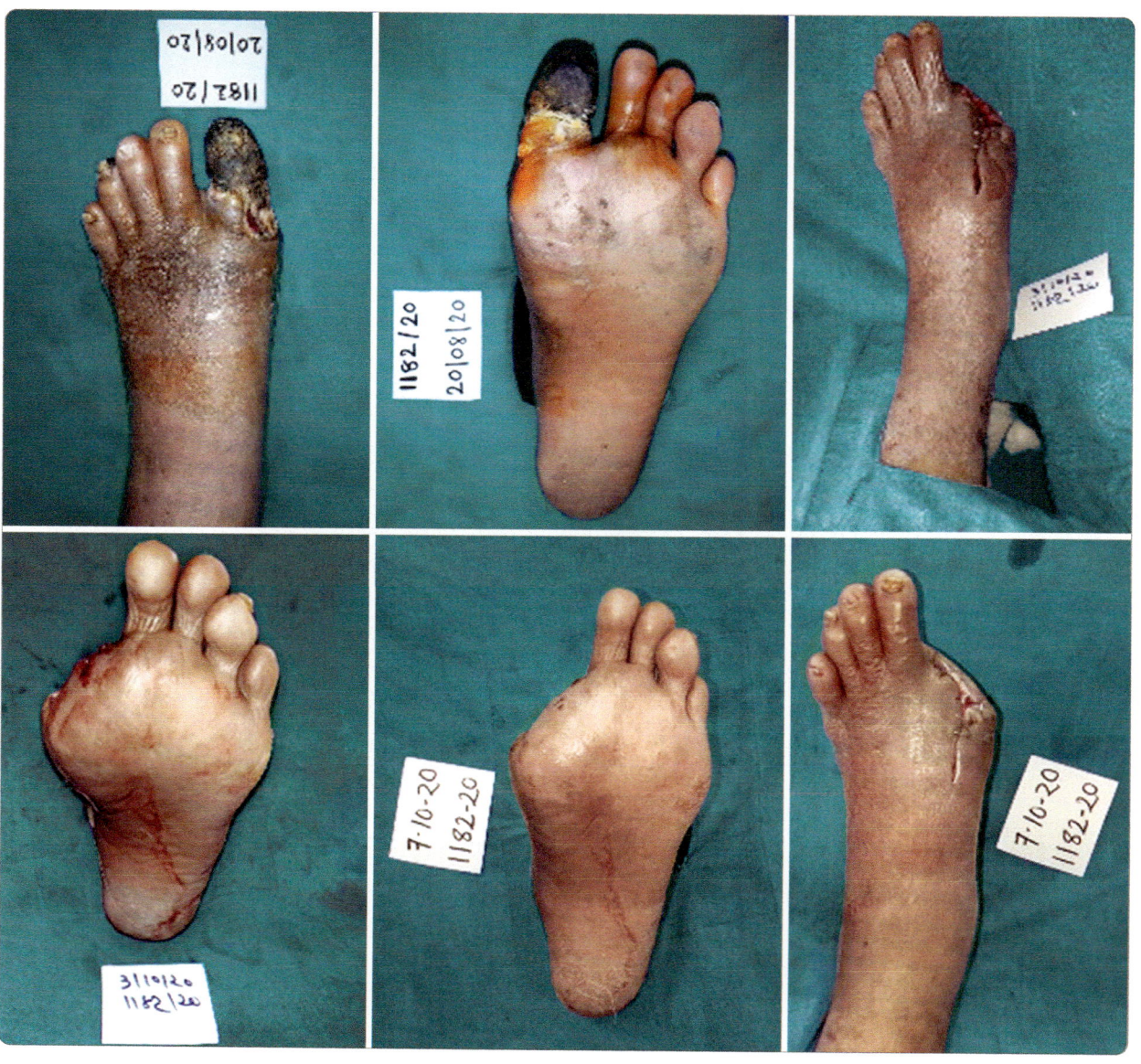

CASE 3

A male patient aged 53 years had an infected blister on right dorsum of foot. He had diabetes of 13 years duration. He had no HTN and no IHD. He had no rest pain and no claudication pain. There was a positive history of smoking 20 *bidis* per day for 25 years. He had normal Hb 11.8 g/dL, HbA1c 10.2%, and serum creatinine 0.6 mg/dL. Serum cholesterol and serum electrolytes were normal. His arterial color Doppler study was suggestive of 60% block in femoropopliteal area with good collateral flow in below-knee vessels. His ABI was 0.6 on right side and 1.1 on left side. His LVEF was 38%. The patient had neuropathy with vibration perception threshold (VPT) > 20 on both feet.

As the patient was not willing for endovascular procedure, we did debridement under ankle block anesthesia on October 6, 2020. Perioperatively there was comparatively less bleeding and postoperative wound reading was suggestive of ischemia. We again requested the patient to undergo endovascular procedure, which he then agreed. Balloon angioplasty was done at femoropopliteal level on October 14, 2020. The wound healing was better and with vacuum dressing, it healed well.

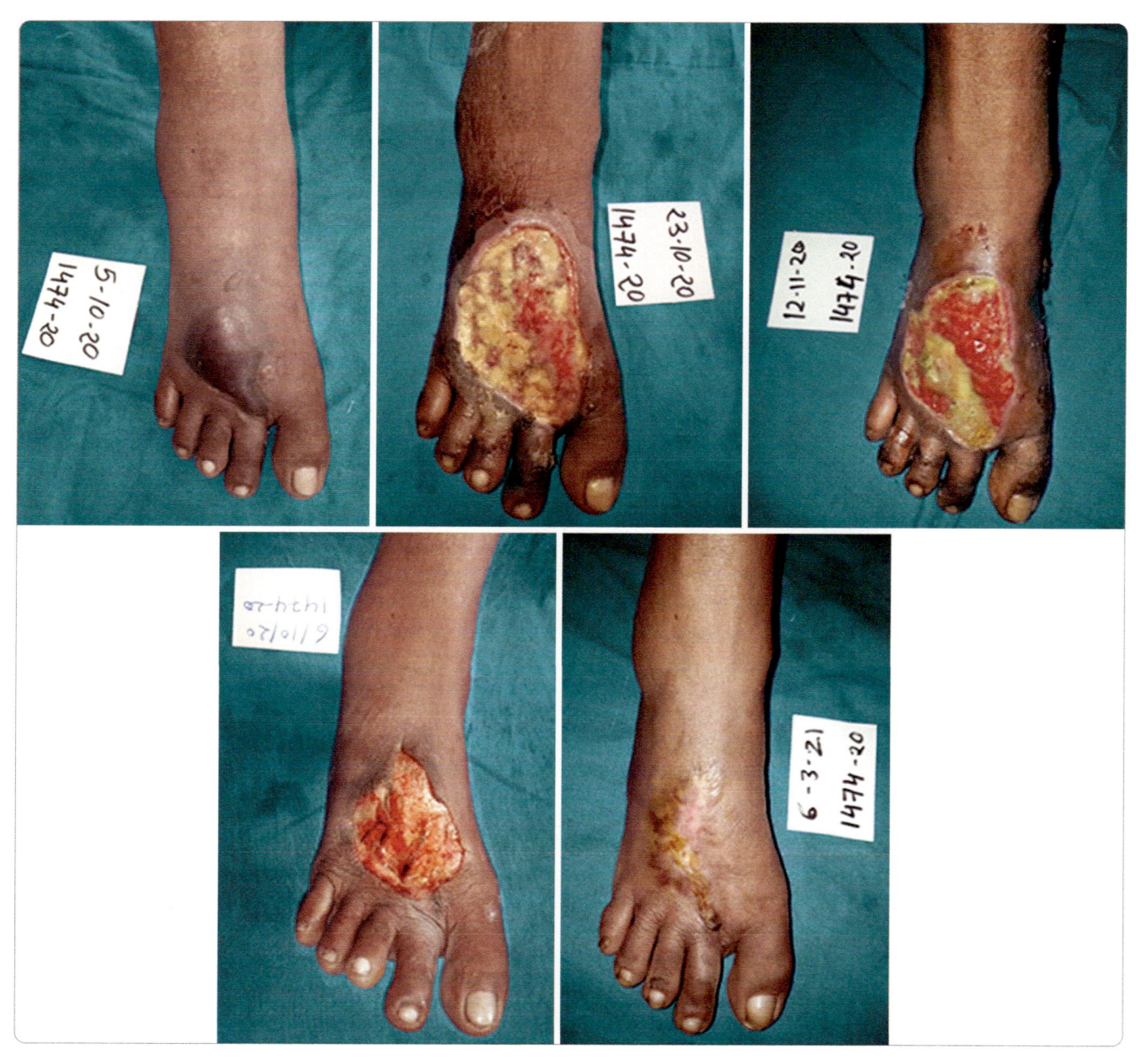

CASE 4

A 55-year-old patient had a history of blackening of great toe of 15 days duration. He had diabetes and HTN of 5 years duration. There was a history of thorn injury. There was no history of claudication pain or rest pain, and he was having no addiction.

He had neuropathy with VPT of >20 bilaterally. He was anemic with Hb 8.4 g/dL, and HbA1c was 8.6% with reasonably good control of diabetes at present. His lipid profile and electrolytes were normal.

His serum creatinine was 2.0 mg/dL with LVEF 20%.

Though his serum creatinine was high we hydrated the patient well and he had undergone balloon angioplasty of peroneal and PTA with a minimum dose of contrast material. Kidney function was well maintained after the use of contrast. Angioplasty was done on June 7, 2021, and we did transmetatarsal amputation on June 15, 2021. Blood transfusions were given.

We kept the wound partially open which then healed secondarily with vacuum dressing, collagen granules, and silver foam dressings. Then we prescribed him specialized footwear.

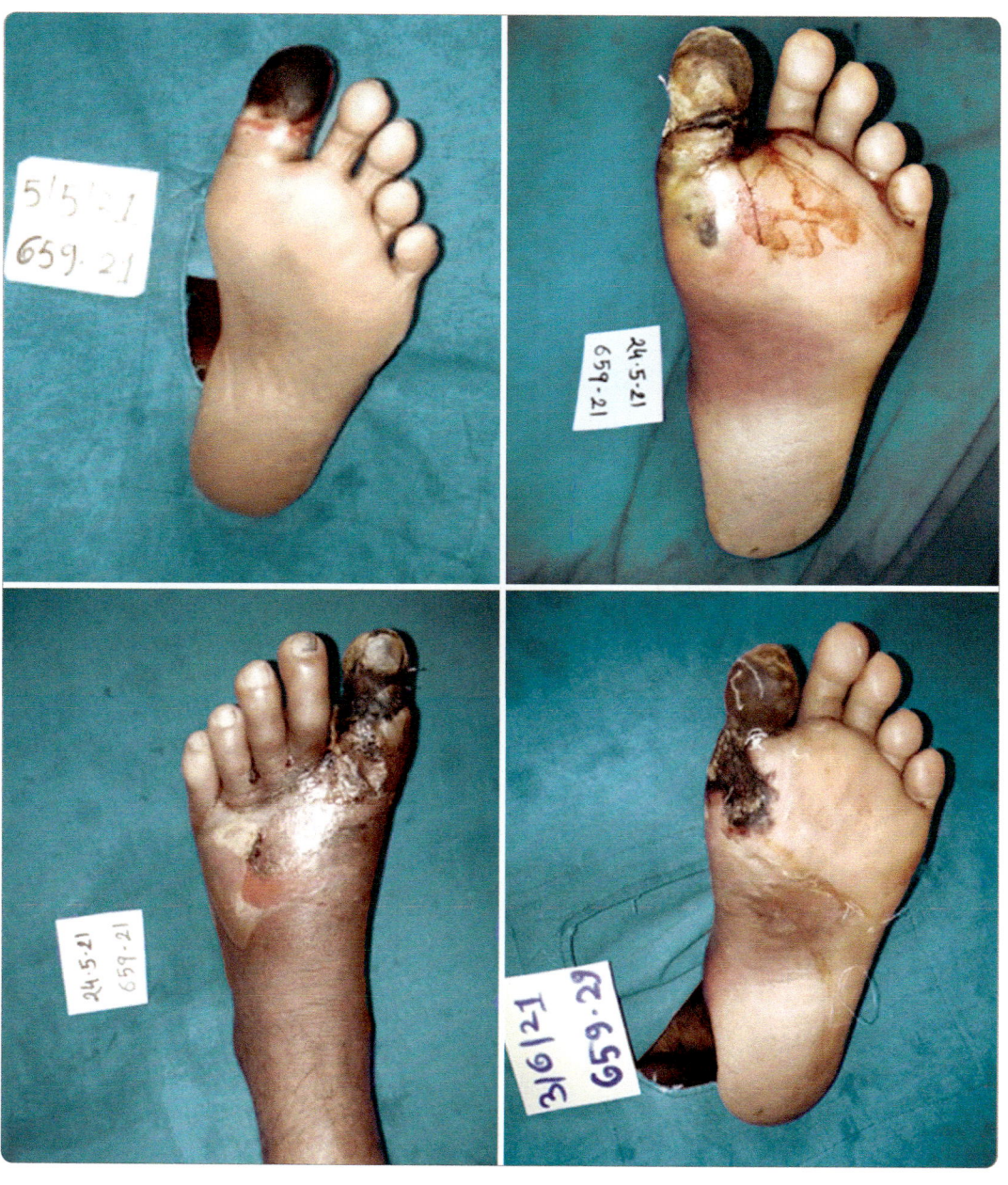

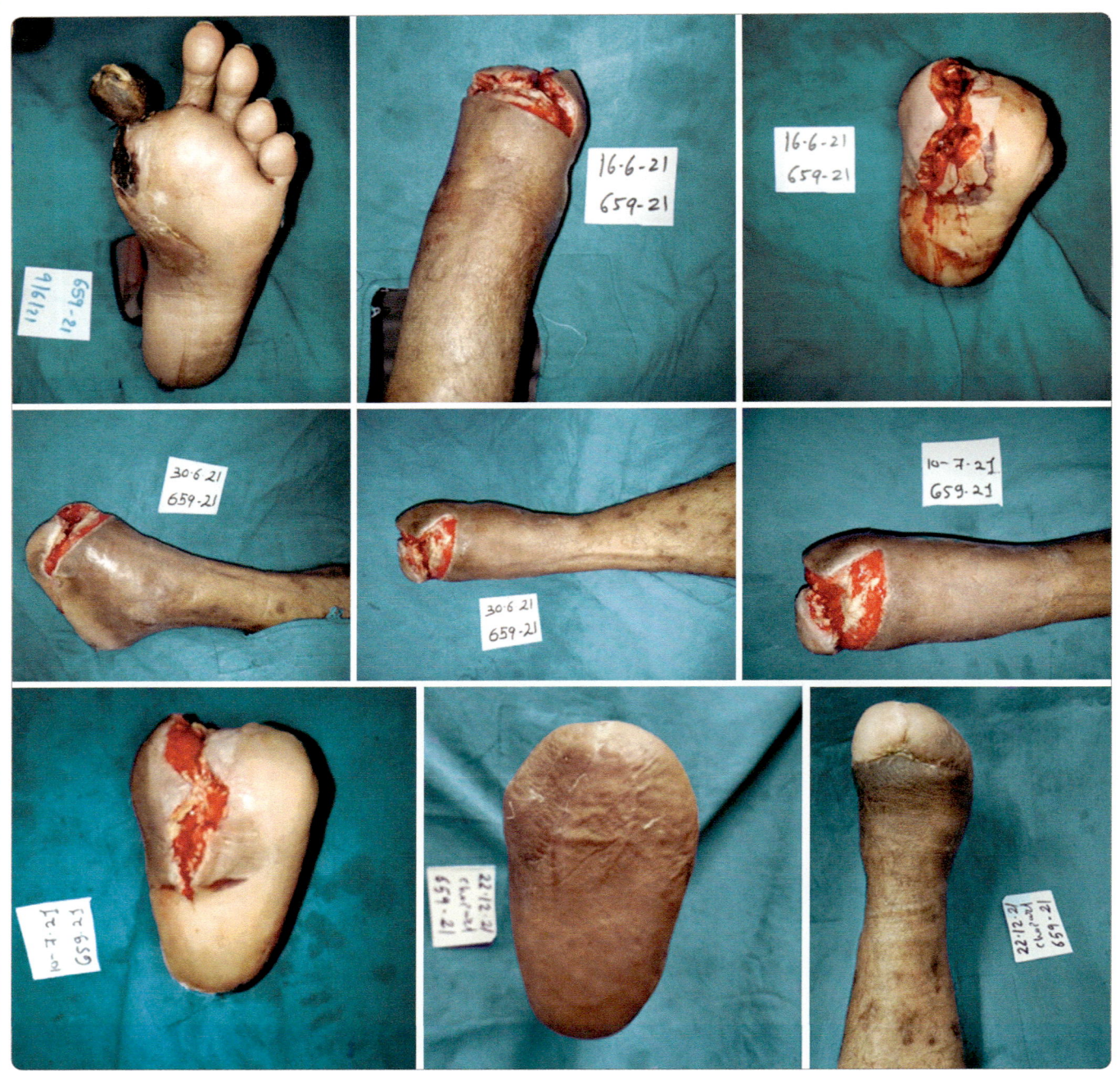

CASE 5

A 90-year-old female patient came to us with blackening of multiple toes bilaterally of 2 months duration. She was recently diagnosed to be having diabetes. She had a history of HTN of 20 years duration and IHD of 20 years duration. There was no neuropathy with VPT of <20. She had claudication pain on 500 feet walk as well as rest pain.

Her Hb was 11.2 g/dL, HbA1c 6.5% with good control of diabetes, and serum creatinine 1.3 mg/dL. Her color Doppler was suggestive of extensive atherosclerotic changes with multiple vessel calcification with no localized stenosis. Her lipid profile and electrolytes were normal and LVEF was 48%. As the relatives were not willing for peripheral angiography, we treated her conservatively. We advised Buerger exercises and foot and ankle exercises to improve microcirculation. There was autoamputation of all the gangrenous toes in 1 year, without pain and with good sleep. In June 2022, there was good healing with autoamputation and in May 2023, she came for follow-up and was asymptomatic with normal feet.

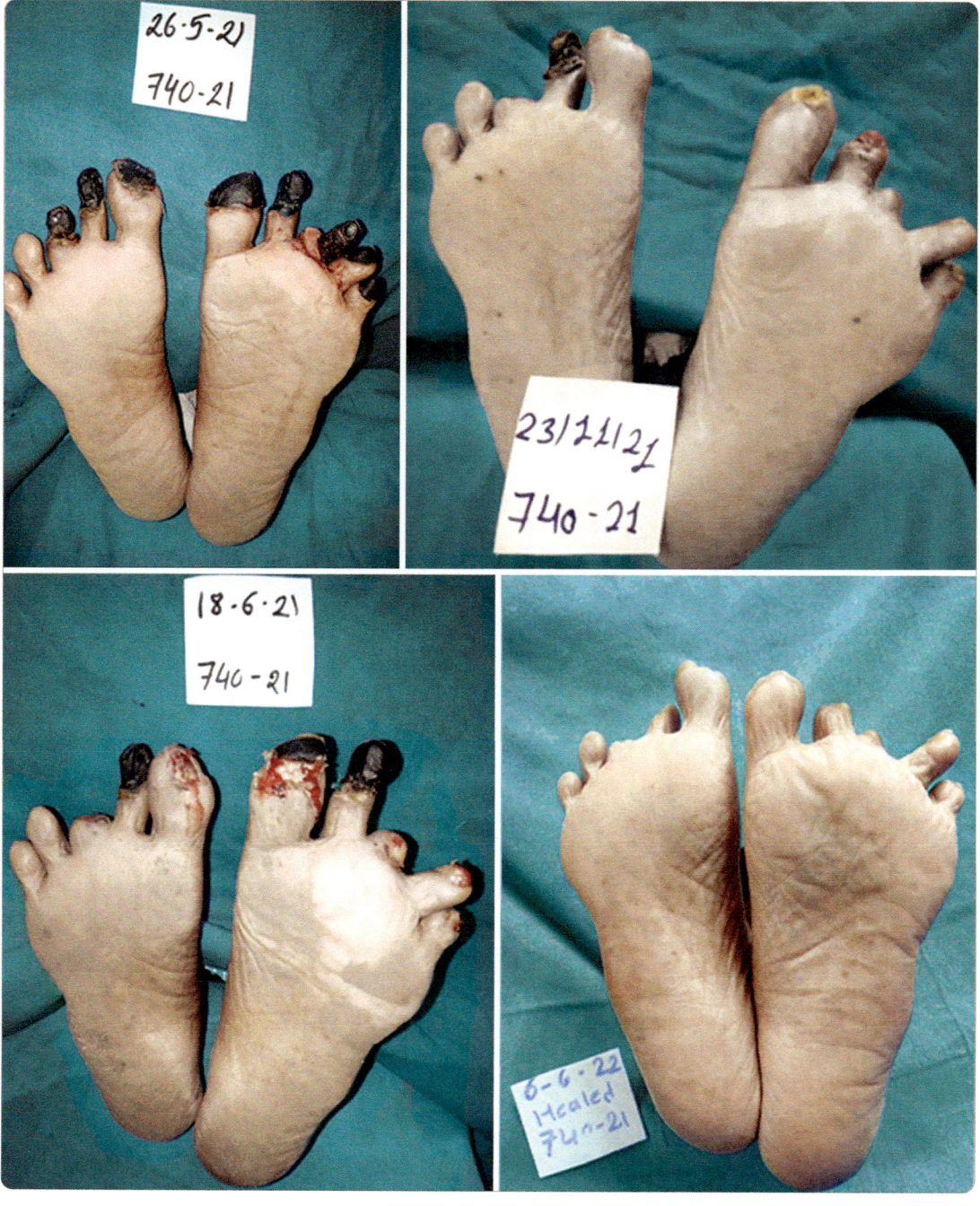

TAKE-HOME MESSAGES

- Diabetes is a polyvascular disease
- Good glycemic control is the most rewarding for all limb-related events
- Structured exercise is an useful modality to improve QOL and to reduce leg symptoms
- Anti-platelets, statins and ACEI/ARBs are effective in symptomatic PAD
- Dual antiplatelet agents are useful for reducing recurrence after lower limb angioplasty
- Rivaroxaban has proven efficacy in reducing MACE and limb events in patients with PAD after endovascular intervention.
- Below the knee angioplasty is technically successful in majority of patients with good clinical outcome and minimal complications.

FURTHER READINGS

1. Bracale UM, Ammollo RP, Hussein EA, Hoballah JJ, Goeau-Brissonniere O, et al. Managing Peripheral Artery Disease in Diabetic Patients: A Questionnaire Survey from Vascular Centers of the Mediterranean Federation for the Advancing of Vascular Surgery (MeFAVS). Ann Vasc Surg. 2020;64:239-45.
2. Marco M, Valentina I, Daniele M, Valerio DR, Andrea P, Roberto G, et al. Peripheral Arterial Disease in Persons with Diabetic Foot Ulceration: a Current Comprehensive Overview. Curr Diabetes Rev. 2021;17(4):474-85.
3. Lin JHX, Papanas N, Zayed H, Vas PRJ. Revascularisation Options for Chronic Limb Threatening Ischaemia in Diabetes: Implications From Two Recent Trials. Int J Low Extrem Wounds. 2023:15347346231188874.
4. International Working Group on the Diabetic Foot (IWGDF) Guidelines 2019
5. International Working Group on the Diabetic Foot (IWGDF) Guidelines 2023
6. Gerhard-Herman MD, Gornik HL, Barrett C, Barshes NR, Corriere MA, Drachman DE, et al. 2016 AHA/ACC Guideline on the Management of Patients With Lower Extremity Peripheral Artery Disease: A Report of the American College of Cardiology/American Heart Association Task Force on Clinical Practice Guidelines. Circulation. 2017;135(12):e726-779.
7. Parvar SL, Fitridge R, Dawson J, Nicholls SJ. Medical and lifestyle management of peripheral arterial disease. J Vasc Surg. 2018;68(5):1595-1606.

Charcot Neuroarthropathy of the Foot

Jayaditya Ghosh, Ashu Rastogi

INTRODUCTION

Charcot neuro-osteoarthropathy (CN) is a condition which is prevalent among patients with neuropathy. It has been documented in conditions such as leprosy, syringomyelia, syphilis, alcoholism, spinal injuries, and mostly in patients with diabetes.[1] It was first described in patients of tabes dorsalis, but later in 1883, Jean-Martin Charcot described this in patients with diabetic neuropathy. It primarily affects the bones and the joints. The prevalence of Charcot foot ranges from 0.5% in individuals with diabetes to high as 8% in patients with diabetic neuropathy.[2] The presentation of Charcot neuroarthropathy can be an acute, acute-on-chronic or chronic type depending upon the temperature difference between the 2 feet, i.e., >2°C and the bony changes.[3,4] Acute Charcot neuroarthropathy presents with signs of redness, swelling, and raised temperature of the involved area, whereas chronicity is based on bony deformities.[5]

The patient if not detected in the acute condition leads to chronic changes in the joints, which lead to joint dislocation, fractures, and the development of rocker-bottom foot. These deformities ultimately lead to the development of ulcers. These ulcers if left untreated or neglected can lead to a state where amputation of the affected foot is needed. The presence of neuropathy is an integral part of the development of Charcot neuroarthropathy.[6]

PATHOPHYSIOLOGY

The pathophysiology of Charcot neuroarthropathy has two main postulates. One is the neurovascular theory in which it is thought to have nerve damage, which results in loss of sympathetic tone in the precapillary arterioles and resulting vasodilatation. It leads to increased local vascularity, which leads to activation of increased osteoclastic activity with the development of secondary osteopenia, fractures, and deformity.[7] The other theory is the more accepted one and has attracted a lot of recent research around it. This involves the neurotraumatic theory where due to the presence of neuropathy in these diabetic patients, they are not able to realize the microtrauma that they sustain. This leads to the development of a state of inflammation resulting in the raised levels of raised interleukin-6 (IL-6) and tumor necrosis factor alpha (TNF-α). There is also activation of the receptor activator of NF-κB ligand (RANKL) and osteoprotegerin (OPG) pathways, leading to bone destruction.[8] This highlights the importance of RANKL in the pathogenesis of acute Charcot neuroarthropathy. It is evident that in the presence of diabetes, the development of neuropathy is an important predisposing factor that starts the cascade of acute Charcot neuroarthropathy. The presence of diabetes leads to increased levels of advanced glycation end products, and this increases the levels of RANKL.[9] Levels of OPG are also low in these patients. There is an increase in the ratio of RANKL/OPG. The neuropathy leads to the low levels of calcitonin gene-related peptide (CGRP) and endothelial nitric oxide synthase (NOS). All this leads to unopposed action of RANKL and increased osteoclastic activity leading to the development of bone resorption, fractures, and dislocation.[10]

CLASSIFICATION OF CHARCOT NEUROARTHROPATHY

Depending on the Phases of Charcot Neuroarthropathy[11]

- *Stage 0*: Pre-Charcot/prodromal—
  - Clinically red, hot, and swollen foot
  - No radiographic deformity

- *Stage 1*: Development/destruction—
  - Clinically red, swollen, and raised temperature
  - Bone destruction changes present in radiograph
- *Stage 2*: Coalescence—
  - Less signs of inflammation
  - There is a worsening of the joints than the previous stage with the presence of coalescence of the large joints.
- *Stage 3*: Consolidation—
  - There is a complete change of the foot architecture and there is no sign of inflammation.
  - Complete remodeling of the affected joints

Depending on the Location of Involvement

Sanders and Frykberg classification is as follows:[12]
- Metatarsophalangeal to interphalangeal joints
- Tarsometatarsal joints
- Intertarsal joints (naviculocuneiform joint, talonavicular, and calcaneocuboid joint)
- Ankle and subtalar joints
- Calcaneus

PRESENTATION AND DIAGNOSIS

Charcot neuroarthropathy of the foot can be unilateral or bilateral. Unilateral Charcot is the most common presentation. The most common presentation is foot swelling along with deformities, as the diagnosis is generally missed initially. In case of acute Charcot neuroarthropathy, apart from swelling of the foot there are associated signs of inflammation like redness and raised local temperature. Midfoot involvement is the most common with 62.3%, followed by forefoot (22.6%) and then hindfoot (12.3%) involvement.[14] In chronic stage, there is deformity of the foot which if untreated for a long duration may lead to the development of ulceration. Bilateral Charcot neuroarthropathy is not uncommon, and it can also present in the same way with swelling along with deformities of the foot.

For the diagnosis of acute Charcot neuroarthropathy of the foot requires a high index of suspicion in diabetic patients. The common presentation of foot swelling with local signs of inflammation could be a close mimic of cellulitis and deep venous thrombosis. Osteomyelitis can also be a possibility in these scenarios but in that case the presence of a sinus or an ulcer is generally seen.

Diagnosis of acute Charcot is mainly clinical. The presence of neuropathy is a key pointer toward suspecting patients with Charcot foot. In the background of foot swelling and neuropathy if there are signs of local inflammation with or without deformity in a diabetic patient, then Charcot neuroarthropathy should be suspected. In case of chronic Charcot neuroarthropathy, the development of deformity with a history of numbness of the lower limbs in a diabetic patient should raise the suspicion of the underlying condition. Rocker-bottom foot is the most common form of deformity seen in Charcot neuroarthropathy where there is midfoot collapse along with loss of the foot arches.

When there is a clinical suspicion of acute Charcot, an infrared thermometer is used to measure the temperature difference between the 2 feet. The patient should be made to sit with both the feet on the ground for some time and then the temperature reading is to be taken. In the case of acute Charcot neuroarthropathy, there is a temperature difference of >2°C. In the case of bilateral Charcot foot, the temperature gradient is seen from the distal to the proximal part of the foot to the leg and then compared, and this gradient is used for monitoring of remission.

CASE 1

A 27-year-old female patient, a known case of type 1 diabetes mellitus for the last 10 years, presented with a history of swelling of the left foot with redness over the dorsal aspect of the foot, which was gradually increasing in nature for the last 3 months **(Fig. 1A)**. She had an occasional history of localized pain over the area. There was a history of numbness of the bilateral lower limbs for the last 6–7 months. She had taken antibiotics for swelling, redness, and edema of the foot in view of cellulitis. On examination, it was found to have increased temperature of the left foot (5°C) with signs of inflammation. The vibration perception threshold was >50/msec. All the peripheral pulses were palpable with ankle–brachial index of 1.1 and 1.02 in the left and right foot. She underwent an X-ray of the feet, which showed destruction of the calcaneum, navicular, and cuboid **(Fig. 1B)**. Magnetic resonance imaging (MRI) of the foot, which is considered the gold standard for diagnosis of Charcot, was done, which showed periarticular edema along with bone marrow edema along with the destruction of the midfoot and hindfoot **(Fig. 1C)**. She was started on total contact cast for off-loading. The patient was then followed up monthly to check for clinical and radiological remission.

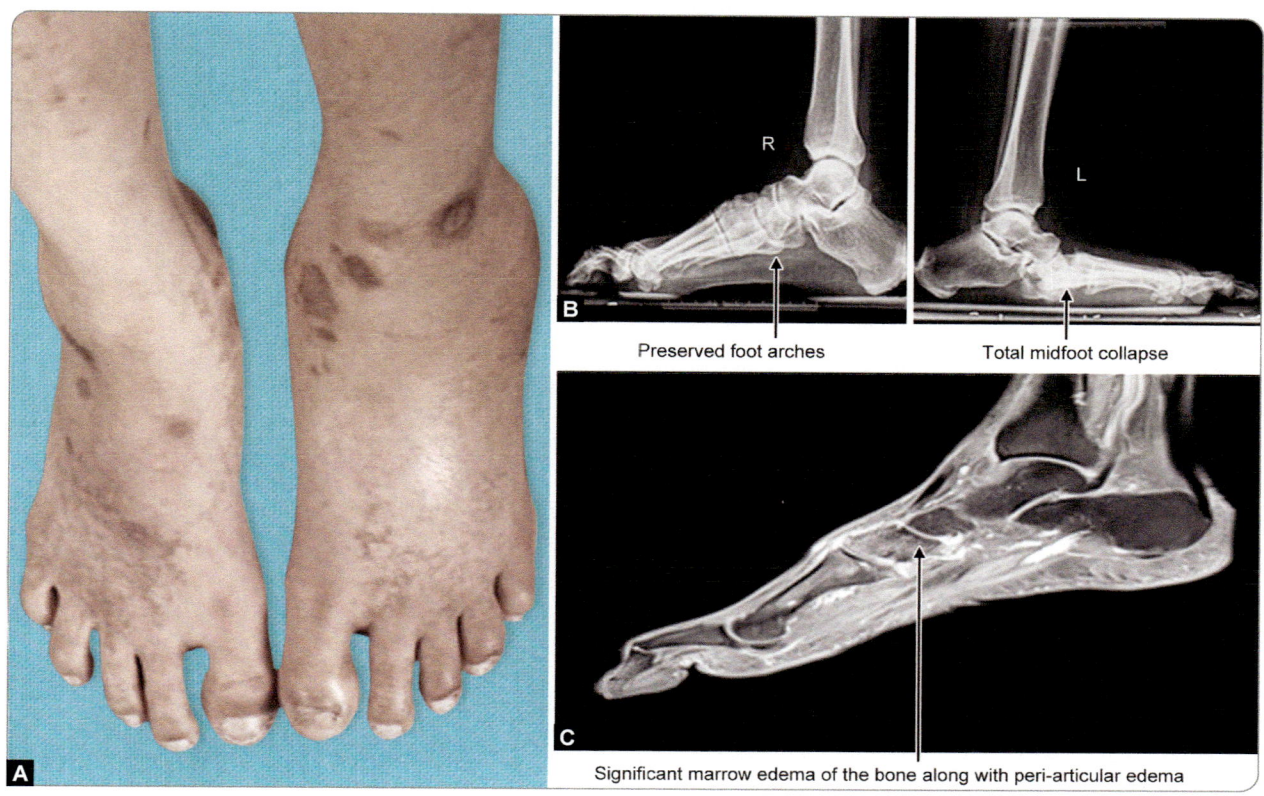

Figs. 1A to C: Asymmetric foot swelling with an X-ray showing midfoot collapse with bone marrow edema in magnetic resonance imaging (MRI).

CASE 2

A 50-year-old female presented with a history of swelling of the right foot for 4 months after twisting of the ankle while walking. She was having no pain in that area and as a result she continued to walk with the swelling. Over the period of 2 months, she gradually developed progressive deformity of the right foot along with redness over the area. She was given antibiotics in view of cellulitis in the initial 2 months but because of the deformity, she sought further assistance. On examination, there was significant deformity with swelling and raised temperature of the right foot compared to the left. X-ray of the foot was done, which showed complete collapse of the right midfoot. MRI of the foot was also done, which showed periarticular edema along with bone marrow edema with destruction of navicular and cuboid **(Figs. 2A to C)**. She was diagnosed as acute-on-chronic Charcot and was put on total contact cast.

86 Charcot Neuroarthropathy of the Foot

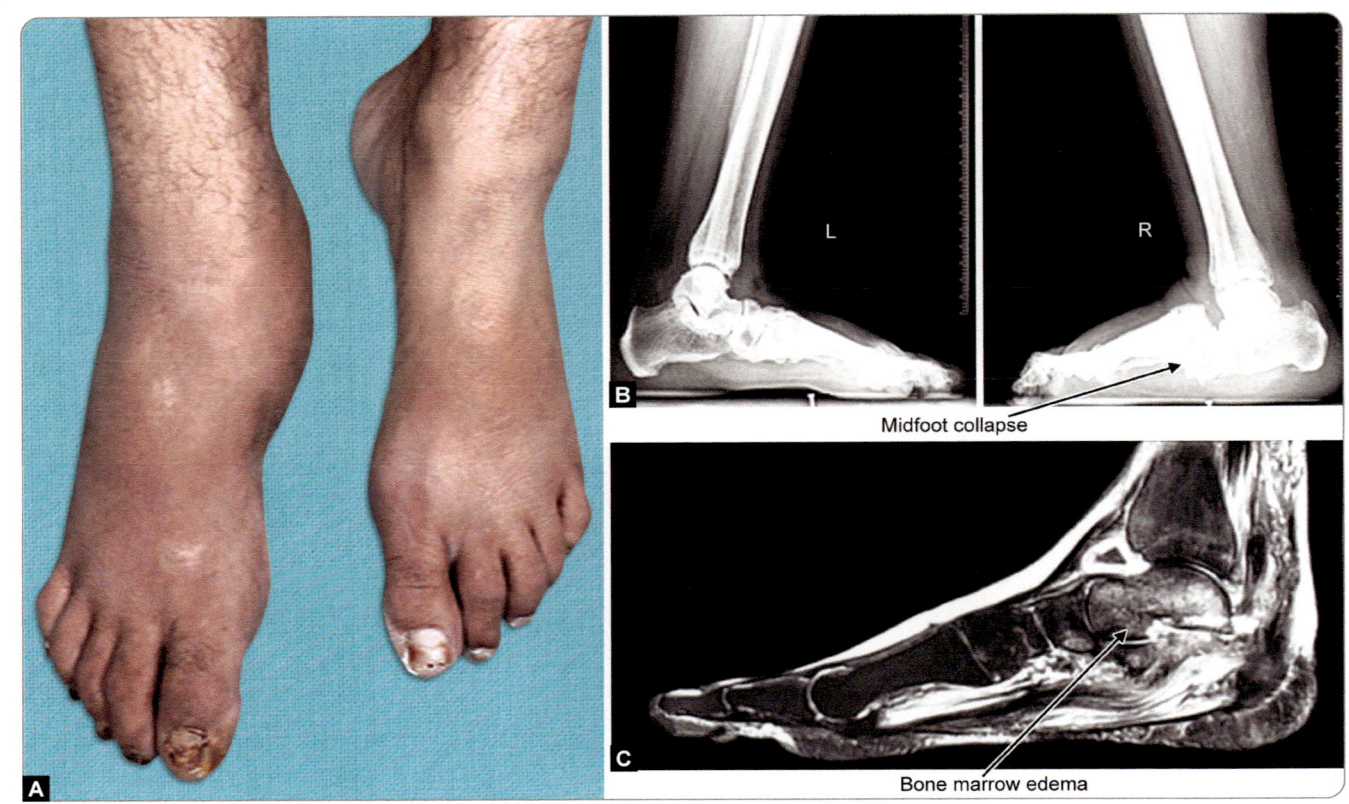

Figs. 2A to C: (A) Asymmetric swelling of the right foot; (B) X-ray showing mid foot collapse with fracture and bone destruction of navicular and cuboid; (C) MRI suggestive of marrow edema involving mid foot bones.

TABLE 1: Magnetic resonance imaging (MRI) and computed tomography (CT) based classification.		
Stage	**Clinical features**	**CT and MRI grading**
Active stage, grade 0	Mild inflammation (swelling, warmth, pain, increased by unprotected walking), no gross deformity	• *Obligatory*: Diffuse BMO and STO (Kiuru Grade I–III), no cortical disruption • *Facultative*: Subchondral trabecular microfractures (bone bruise), ligament damage
Active stage, grade 1	Severe inflammation (swelling, warmth, pain, increased by unprotected walking), gross deformity, increased by unprotected walking	• *Obligatory*: Fracture(s) with cortical disruption, BMO and STO (Kiuru grade IV) • *Facultative*: Osteoarthritis, cysts, cartilage damage, osteochondrosis, joint effusion, fluid collection, bone erosion/necrosis, bone lysis, debris, bone destruction, joint luxation/subluxation, ligament damage, tenosynovitis, and bone dislocation
Inactive stage, grade 0	No inflammation, no gross deformity	No abnormal imaging, or minimal residual BMO; subchondral sclerosis, bone cysts, osteoarthrosis, and ligament damage

Source: With permission from Chantelau EA et al (2014).[13]

RADIOLOGICAL IMAGING

Imaging in the form of X-ray of the foot is the initial investigation of choice. X-ray of the foot with ankle with lateral view and anteroposterior view is generally done. Bony destruction and joint changes of subluxation and dislocation are generally seen in advanced case of Charcot neuroarthropathy. Though in stage 0, there is no change seen in the X-ray, only clinical signs of foot swelling with local signs of inflammation are present.

The other known modality used for diagnosis is MRI of the foot. In MRI, subchondral cysts are seen in the initial stages followed by periarticular changes with bone marrow edema **(Table 1)**.

Other modalities that can be done in cases where MRI is contraindicated are single-photon emission computed tomography (SPECT), computed tomography (CT) scan of the foot and ankle, and nuclear scan in the form of fludeoxyglucose ^{18}F positron emission tomography (FDG PET) scan.

TREATMENT

For acute Charcot neuroarthropathy of the foot, off-loading is the only accepted modality of treatment. It is done with the help of total contact cast **(Figure 3)**. The total contact cast has to be changed every 2–4 weeks depending on the loosening of the cast. Every monthly temperature monitoring of the bilateral feet has to be done and it has to be continued till the temperature difference between the 2 feet is <2°C. Once the temperature difference is <2°C then the total contact cast is discontinued, and it is considered as clinical remission.[15] But certain studies have shown that discontinuation of the total contact cast at this point of clinical remission can lead to a recurrence of around 12–33%.[16] So multiple studies have been done to monitor the remission of acute Charcot. Magnetic resonance (MR) spectroscopy has been done to see quantitative remission of acute Charcot. Nuclear scans in the form of triple-phase bone scan and ^{18}F-FDG PET have been done to see the remission process and serial MRI of the foot.

Time period to remission varies according to different regions. In the UK, there are studies indicating a treatment period of 9–12 months for acute Charcot neuroarthropathy.[5]

While in the US, Europe, and certain parts of Asia, studies showed a duration of 3–9 months for acute Charcot neuroarthropathy.[17]

Postclinical remission patients are generally advised to use air walkers or customized footwear to prevent microtrauma and callus or ulcer formation.

Medical Therapy

This has also been tried in case of acute Charcot to decrease the time to remission but none of the treatment modalities has gained much success. Bisphosphonates, denosumab,[18] and methylprednisolone[19] have been tried to decrease the time to remission but the results are equivocal. In a systematic review on the use of bisphosphonates, there are contradictory results, and long-term studies are still required.[20] Denosumab single-dose injection has been shown to decrease the time to remission as well decrease the misalignment in Chopart–Lisfranc joint post total contact cast.[18] Teriparatide has also been tried in acute Charcot but in that too no significant benefit regarding the time to remission as compared to placebo.[21] But another study used teriparatide in inactive Charcot foot, and it showed that there was significant increase in bone remodeling as evidenced by an increase in bone turnover markers and increased uptake in ^{18}F-PET scan during follow-up of 12 months.[22]

In case of chronic Charcot, off-loading with the help of air walker or customized footwear is advised to prevent reactivation. Surgical intervention is also important for chronic Charcot as corrective surgery can be done. It helps in the rehabilitation process and walking of the patients with therapeutic footwear.

Apart from all these interventions, regular calcium and vitamin D supplementation are given in all patients of Charcot foot.

FOLLOW-UP

Acute Charcot Neuroarthropathy

The follow-up strategy for patients with active Charcot neuroarthropathy of foot is provided in **Flowchart 1**.

Chronic Charcot

In case of chronic Charcot neuroarthropathy of the foot, specialized footwear and application of air walker or surgical intervention are the only form of treatment, and

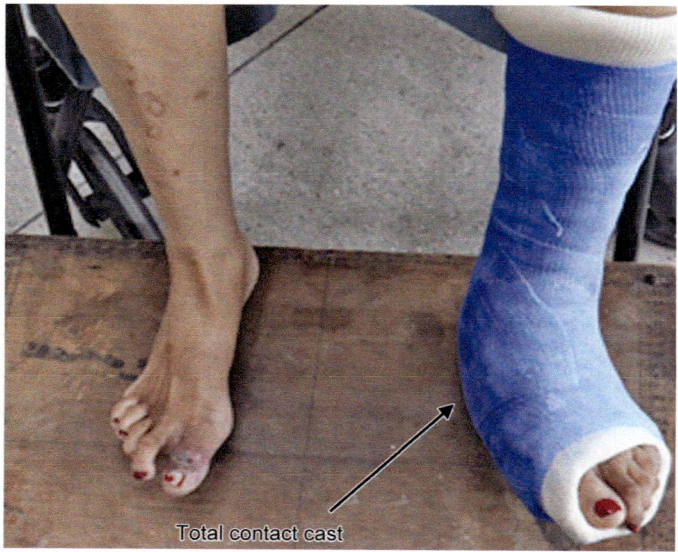

Fig. 3: Total contact cast applied on the left foot.

Asymmetric foot swelling with signs of inflammation i.e., redness, swelling and increased temperature
↓
Temperature difference of >2°C between the two feet
↓
X-ray of the foot to see for joint dislocation or degenerative changes MRI of the foot for confirmation of diagnosis in doubtful cases or in-case of suspected osteomyelitis
↓
Application of total contact cast (TCC) **(Fig. 3)** in case of acute Charcot
↓
2–4 weekly temperature monitoring of the bilateral foot and TCC changing till temperature difference <2°C between the two feet
↓
Temperature difference <2°C documented 2–4 weeks apart on two occasions, clinical remission
↓
TCC discontinuation and putting the patient on specialized footwear (air walker)

Flowchart 1: A guide to assessment and follow-up of patient with active Charcot neuroarthropathy.

regular foot examination should be done at least twice a year to see for any development of further deformity or development of acute component of Charcot.

LONG-TERM COMPLICATION

There are some well-known long-term complications of Charcot neuroarthropathy of the foot. The most common being the development of deformity of the foot. When the diagnosis of Charcot is delayed it generally results in the development of deformity of the foot. All cases of chronic Charcot foot generally have some degree of deformity of the foot associated with it. In case acute Charcot foot is not properly immobilized then also the development of deformity is also very high.

As these patients of Charcot foot have an underlying neuropathy associated with it, the development of neuropathic ulcers is also very common as there is loss of the normal architecture of the foot and there is malfunction of the weight bearing of the body on the foot bones. Larsen et al. showed that 37% of the patients with diabetic Charcot foot had developed ulcers in the foot during follow-up of around 1–14 months in his study.[23] Another study showed that the prevalence of prior or incident foot ulcer was 39.8% in Charcot foot patients.[14]

Infection of these ulcers is also common. As around 50% had developed infection of the ulcers.[24] Treatment of these included antibiotics as well as proper off-loading **(Figs. 4A and B)**. Surgical debridement may also be required in some cases to excise the necrotic components.

The next complication that happens is the requirement of amputation of the foot. This happens because of the lack of adherence to the treatment or because of delayed diagnosis. The rate of amputation in patients of Charcot is around 14.7%.[25]

Because of all these things, ultimately the patient has a decline in the overall quality of life, and surgical correction of the deformity has been shown to improve the overall quality of life.[26]

The ultimate effect of all these is that the mortality rate of patients with Charcot foot is increased. A study done in the UK had shown that there is a decrease of around 14.4 years of life in such patients compared to the normative data of the region.[27] In another study done in India, it was seen that people affected with Charcot neuroarthropathy had almost three times more risk of mortality as compared to age-matched population.[14]

CONCLUSION

Charcot neuroarthropathy of the foot is a disorder which has less awareness among the people as well as physicians. If not detected at an appropriate time then it can lead to severe complications, which can lead to increased morbidity as well as mortality. If not detected at the acute state, then it can progress to chronic deformity and decrease in the quality of life. Even at this state if the progress is not arrested then the person usually lands in the amputation of the foot. Thus, it is very crucial to have a very high index of suspicion of Charcot foot in diabetic patients with neuropathy having asymmetric foot swelling with signs of inflammation with or without deformity.

TAKE-HOME MESSAGES

- Charcot is a relatively uncommon complication of diabetes affecting foot.
- The diagnosis requires keen clinical examination and plain weight bearing radiograph.
- Total contact cast is the gold standard for treatment
- Follow-up requires infrared thermometry for charcot remission
- Missing the diagnosis of CN has devastating consequences in terms of limb amputation and mortality.

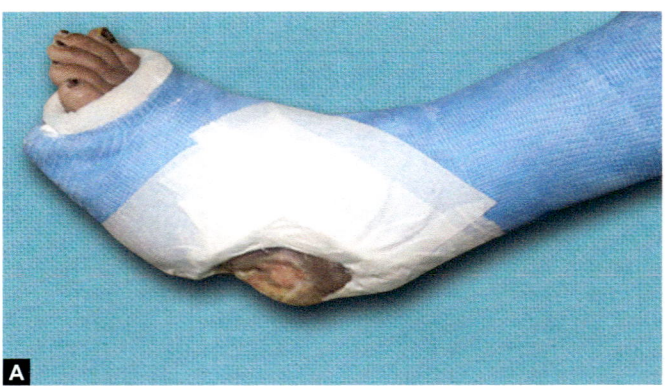
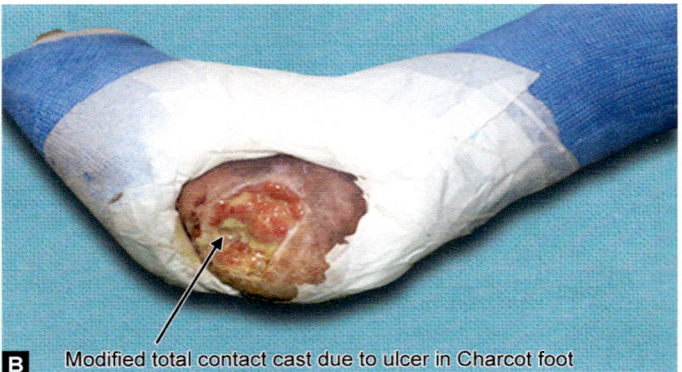

Figs. 4A and B: Ulcer development in Charcot foot.

REFERENCES

1. Yousaf S, Dawe EJC, Saleh A, Gill IR, Wee A. The acute Charcot foot in diabetics: Diagnosis and management. EFORT open Rev. 2018;3(10):568-73.
2. Rosskopf AB, Loupatatzis C, Pfirrmann CWA, Böni T, Berli MC. The Charcot foot: a pictorial review. Insights Imaging. 2019;10(1):77.
3. Armstrong DG, Lavery LA, Liswood PJ, Todd WF, Tredwell JA. Infrared dermal thermometry for the high-risk diabetic foot. Phys Ther. 1997;77(2):169-75.
4. Rajbhandari S, Jenkins R, Davies C, Tesfaye S. Charcot neuroarthropathy in diabetes mellitus. Diabetologia. 2002;45(8):1085-96.
5. Game FL, Catlow R, Jones GR, Edmonds ME, Jude EB, Rayman G, et al. Audit of acute Charcot's disease in the UK: The CDUK study. Diabetologia. 20128;55(1):32-5.
6. Rogers LC, Frykberg RG, Armstrong DG, Boulton AJ, Edmonds M, Van GH, et al. The Charcot foot in diabetes. Diabetes Care. 2011;34(9):2123-9.
7. Shapiro SA, Stansberry KB, Hill MA, Meyer MD, McNitt PM, Bhatt BA, et al. Normal blood flow response and vasomotion in the diabetic Charcot foot. J Diabetes Complications. 1998;12(3):147-53.
8. Jeffcoate WJ, Game F, Cavanagh PR. The role of proinflammatory cytokines in the cause of neuropathic osteoarthropathy (acute Charcot foot) in diabetes. Lancet. 2005;366(9502):2058-61.
9. Das L, Rastogi A, Jude EB, Prakash M, Dutta P, Bhansali A. Long-term foot outcomes following differential abatement of inflammation and osteoclastogenesis for active Charcot neuroarthropathy in diabetes mellitus. PLoS One. 2021;16(11):e0259224.
10. Larson SA, Burns PR. The pathogenesis of Charcot neuroarthropathy: current concepts. Diabet Foot Ankle. 2012;3.
11. Rosenbaum AJ, DiPreta JA. Classifications in brief: Eichenholtz classification of Charcot arthropathy. Clin Orthop Relat Res. 2015;473(3):1168-71.
12. Harris A, Violand M. Charcot Neuropathic Osteoarthropathy. Treasure Island (FL): StatPearls Publishing; 2023.
13. Chantelau EA, Grützner G. Is the Eichenholtz classification still valid for the diabetic Charcot foot? Swiss Med Wkly. 2014;144:w13948.
14. Chaudhary S, Bhansali A, Rastogi A. Mortality in Asian Indians with Charcot's neuroarthropathy: a nested cohort prospective study. Acta Diabetol. 2019;56(12):1259-64.
15. Griffiths DA, Kaminski MR. Duration of total contact casting for resolution of acute Charcot foot: a retrospective cohort study. J Foot Ankle Res. 2021;14(1):44.
16. Osterhoff G, Böni T, Berli M. Recurrence of acute Charcot neuropathic osteoarthropathy after conservative treatment. Foot Ankle Int. 2013;34(3):359-64.
17. Pinzur MS. An Evidence-Based Introduction to Charcot Foot Arthropathy. Foot and Ankle Orthop. 2018;3(3):247301141877426.
18. Busch-Westbroek TE, Delpeut K, Balm R, Bus SA, Schepers T, Peters EJ, et al. Effect of Single Dose of RANKL Antibody Treatment on Acute Charcot Neuro-osteoarthropathy of the Foot. Diabetes Care. 2018;41(3):e21-2.
19. Das L, Bhansali A, Prakash M, Jude EB, Rastogi A. Effect of Methylprednisolone or Zoledronic Acid on Resolution of Active Charcot Neuroarthropathy in Diabetes: A Randomized, Double-Blind, Placebo-Controlled Study. Diabetes Care. 2019;42(12):e185-6.
20. Richard JL, Almasri M, Schuldiner S. Treatment of acute Charcot foot with bisphosphonates: a systematic review of the literature. Diabetologia. 2012;55(5):1258-64.
21. Petrova NL, Donaldson NK, Bates M, Tang W, Jemmott T, Morris V, et al. Effect of Recombinant Human Parathyroid Hormone (1-84) on Resolution of Active Charcot Neuro-osteoarthropathy in Diabetes: A Randomized, Double-Blind, Placebo-Controlled Study. Diabetes Care. 2021;44(7):1613-21.
22. Rastogi A, Hajela A, Prakash M, Khandelwal N, Kumar R, Bhattacharya A, et al. Teriparatide (recombinant human parathyroid hormone [1-34]) increases foot bone remodeling in diabetic chronic Charcot neuroarthropathy: a randomized double-blind placebo-controlled study. J Diabetes. 2019;11(9):703-10.
23. Larsen K, Fabrin J, Holstein PE. Incidence and management of ulcers in diabetic Charcot feet. J Wound Care. 2001;10(8):323-8.
24. Edmonds M, Manu C, Vas P. The current burden of diabetic foot disease. J Clin Orthop Trauma. 2021;17:88-93.
25. Sohn MW, Stuck RM, Pinzur M, Lee TA, Budiman-Mak E. Lower-extremity amputation risk after Charcot arthropathy and diabetic foot ulcer. Diabetes Care. 2010;33(1):98-100.
26. Kroin E, Chaharbakhshi EO, Schiff A, Pinzur MS. Improvement in Quality of Life Following Operative Correction of Midtarsal Charcot Foot Deformity. Foot Ankle Int. 2018;39(7):808-11.
27. Van Baal J, Hubbard R, Game F, Jeffcoate W. Mortality associated with acute Charcot foot and neuropathic foot ulceration. Diabetes Care. 2010;33(5):1086-9.

13 CHAPTER

Infected Diabetic Foot Ulcer: Case Scenario and Management Considerations

Manisha Singh Jadaun

CASE 1

Case Presentation
A 70-year-old male presented with type 2 diabetes mellitus, hypertension (HTN), and chronic kidney disease (CKD). Duration of diabetes was 28 years. He was regularly on antihypertensives and oral hypoglycemic agents with uncontrolled diabetes mellitus. He had no previous history of foot problems and foot examination. He accidently collided with dining table and had blunt injury to left great toe 20 days back. Gradually, he developed swelling, occasional fever with chills followed by recent duskiness of toe when he reported to us.

Past Medical and Family History
Diabetes mellitus since 28 years, HTN 20 years, CKD 6 years

Family history: None

Initial Assessment/Physical Examination
He was 178 cm tall and 67 kg by weight. On local examination, there was nonhealing ulcer with surrounding scab and duskiness of right great toe with tenderness. Dorsalis pulse, anterior tibial, posterior tibial, and popliteal and femoral pulses were palpable on right side. Ankle–brachial index (ABI) was 1.27 on the right and 1.36 on the left; 10-g monofilament test was positive on the both sides. Vibration perception threshold (VPT) was 23.7 volt on the right and 26.4 on the left side. Tip therm test on both sides was nonresponsive.

Right great toe nail was dusky with scabs on ulcer and duskiness overlying terminal phalanx of great toe; swelling of great toe was present, no active signs of inflammation, wet gangrene on plantar aspect of great toe was present with foul smell and fluctuations.

Laboratory Investigations
- Glycated hemoglobin (HbA1c) was 8%, blood urea 68 mg/dL, serum creatinine 1.2 mg/dL
- Total leukocyte count (TLC) 15,400, plasma (P) 71%, leukocytes (L) 24%, erythrocytes (E) 2%, monocytes (M) 2%, and random blood sugar (RBS) 289 mg%

Management
The debridement was done under the local great toe block anesthesia, followed by systemic antibiotics and local dressings. However, entire soft tissue envelope was destroyed due to infection, and partial toe amputation was done. Around 10 days later another drainage debridement was done for fluctuant swelling on medial plantar aspect of the toe; after 3 weeks patient again developed swelling of foot and ankle with an infected wound around lateral aspect of

ankle along with loss of appetite and fever with chills. Within 2 days swelling spread to leg with induration and warmth ascending up to the upper part of leg and lower thigh. Emergent exploration of right leg, ankle, and lower thigh was carried out. Large amount of pus was drained, fasciotomy with fasciectomy done, and muscles were healthy. Patient stood well after surgery. Two days after surgery patient had a severe life-threatening cardiac event and he expired.

Wound Images

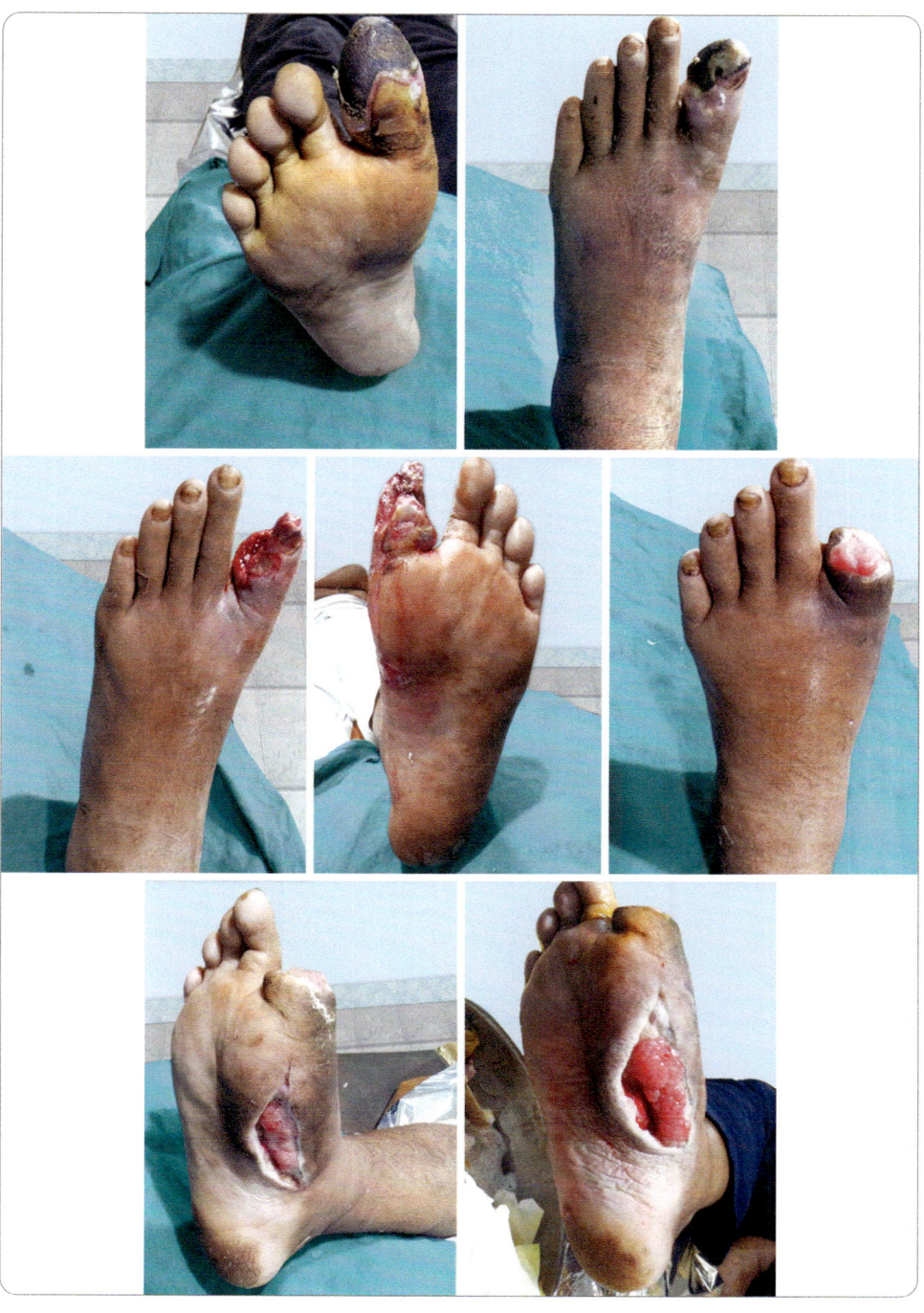

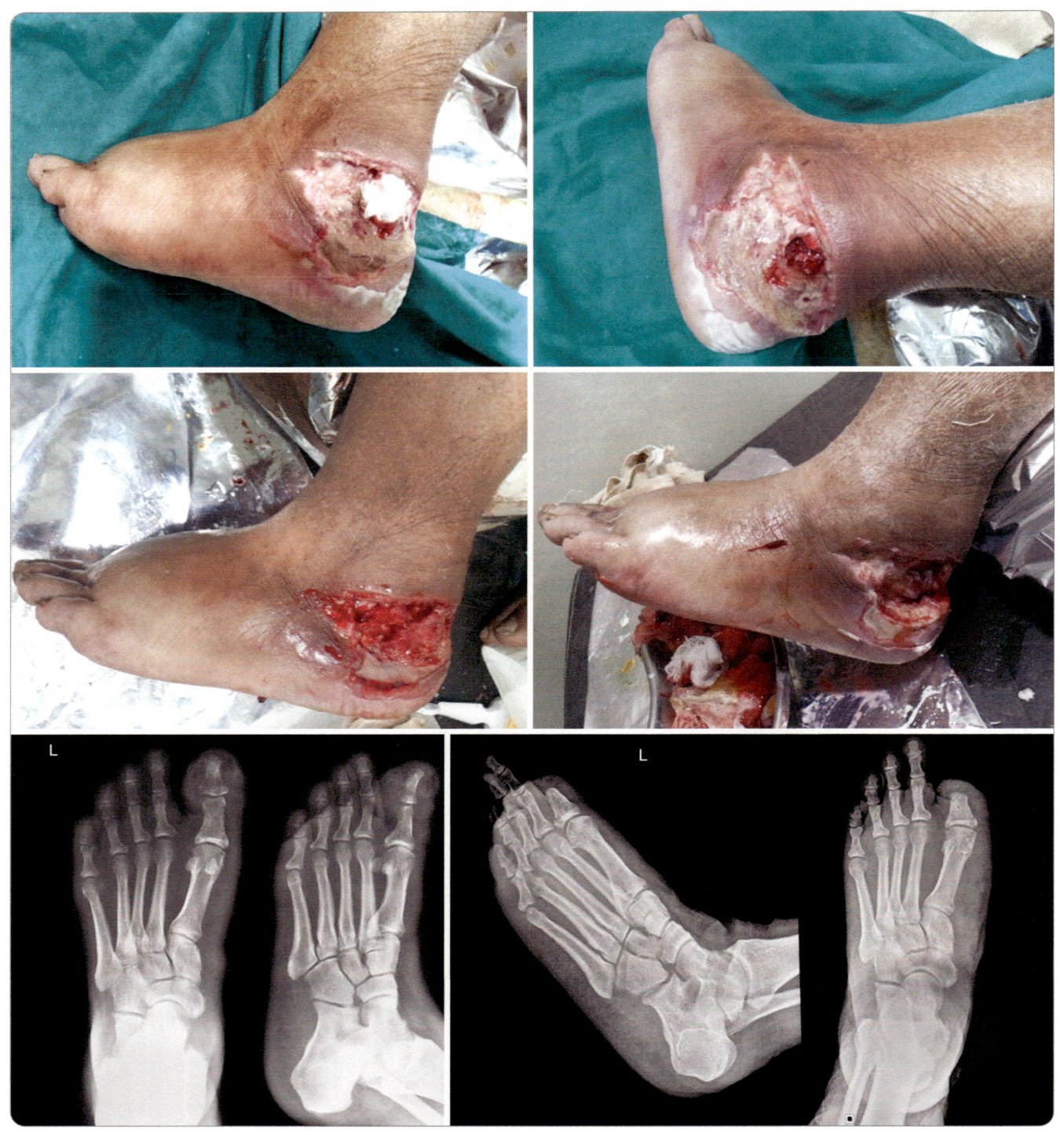

Infected Diabetic Foot Ulcer: Case Scenario and Management Considerations

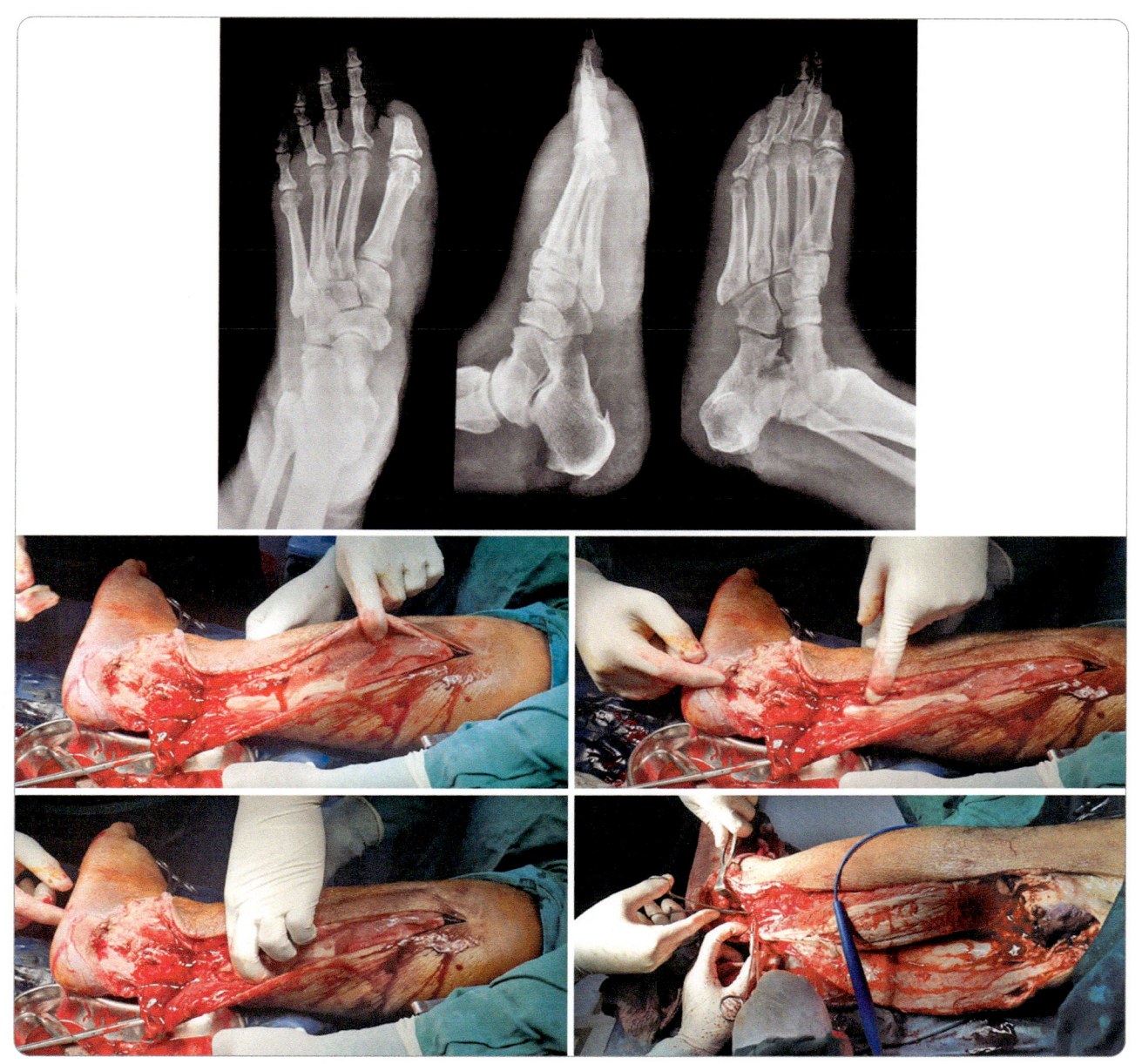

CASE 2

Case Presentation

A 57-year-old male presented with type 2 diabetes mellitus. Duration of diabetes was 12 years and was on oral hypoglycemic agents for last 5–6 years irregularly with uncontrolled diabetes mellitus. He gives history of surgical intervention elsewhere around 3 or 4 weeks back following a weeklong sudden-onset swelling of right foot with prior nonhealing trophic ulcer on the plantar aspect of forefoot for almost 6 months. Wound care and medical management was poor for last 6 months. After surgery he developed infective gangrene of toes gradually with foul smell when he reported to foot specialist. A fresh X-ray was taken and his color arterial Doppler study reported normal vascularity.

Past Medical and Family History

Diabetes mellitus for last 12 years after which he tried some alternative medicines but poor diet control. Being a farmer, he preferred walking bare foot. He sustained injury by stone in right foot. There was an ulcer in forefoot, which gradually increased in last 6 months. He dressed his wound himself.

Family history: None

Personal history: He consumed alcohol occasionally but was a chronic *bidi* smoker (approximately 10 per day) for last 20 years.

Initial Assessment/Physical Examination

He was 164 cm tall and 69.5 kg by weight. On examination, right foot had infected fossa of recently amputated fifth toe, partial gangrene of third and fourth toes, large, debrided wound on plantar aspect of forefoot, swelling on dorsum, and foul smell from wound. All pedal pulses were palpable in right foot. ABI was 1.3 on the right and 1.2 on the left. Monofilament test was positive in both the feet. Biothesiometry was not possible due to large forefoot and plantar wound.

Laboratory Investigations

- HbA1c 8.9%, TLC 19,400, P 76%, L 20, E 3%, and M 01%. Blood urea 48 mg/dL, serum creatinine 1.9 mg/L, and serum bilirubin 1.1
- Color arterial Doppler study of both lower limbs—normal study

Pre- and Post-treatment Images

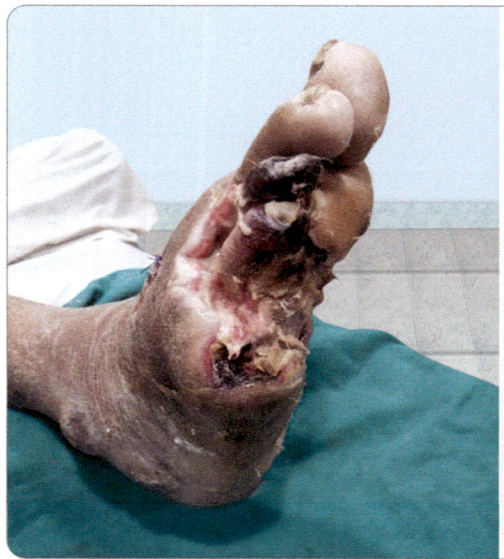
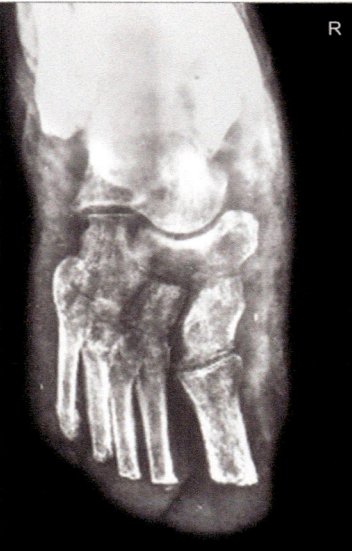
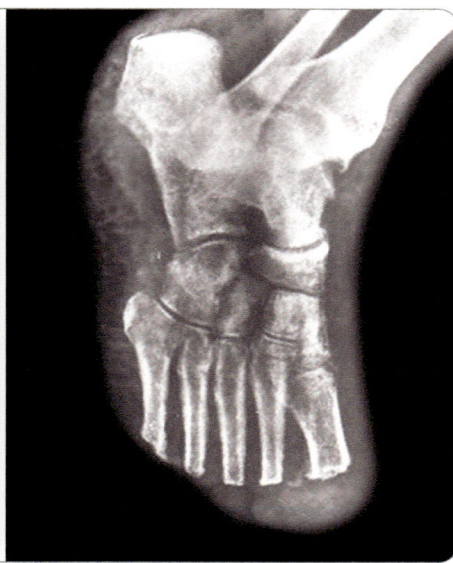

Infected Diabetic Foot Ulcer: Case Scenario and Management Considerations

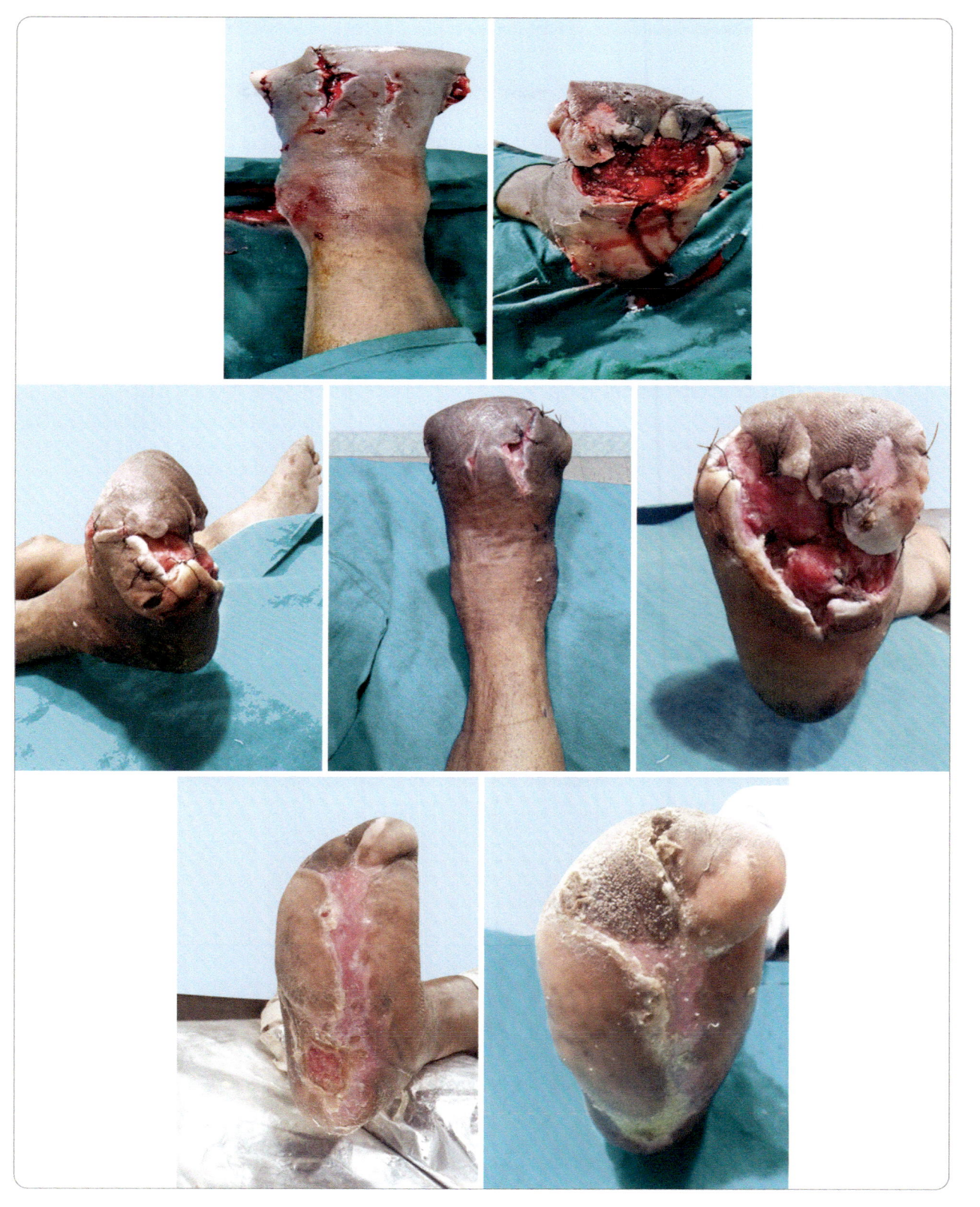

CASE 3

Case Presentation

A 56-year-old female having type 2 diabetes mellitus, coronary artery disease (CAD), HTN, and cerebrovascular accident (CVA) episode with left-sided resolving weakness. Duration of diabetes was 22 years and she was on antihypertensives, insulin, oral hypoglycemic agents with uncontrolled diabetes mellitus. She had valgus deformity of foot with shortening and postaccident orthopedic surgery at the age of 28 years. She gives history of recurrent nonhealing trophic ulcer on the plantar aspect of left forefoot. She only ties a thick padded cloth underneath after wound toilet and does not use any special footwear. Currently reported with foul smell and increasing size of ulcer because of which she is unable to walk.

Past Medical and Family History

Diabetes mellitus since 22 years, HTN 20 years, CAD 8 years, CVA 6 years back, now recovered.

Family history: None

Initial Assessment/Physical Examination

Height is 150 cm tall and weight 77 kg. On examinations, there was nonhealing ulcer at the medial malleolus of the right foot. All pulses were palpable. ABI was 1.1 on the right and 1.16 on the left; 10-g monofilament test was positive on the right side and was negative on the left side. VPT was 12.7 volt on the right and 10.4 on the left side.

Laboratory Investigations

HbA1c 9.9%, TLC 12,400, blood urea 31 mg/dL, and serum creatinine 1 mg/dL

Management

Minor debridement was done followed by systemic oral antibiotics and dressings.

Wound Images

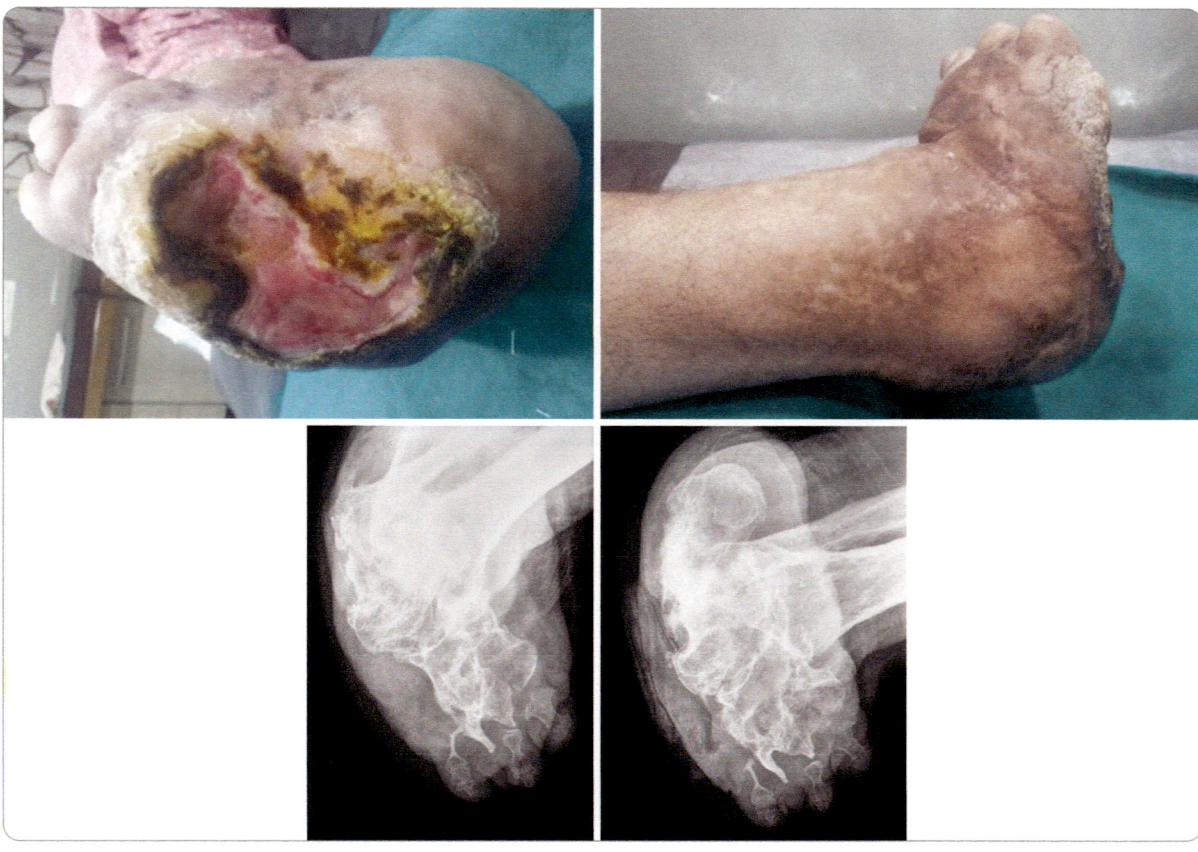

Infected Diabetic Foot Ulcer: Case Scenario and Management Considerations | 97

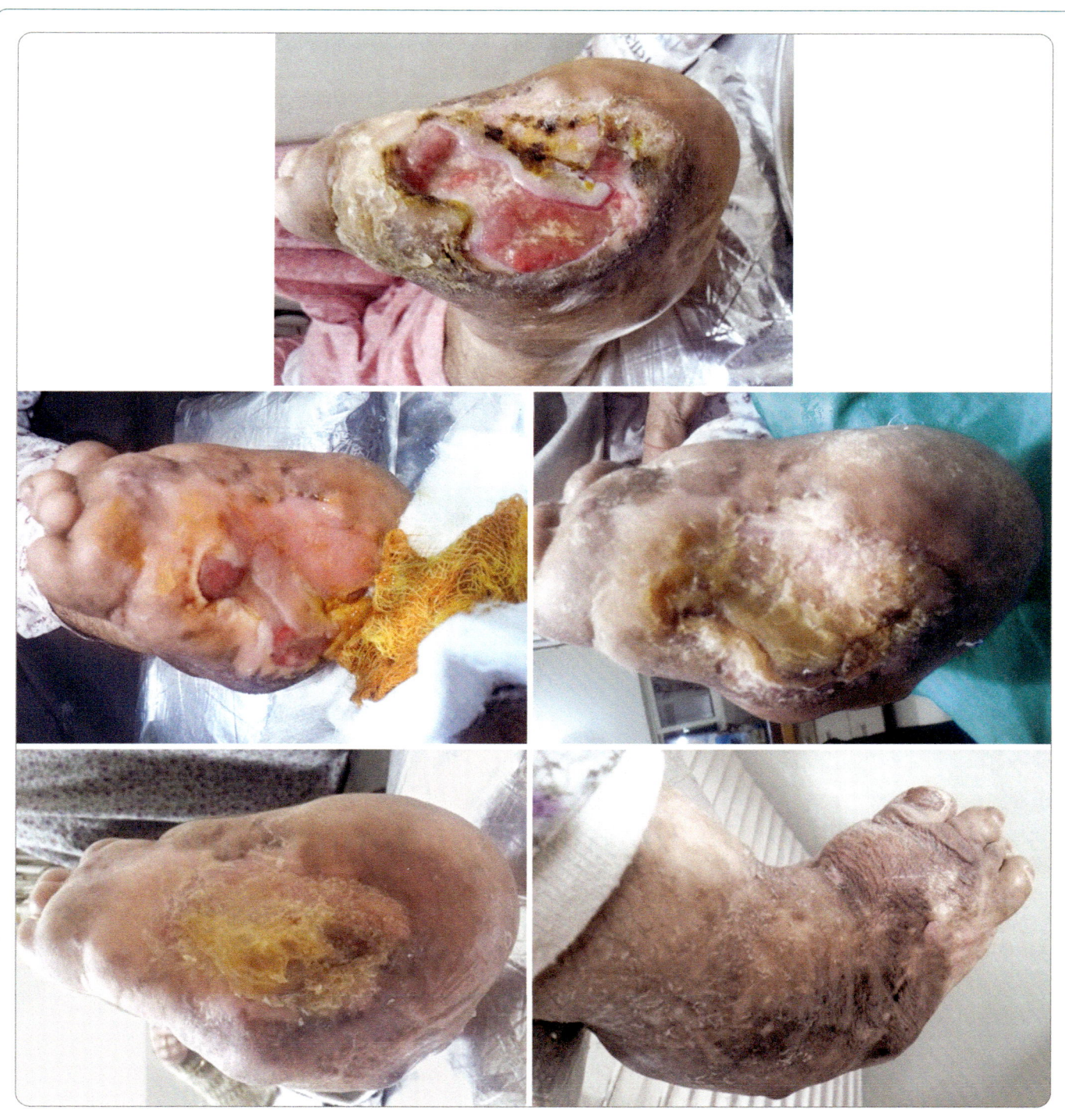

Infected Diabetic Foot Ulcer: Case Scenario and Management Considerations

CASE 4

Case Presentation
A 65-year-old male, a known case of type 2 diabetes mellitus, gave history of spontaneous swelling in left great toe for one and half months. For last 1 week, increase in swelling noted and pus was discharging from multiple points on plantar and lateral aspect of great toe. He was also not advised offloading antibiotics randomly with home dressings. He took alternative therapies also to control blood sugar apart from insulin. His diet control was poor and also skipped insulin.

Past Medical and Family History
A 65-year-old male, a known case of type 2 diabetes mellitus 15 years, HTN 18 years, diabetic polyneuropathy (DPN) 5 years.

Initial Assessment/Physical Examination
The patient's foot were well perfused. Probe-to-bone test was positive, and through and through wound on plantar aspect of toe to dorsum of toe. Multiple pus was discharging from sinuses; all intercommunicating seen on lateral and plantar aspect of great toe. A fluctuant inflammatory swelling with erythema and warmth was seen on plantar aspect of first metatarsal (MT). Entire right foot appeared swollen. ABI showed right side 1.2 and left side 1.3. VPT was recorded by biothesiometry—right and left side >25 volts. Monofilament test was positive in both feet.

Laboratory Investigations
HbA1c 8.7%, TLC 13,800, P 68%, L 28%, E 2%, basophils (B) 2%, blood urea 46 mg/dL, and serum creatinine 1.2 mg/dL

Management
On contrast MRI scan of foot, septic arthritis of great toe with interphalangeal (IP) and metatarsophalangeal (MTP) joints was found along with osteomyelitis of great toe.

On exploration of foot under popliteal block anesthesia, right great toe disarticulation with first MT of head resection with sesamoidectomy and drainage of pus with minor debridement necrosectomy was done on plantar aspect of first MT of head. Dorsal skin of great toe was rotated to cover the great toe stump, which was excised after it became dusky. The wound healed by secondary intention over a period of 45 days. In sandal offloading was done with samadhan technique.

Wound Images

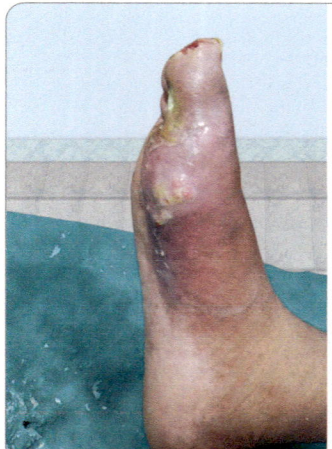 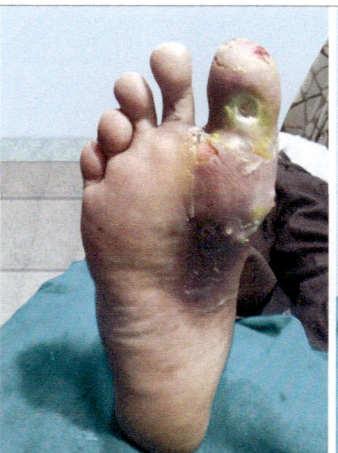 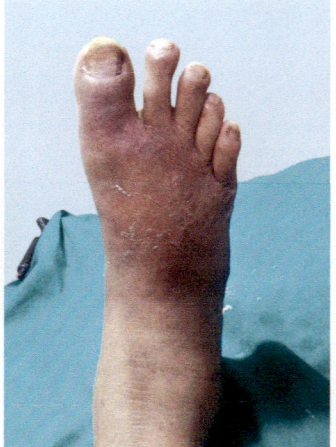 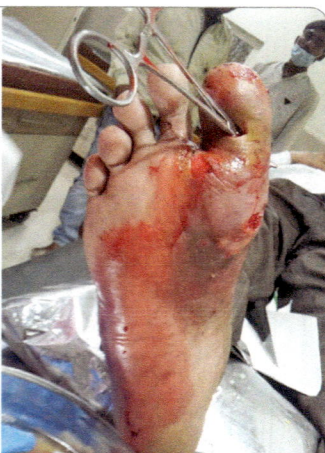

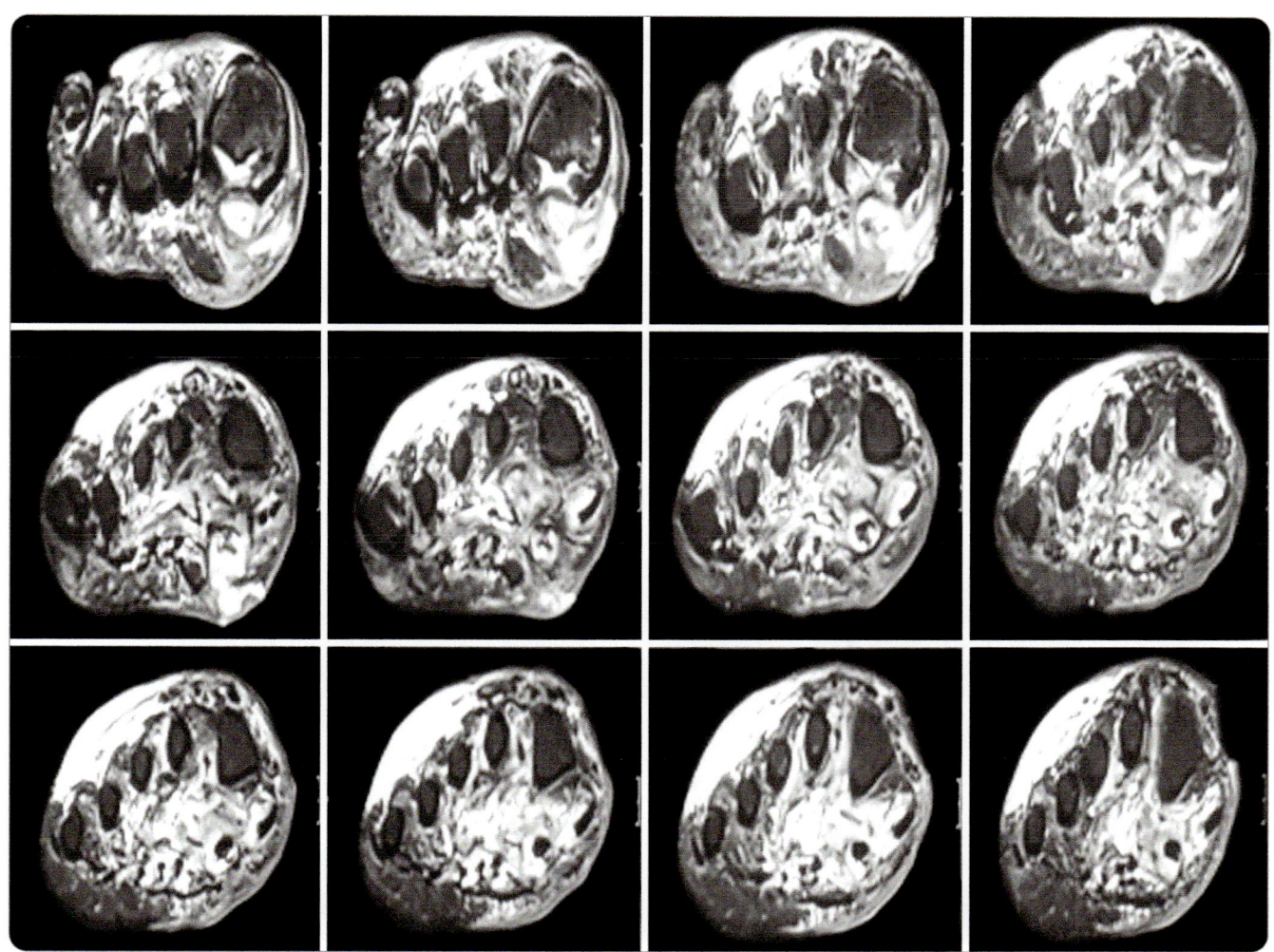

Opinion

Reduced inter phalangeal joint space of great toe with articular surface irregularity/erosion, small interphalangeal joint effusion and abnormal edema signal in the form of T2W and STIR hyperintensity and T1W hypointensity in great toe phalanges – Osteomyelitis with great toe interphalangeal joint septic arthritis.

Abnormal predominantly organized collection/abscess of volume approximately 8 cc along plantar aspect of great toe phalanges and contiguous involvement of flexor hallucis longus tendon associated with extension of edema signals in deep foot adipose tissue.

Collection/abscess has contiguous extension upto plantar surface by few superficial erosions/discharging sinuses.

CHAPTER 13
100 Infected Diabetic Foot Ulcer: Case Scenario and Management Considerations

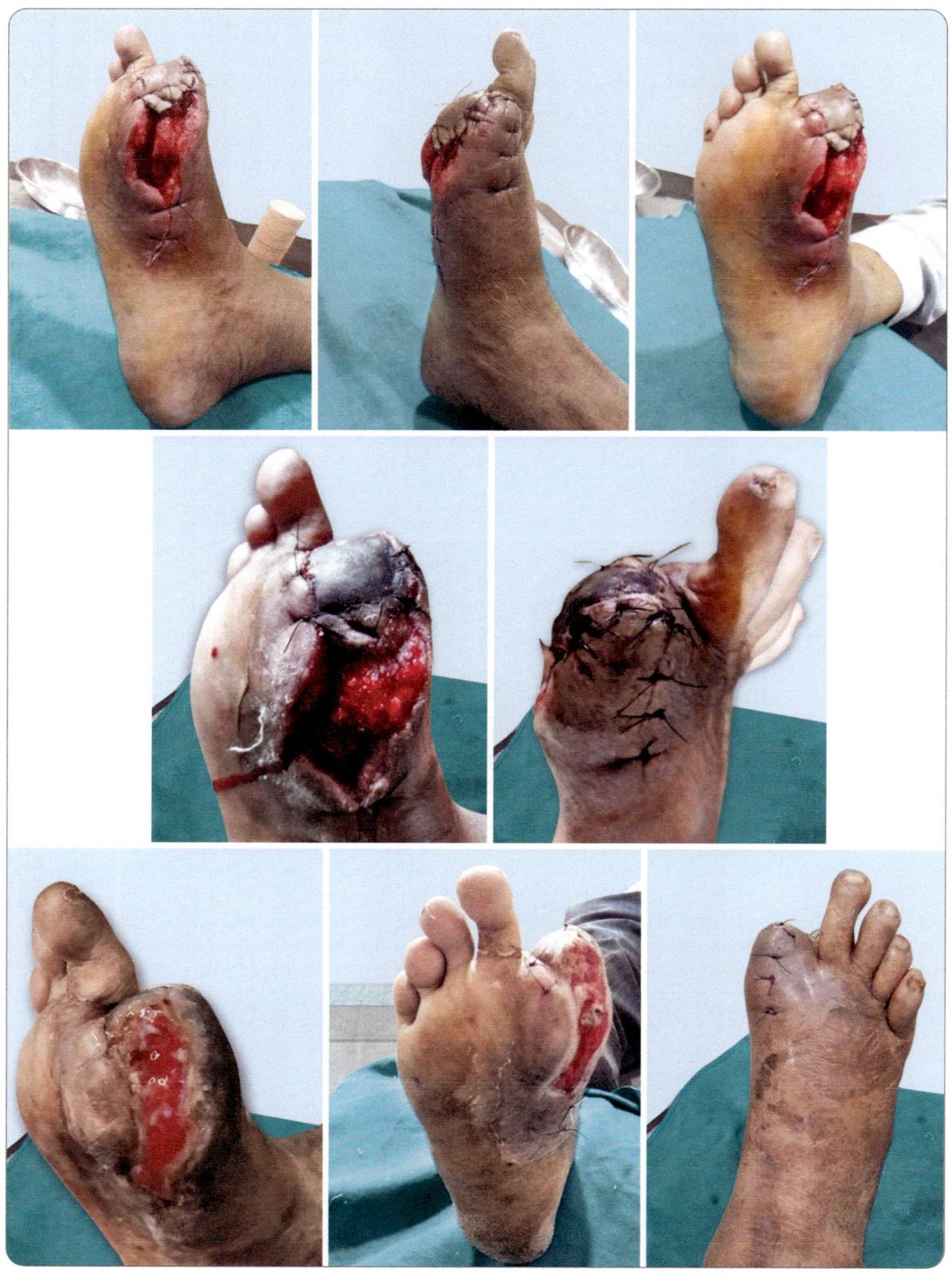

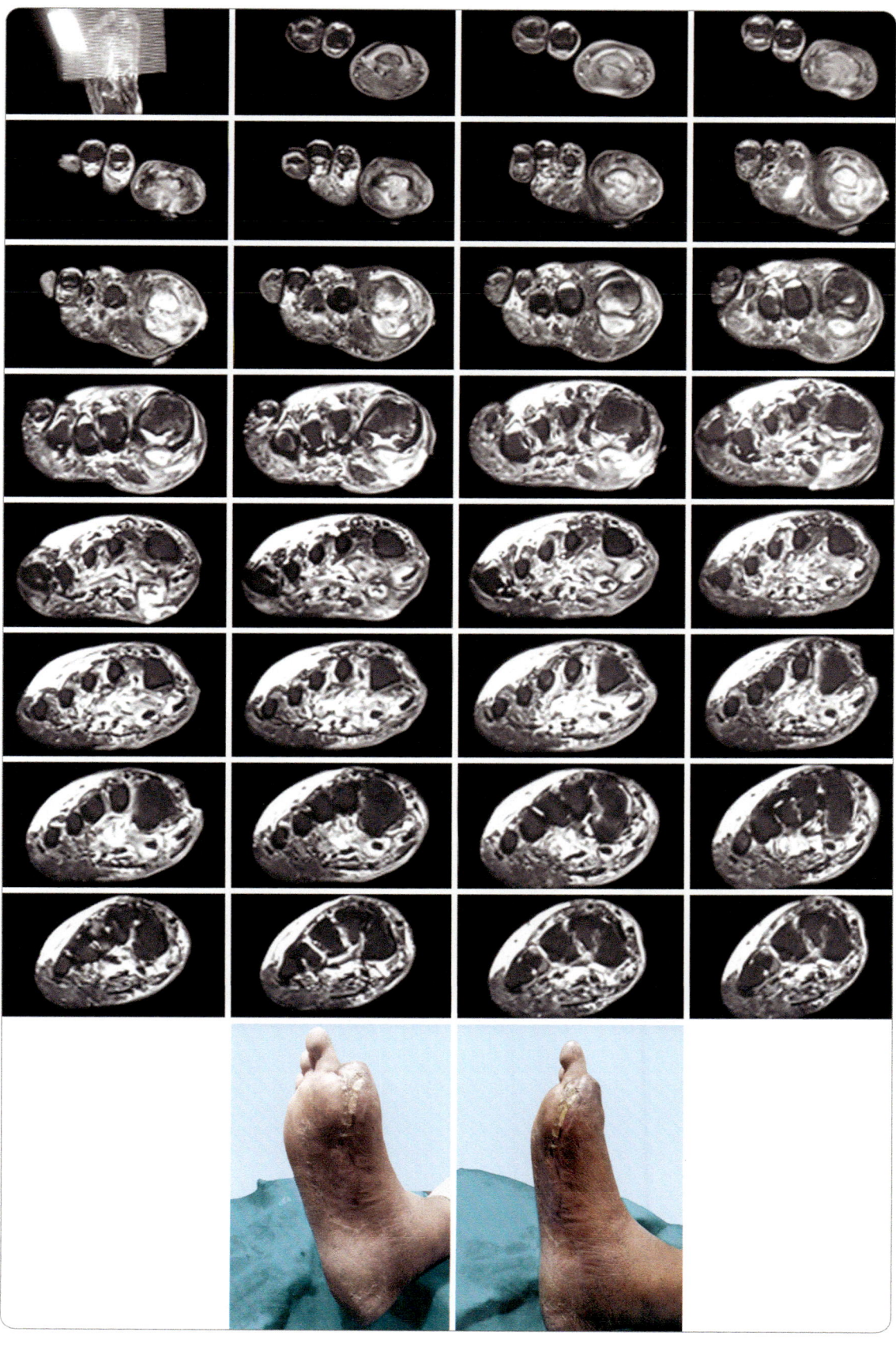

CASE 5

Case Presentation
A 56-year-old female presented with type 2 diabetes mellitus, CAD, HTN, and CVA episode with left-sided resolving weakness. Duration of diabetes was 22 years and she was on antihypertensives, insulin, and oral hypoglycemic agents with uncontrolled diabetes mellitus. She had valgus deformity of foot with shortening and postaccident orthopedic surgery at the age of 28 years. She gives history of recurrent nonhealing trophic ulcer on the plantar aspect of left forefoot. She only ties a thick padded cloth underneath after wound toilet and does not use any special footwear. Currently reported with foul smell and increasing size of ulcer because of which she is unable to walk.

Past Medical and Family History
Diabetes mellitus since 22 years, HTN 20 years, CAD 8 years, CVA 6 years back, now recovered.

Family history: None

Initial Assessment/Physical Examination
Height is 168 cm tall and weight 61 kg. On examination, there was fluctuant swelling with inflammatory erythema, local warmth on dorsum of left foot with thick foul smelling pus discharge and duskiness of second toe. Pedal pulses were well palpable. ABI was 1.1 on the right 1.26 on the left; 10-g monofilament test was positive on both sides. VPT was 18 volt on the right and 16.4 volt on the left side.

Laboratory Investigations
- HbA1c 8.1%, TLC 17,200, P 82%, L 15%, E1%, and M 2%
- Blood urea 58 mg/dL and serum creatinine 1.3 mg/dL

Management
Debridement was done on dorsum of toe under the local ankle block anesthesia with disarticulation of second toe followed by systemic antibiotics and wound dressings. Wound healed in approximately 17 weeks.

Wound Images

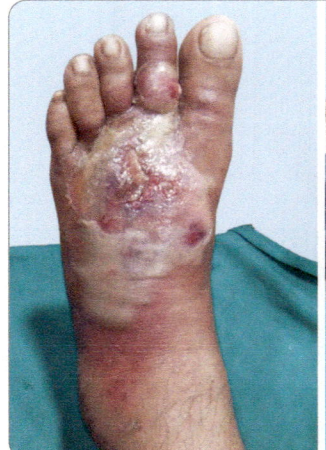 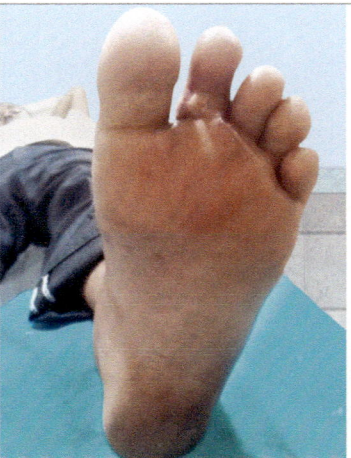 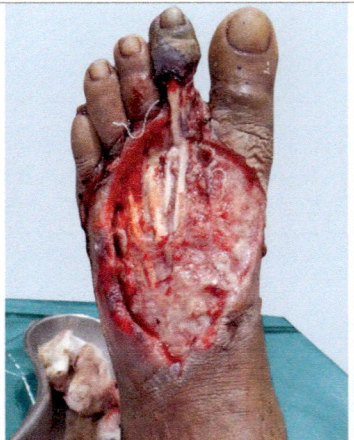 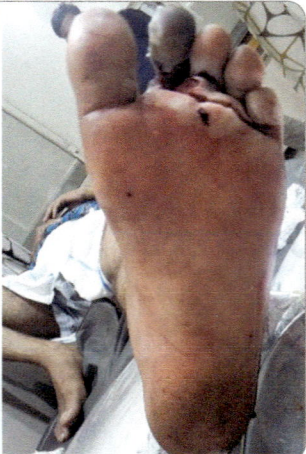

Infected Diabetic Foot Ulcer: Case Scenario and Management Considerations

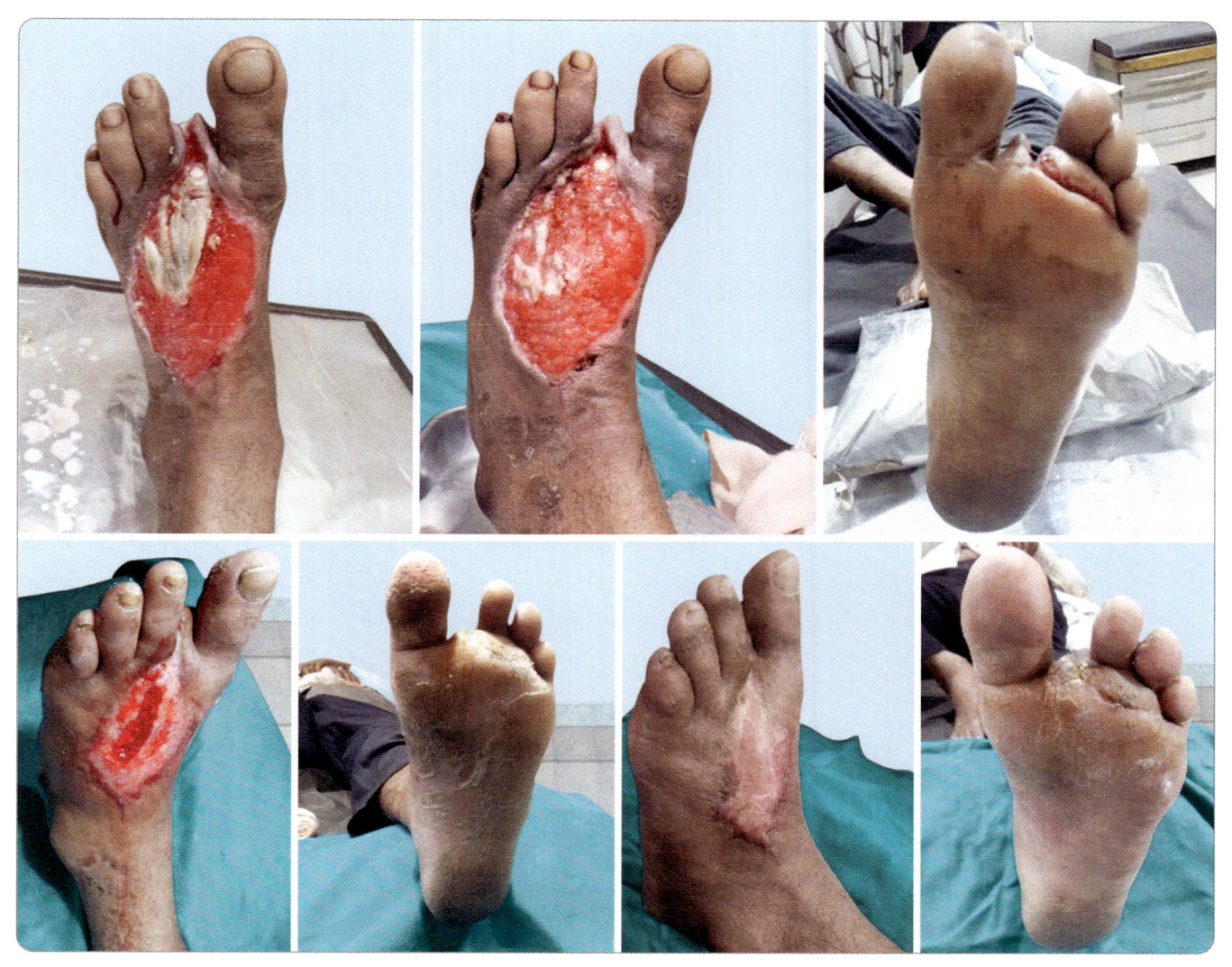

CASE 6

Case Presentation
A 49-year-old female having type 2 diabetes mellitus, HTN, and hypothyroidism sustained scald injury with hot water spillage on feet on same day of visit. The blisters formed consequent to dermoepidermal burn on dorsum of foot were deroofed and dressings were done.

Past Medical and Family History
Diabetes mellitus and HTN for last 6 years, hypothyroidism for 12 years.

Family history: Mother and father both have type 2 diabetes mellitus.

Infected Diabetic Foot Ulcer: Case Scenario and Management Considerations

Initial Assessment/Physical Examination

He was 160 cm tall with 70 kg weight. On examinations, there were blisters on dorsum of foot with erythema around the blisters. Pedal pulses were palpable. ABI was 1.0 on the right and 1.1 on the left; 10-g monofilament test was positive bilaterally. VPT was 22 volt on the right and 24 on the left side.

Laboratory Investigations—Tests and Reports (If, Any)

HbA1c 8.9%, TLC 19,400, P 59%, L 29, E 5%, M 3%, B 2%, blood urea 26 mg/dL, and serum creatinine 0.9 mg/dL

Management

The blisters were deroofed and dressings were done.

Wound Images

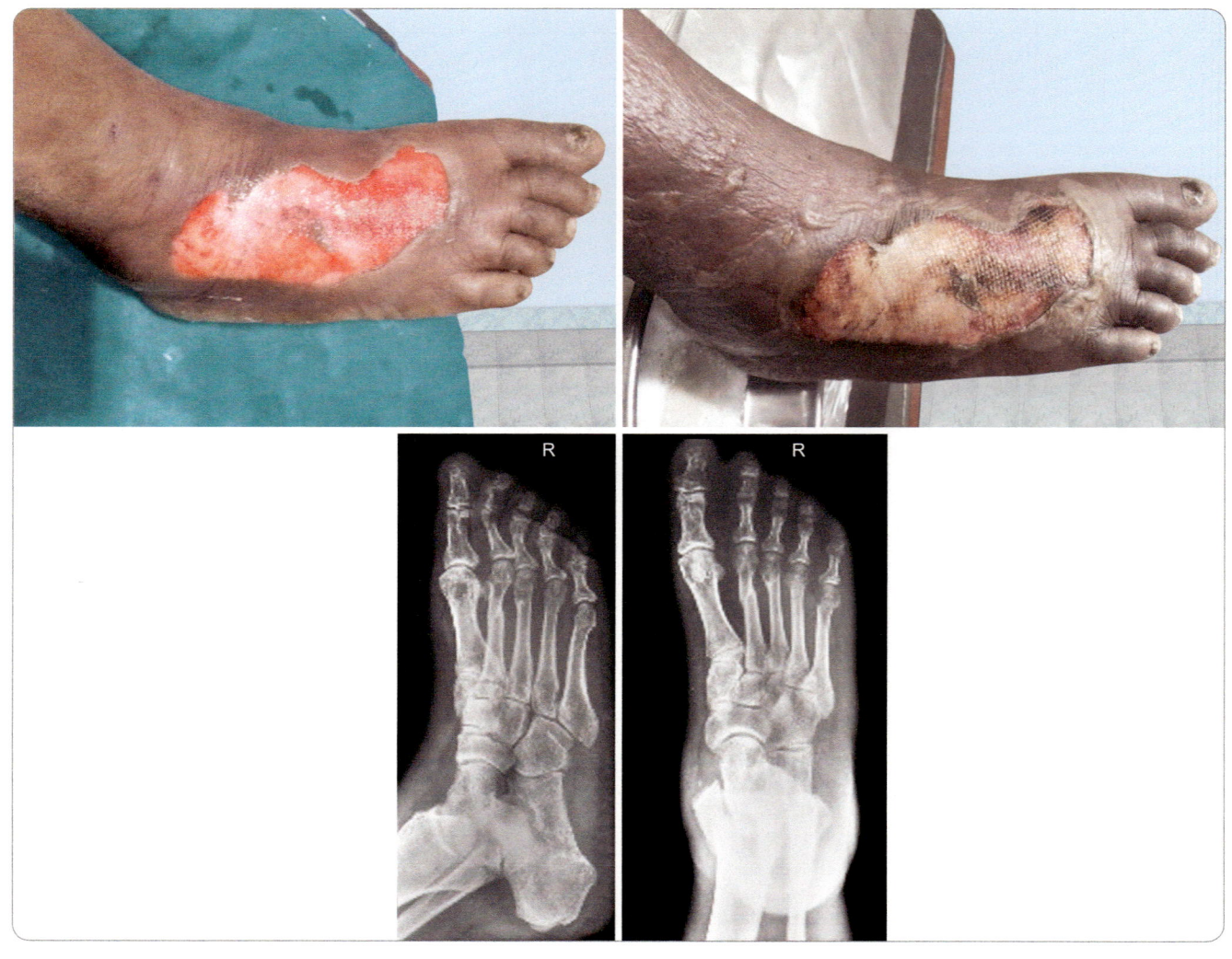

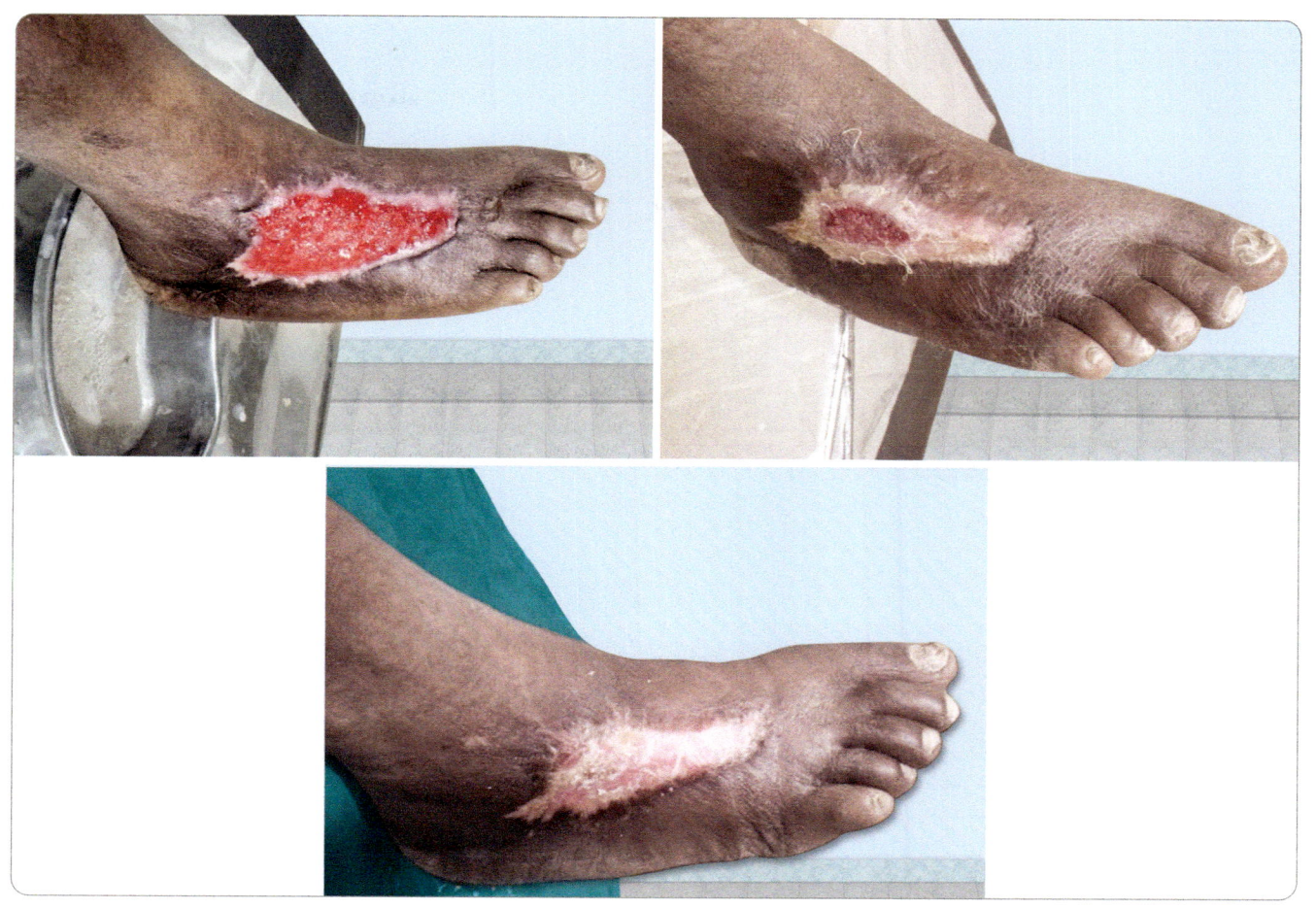

Case Discussion

The diabetic ulcers are very sensitive to heal; it requires adequate assessment in terms of the vascularity of lower limb, neuropathy and blood sugar control, and sign of infections.

Adequate blood sugar control, with treatment of infection and improve vascularity, is the key of management. The topical antibiotics have a role only after removal of biofilm either by mechanically or chemically. The Cadexomer has special property to release the iodine slowly and remove the biofilm. Therefore, it helps in healing faster in diabetic ulcers.

TAKE-HOME MESSAGES

- Diabetic foot infection lead to limb amputation and mortality
- Early surgical debridement of infected ulcer is key to prevent amputation
- Surgical debridement also removes biofilm and aids in wound healing

CHAPTER 14

Imaging of Diabetic Foot

Ragghuraman Soundararajan, Ashu Rastogi

INTRODUCTION

Diabetes mellitus is a major health problem worldwide with growing incidence rates and a projected global prevalence of 7.1% in 2030. Diabetes affects multiple organ systems, thus leading to end organ damage. One dysfunction is diabetic foot and its complications, which poses significant morbidity and mortality. Ischemia, neuropathy, and infection are the three main pathophysiological processes complicating diabetic foot. Complications of diabetic foot comprise a spectrum of involvement of various bones, joints, muscles, tendons, and other soft tissue structures.[1]

Infection of the bones and soft tissues is common with diabetic foot and early diagnosis is crucial in timely medical/surgical management to reduce morbidity and mortality. Diabetic foot infections are almost always due to the direct spread of infection from an overlying ulcer due to microangiopathy/neuropathy/altered biomechanics. Unrecognized trauma in this background leads to superimposed infections. Hematogenous spread of infection is rare and is seen predominantly in children.

Chronic unrecognized trauma to the foot in the background of angiopathy and neuropathy results in neuroarthropathy, leading to damage of joint and subsequent deformation of foot. Acute and chronic forms of neuroarthropathy have been recognized. Osteomyelitis and neuroarthropathy often coexist and at times it is difficult to differentiate between these two entities clinically and radiologically.

IMAGING MODALITIES IN DIABETIC FOOT[2]

Plain radiography is the initial modality of choice as it is easily available, less expensive, and provides excellent details of the bony changes. However, in a subset of cases, viz. early osteomyelitis, plain radiographs may be normal as they do not show the soft tissue abnormalities adequately. If soft tissue gas is detected, the adjacent joint must be included to assess its extent **(Figs. 1 to 4)**.

Ultrasonography, despite being easily available and noninvasive, its role in the diagnosis of diabetic foot complications is limited. It is useful for the diagnosis of infective/inflammatory changes in the soft tissues, for the localization of foreign bodies, diagnosis of synovitis/tenosynovitis, diagnosis, and localization of fluid collections. It also aids in image-guided aspirations of fluid collections/cystic lesions. However, bony changes are not depicted by ultrasonography.

Computed tomography (CT) though has a limited role, scores over plain radiography due to its three-dimensional capability and good soft tissue resolution. It helps in better detection of bony erosions, small sequestra, gas within soft tissue, calcification, and foreign bodies. However, demarcation between infected and healthy tissues is not well depicted in CT, due to beam hardening artifacts from the closely placed bones with added risk of ionizing radiation.

Magnetic resonance imaging (MRI) is the modality of choice for the assessment of soft tissue and bone marrow involvement due to its high sensitivity and specificity. High soft tissue contrast and multiplanar imaging help in demarcation between the normal and abnormal regions, thus aiding accurate presurgical planning. Hence, radiograph combined with MRI helps in the accurate assessment of osteomyelitis and differentiation from neuroarthropathy. MRI also helps in differentiation of septic arthritis from sterile joint effusions **(Figs. 5A to D)**.

Nuclear scans such as triple-phase bone scan using technetium-99m phosphonates, inflammation scintigraphy, and bone marrow scintigraphy are used for diagnosis of

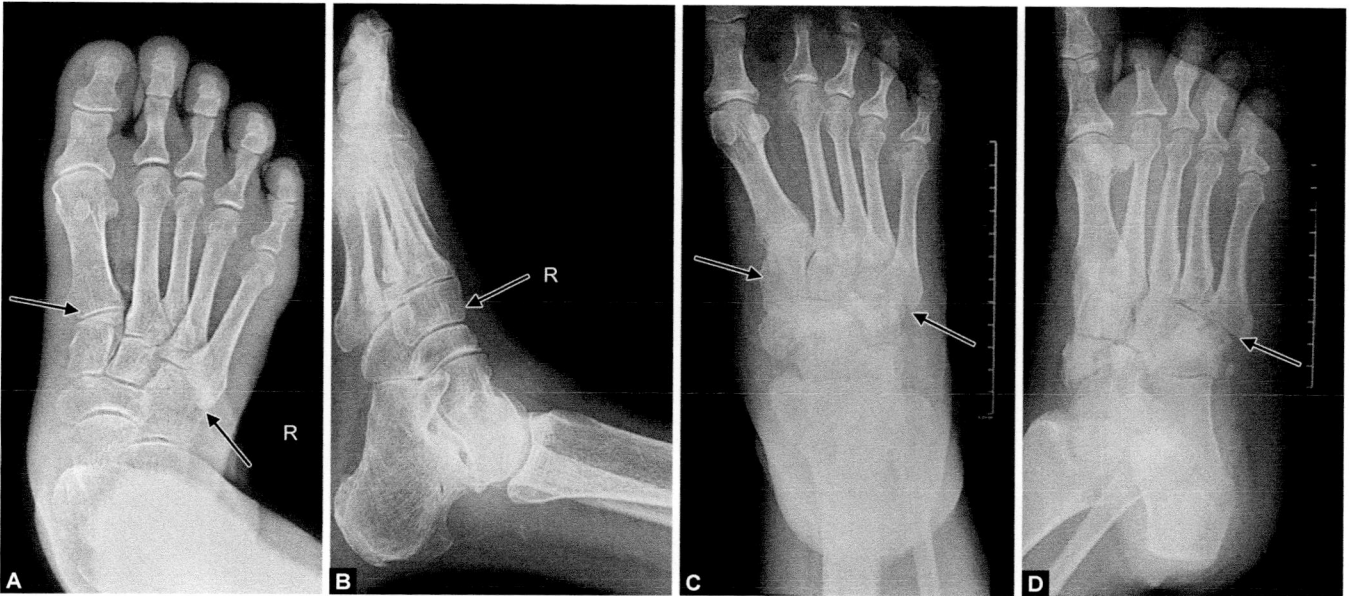

Figs. 1A to D: (A and B) Anteroposterior (AP) and lateral radiographs of foot in a diabetic patient with asymmetrical swelling of foot showing periarticular osteopenia predominantly in the midfoot. No bony fragmentation/dislocations are seen. (C and D) AP and lateral radiographs of foot in another patient showing periarticular osteopenia in midfoot with no bony fragmentation/dislocation. Features are likely to suggest subacute neuroarthropathy.

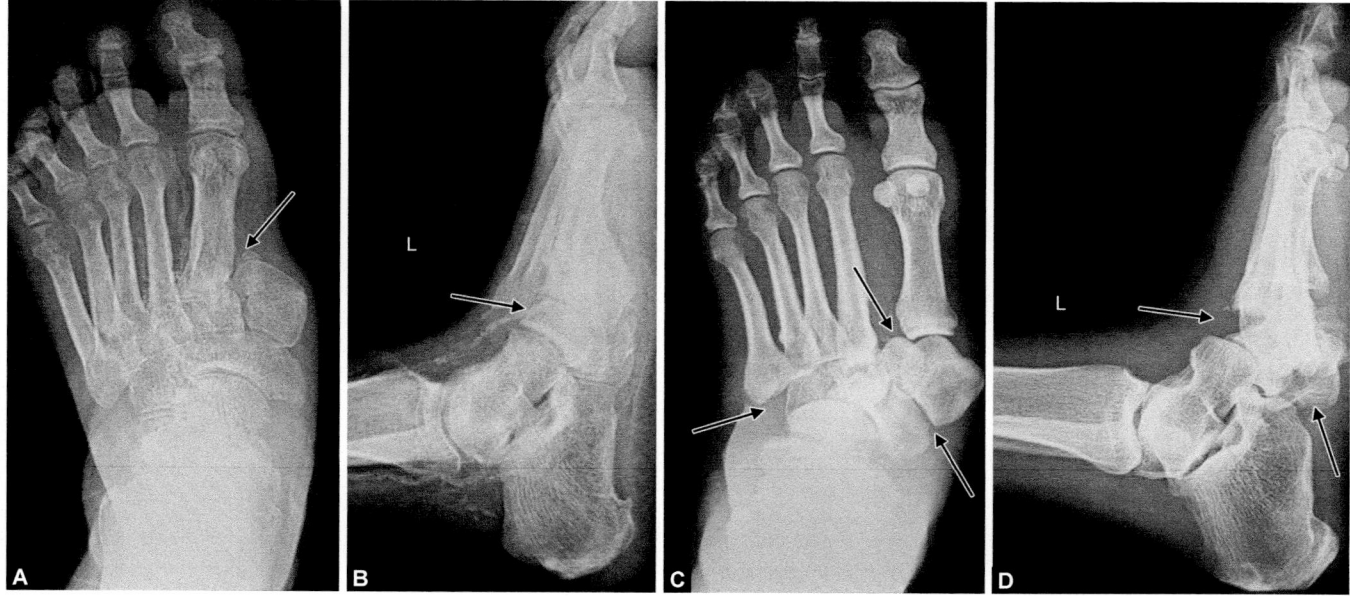

Figs. 2A to D: Anteroposterior (AP) and lateral radiographs of two different patients (A, B and C, D) with asymmetrical swelling of foot showing multiple intertarsal and tarsometatarsal dislocation and subluxation with loss of longitudinal arches of the foot. Features are suggestive of chronic neuroarthropathy.

diabetic foot complications. Triple-phase bone scan has shown to have high sensitivity and specificity to diagnose osteomyelitis in the absence of neuroarthropathy, surgery, or trauma in which specificity is significantly reduced. Inflammation scintigraphy carries high sensitivity and specificity for the detection of pedal osteomyelitis.

Positron emission tomography (PET)/CT with ^{18}F-fluorodeoxyglucose (^{18}FDG) is a highly sensitive and specific investigation for the diagnosis of osteomyelitis as well as neuroarthropathy with better anatomical localization. PET/CT is a good alternative for patients with metallic implants when MRI cannot be performed **(Figs. 6 to 10)**.

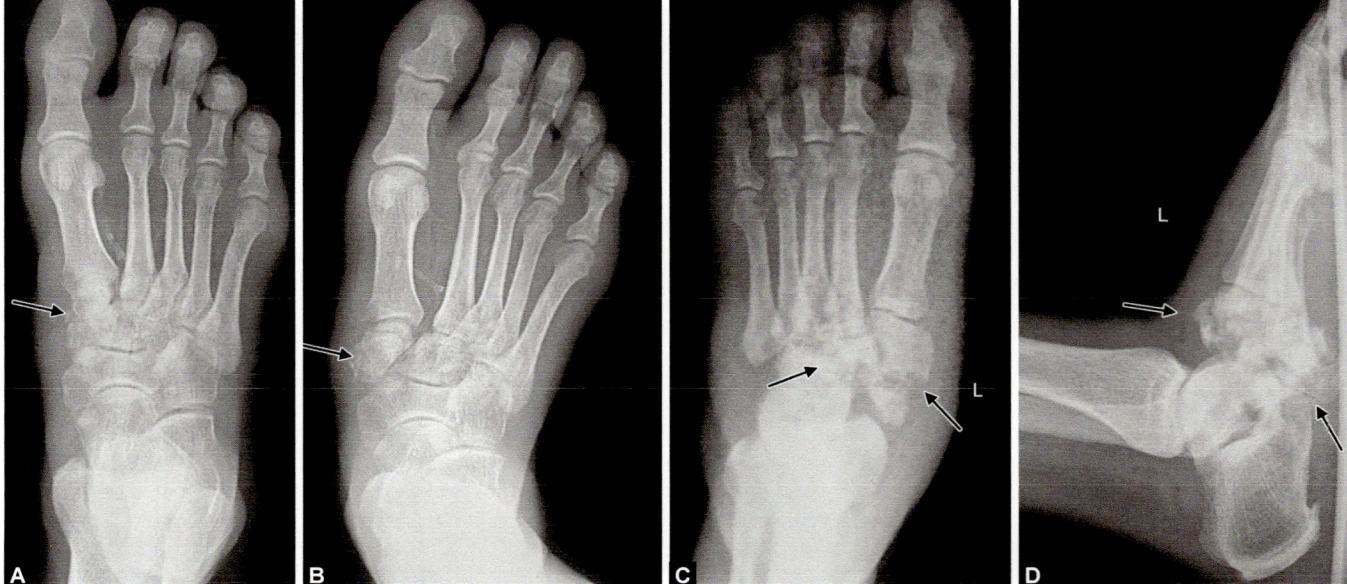

Figs. 3A to D: (A and B) Anteroposterior (AP) and oblique radiographs of a diabetic patient with midfoot swelling showing fragmentation of the medial cuneiform with periarticular osteopenia in midfoot. (C and D) AP and lateral radiographs of another patient showing fragmentation of cuneiforms with intertarsal and tarsometatarsal subluxations. Features are suggestive of chronic neuroarthropathy.

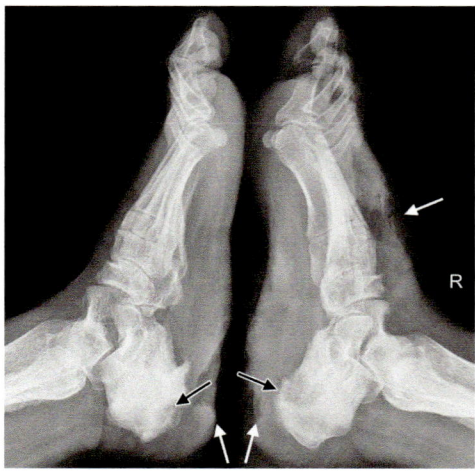

Fig. 4: Lateral radiograph of bilateral feet in a diabetic patient with ulcers in bilateral heels and right dorsal midfoot (white arrows). There is sclerosis with cortical erosions and a geographic lytic area in the plantar aspect of bilateral calcaneum adjacent to the ulcers (black arrows) suggestive of osteomyelitis.

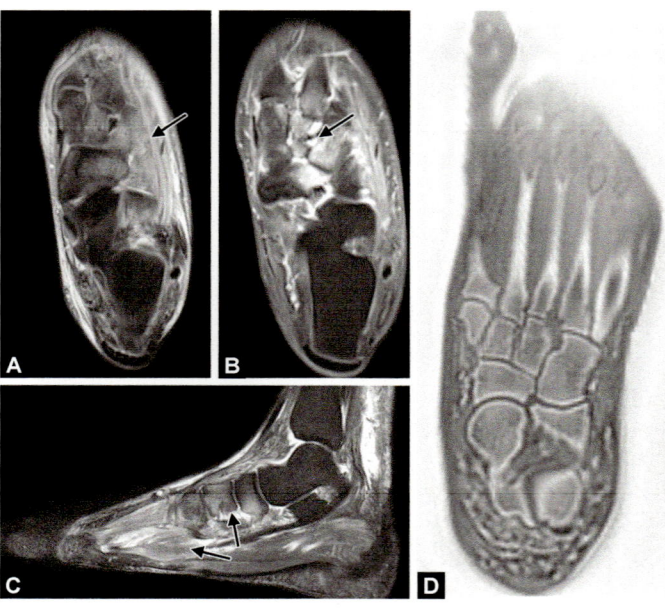

Figs. 5A to D: MRI of a foot of a diabetic patient (A and C). T2FS coronal and sagittal images and PCT1FS (B) showing marrow edema and enhancement involving the navicular, cuneiforms, and cuboid with enhancement; however, no significant bony fragmentations/subluxations are seen on zero TE MR (D). There is diffuse muscle edema in foot. Features are consistent with acute neuroarthropathy.
(MRI: magnetic resonance imaging: PCT1FS: postcontrast T1-weighted fat saturated; T2FS: T2-weighted fat-saturated)

IMAGING OF THE COMPLICATIONS OF DIABETIC FOOT[3]

Soft-tissue Complications

Callus formation at weight-bearing sites is due to the redistribution of subcutaneous fat due to altered biomechanics, exacerbated by ill-fitting footwear. Callus formation occurs over the metatarsal heads (particularly first and fifth), tip of great toes, tarsometatarsal joints, and over cuboid in ambulatory patients. In bed-ridden patients, it is seen over the calcaneum and lateral malleolus. On MRI, they appear as focal T2 intermediate and T1 hypointense subcutaneous lesions without surrounding soft tissue inflammation. Callus may be associated with the formation of adventitious bursae over the bony prominences.

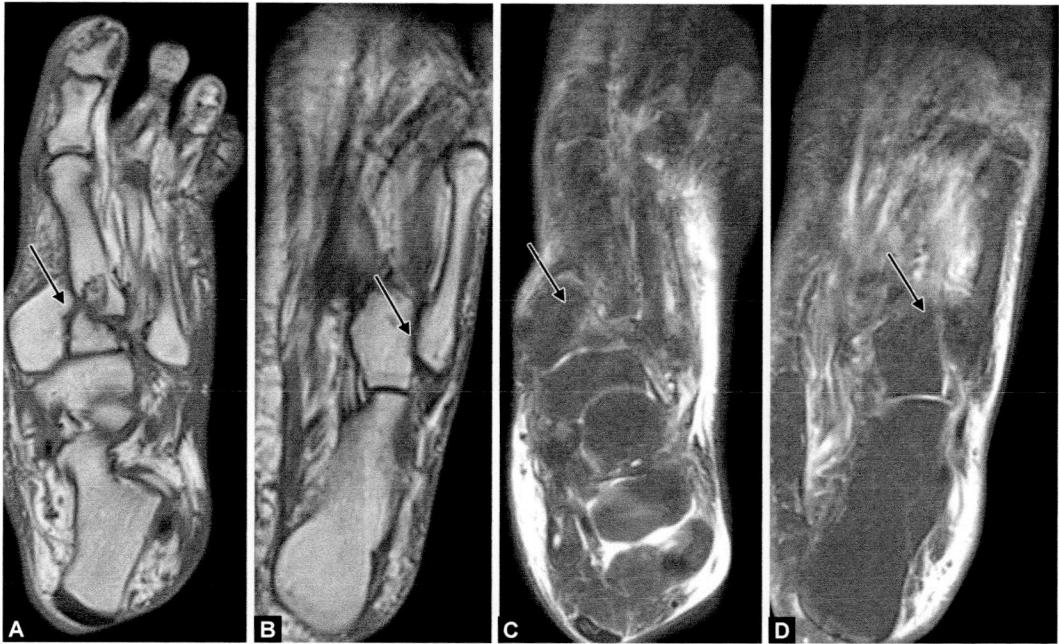

Figs. 6A to D: T1 and T2FS images of a diabetic patient with progressive deformity in foot showing multiple tarsometatarsal dislocations; however, no bone marrow edema is seen in the involved bones. Features are suggestive of chronic neuroarthropathy.
(T2FS: T2-weighted fat-saturated)

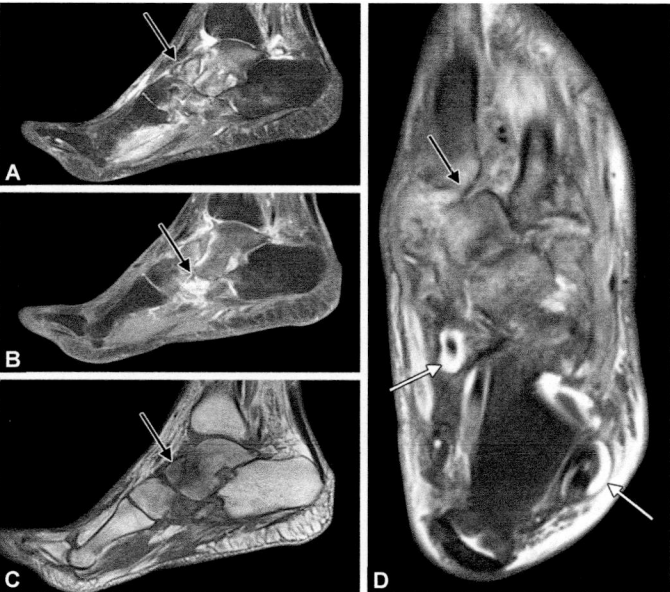

Figs. 7A to D: (A) T2FS, (B) postcontrast, and (C) T1-weighted images of foot in a diabetic patient showing fragmentation of the head of talus and lateral cuneiform. There is periarticular marrow edema and enhancement in the tarsal bones with edema in intrinsic muscles of foot. Mild synovitis is seen in the ankle. (D) T2FS image of another patient showing intertarsal and tarsometatarsal subluxations, marrow edema in tarsals with tenosynovitis of the flexor, and peroneal tendons (white arrows).
(T2FS: T2-weighted fat-saturated)

Breakdown of the callus leads to skin ulceration except in cases of neuropathic midfoot ulcers and toe ulcers due to flexion deformity. Though sensory neuropathy predominantly contributes to the breakdown of callus, autonomic neuropathy leads to dryness, fissuring, and ulceration. On MRI, it is seen as break in the cutaneous line with raised edges and soft tissue defect. Acute ulcerations may show edema and enhancing granulation tissue; however, chronic ulcers are fibrotic. Ulcers deeper than 2 cm are more prone to associated osteomyelitis.

Cellulitis is a non-necrotic inflammatory process involving the skin and subcutaneous tissue with sparing of the deep fascia and muscles. It can often be confused with changes in acute neuroarthropathy. On MRI, cellulitis is seen as diffuse T2 hyperintensity with enhancement, with reticulations in fat. Edema of neuropathic foot is typically nonenhancing.

Abscess formation occurs with chronic infections or in the early phase of aggressive infections. MRI shows rim-enhancing lesion of fluid signal intensity and may be remote from the site of ulceration. Majority of abscesses are small and frequently in communication with sinus tracts, which show tram-track pattern of enhancement.

Gangrene occurs due to microangiopathy causing ischemia. MRI helps in determining extent and helps surgical planning. It is seen as nonenhancing area on MRI. Soft tissue gas may be seen in cases of wet gangrene

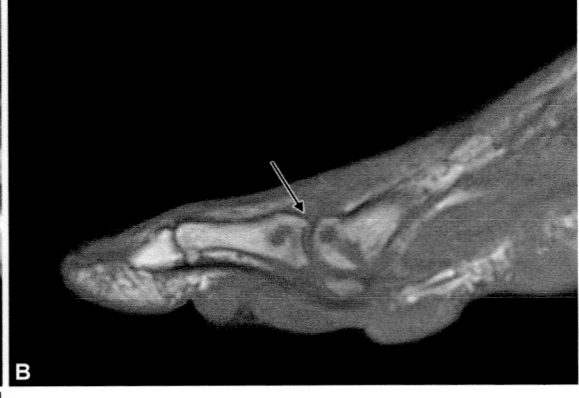
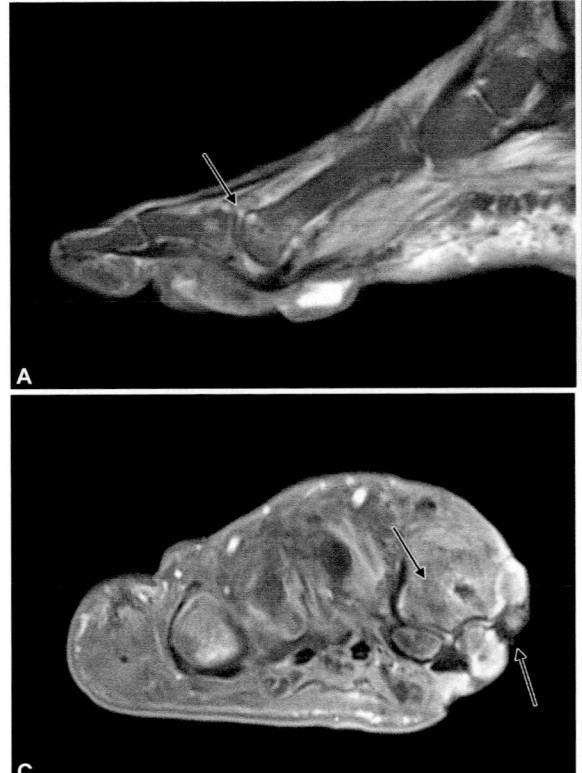

Figs. 8A to C: (A) T2FS, (B) T1-weighted, and (C) postcontrast T1 images of a diabetic patient with nonhealing ulcer in the plantar aspect of ball of great toe showing mild synovitis in first MTP joint with periarticular marrow edema and an intraosseous grossly T1 hypointense peripherally enhancing sinus tract in the head of metatarsal extending up to the skin ulcer. A small peripherally enhancing fluid collection is seen adjacent to the ulcer. Features are suggestive of osteomyelitis of head of first metatarsal with possible septic synovitis of first MTP joint.
(MTP: metatarsophalangeal; T2FS: T2-weighted fat-saturated)

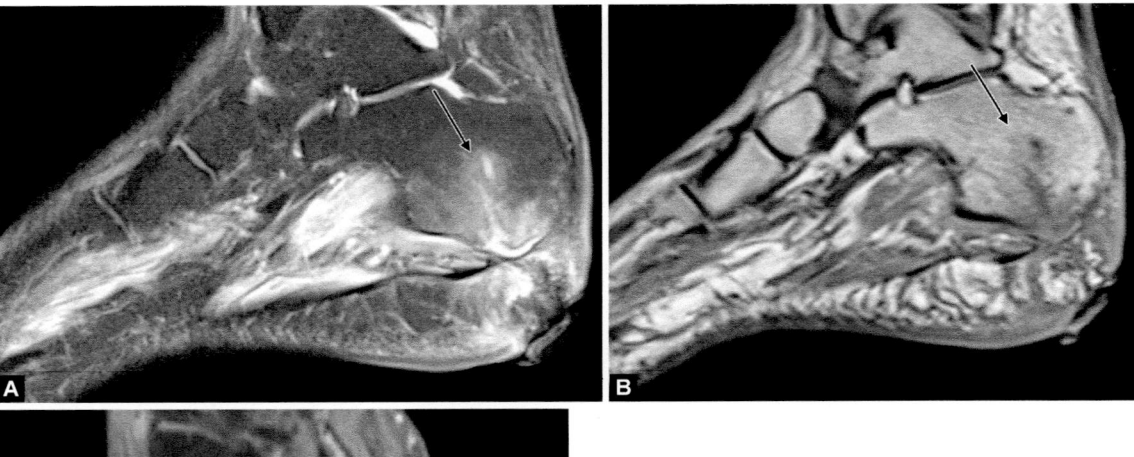
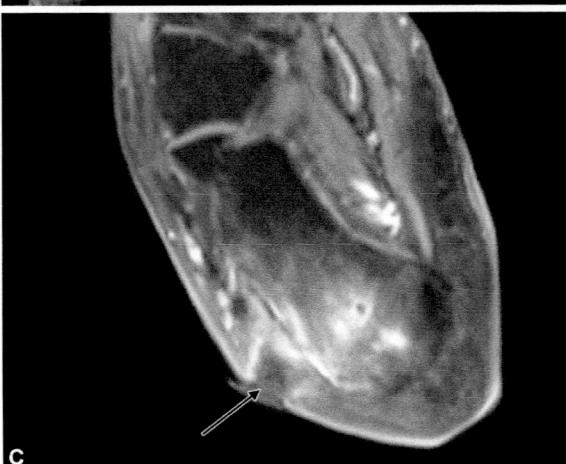

Figs. 9A to C: (A) T2FS, (B) T1-weighted, and (C) postcontrast T1 images of a diabetic patient with nonhealing ulcer in the plantar aspect of the heel showing marrow edema and enhancement in the plantar aspect of calcaneum with a peripherally enhancing, grossly T1 hypointense intraosseous sinus tract extending up to the skin ulcer. Features are suggestive of calcaneal osteomyelitis.
(T2FS: T2-weighted fat-saturated)

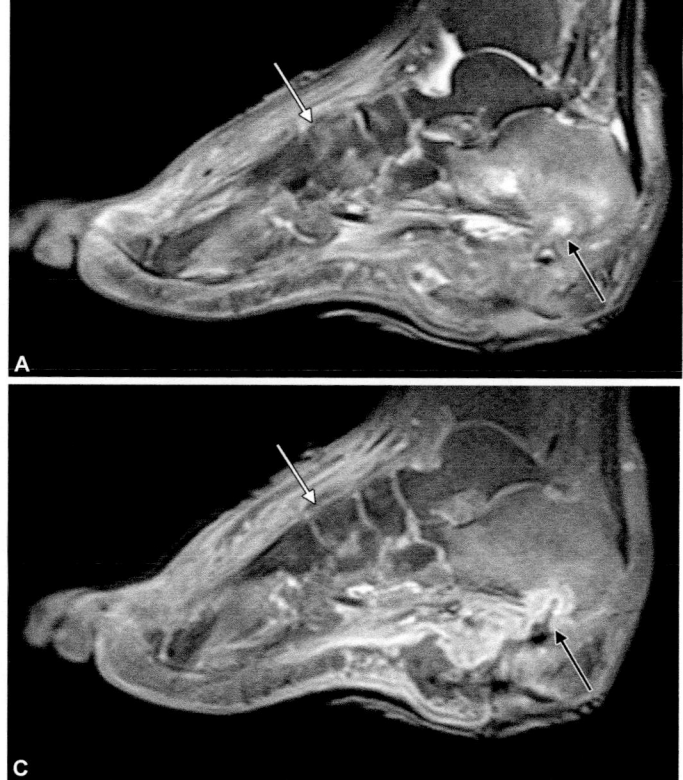
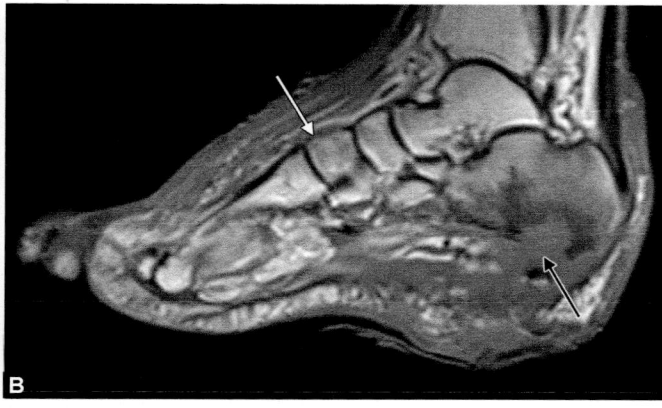

Figs. 10A to C: (A) T2FS, (B) T1-weighted, and (C) postcontrast T1 images of a diabetic patient with nonhealing ulcer in the plantar aspect of the heel showing a large cortical erosion in the plantar aspect of calcaneum with surrounding marrow edema, which is grossly T1 hypointense with enhancement, and showing contiguity with the plantar ulcer (black arrows). In addition, there is periarticular marrow edema in the midfoot, which is mildly T1 hypointense (white arrows). There is edema in the intrinsic muscles of the foot. Features are suggestive of coexisting calcaneal osteomyelitis with acute neuroarthropathy.
(T2FS: T2-weighted fat-saturated)

and gas may not be well seen on MRI. Necrotizing fasciitis, pyomyositis, and myonecrosis may also be identified on MRI.

Foreign bodies are common due to unperceived penetrative trauma and are usually located under the metatarsal heads. They are typically T1/T2 hypointense and show blooming on gradient echo images.

Bone and Joint Complications

Osteomyelitis

Clinical findings of infection are seen in approximately 50% of patients with ulcers and 20–60% of these infections involve the bones. They can be identified by tracing the sinus tract from the skin surface. Marked T1 hypointensity is a key sign of osteomyelitis. Secondary signs of infection such as periosteal reaction and the aforementioned soft-tissue complications suggest infection.

Osteomyelitis should be differentiated from osteitis, which is reactive marrow edema secondary to infection of adjacent soft tissue or cortical bone; however, marked T1 hypointensity is not seen in osteitis. Postdebridement edema may mimic osteomyelitis; however, does not show marked T1 hypointensity.

Neuroarthropathy

Though uncommon, neuroarthropathy is a serious complication of diabetes mellitus with an estimated prevalence of 0.8–8%. It is often difficult to differentiate early neuroarthropathy from osteomyelitis clinically or on MRI/bone scans.

In the acute phase, the radiographs are usually normal. MRI shows soft tissue edema, joint effusions, and periarticular marrow edema, which shows enhancement along with the periarticular soft tissue. In the subacute phase, there is bone resorption. In the chronic phase, there is deformity and bony fragmentation. On MRI, chronic neuroarthropathy may show mild periarticular marrow edema and joint effusion; however, there is no soft tissue enhancement. Hence, chronic neuroarthropathy does not resemble osteomyelitis clinically and any sign of infection should raise possibility of osteomyelitis.

Osteomyelitis versus Neuroarthropathy

Neuroarthropathy is primarily joint centered; however, osteomyelitis almost always occurs at typical sites by direct extension from the skin ulcers. Hence, the presence of periarticular marrow edema without skin ulcers is suggestive of neuroarthropathy. Osteomyelitis involves the bone diffusely, whereas neuroarthropathy involves only the periarticular bone.

Location is a helpful feature where neuroarthropathy involves the tarsometatarsal and metatarsophalangeal joints, whereas osteomyelitis commonly involves calcaneum, distal tibia/fibula, and bones distal to the tarsometatarsal joint.

The biggest diagnostic challenge arises when there is involvement of midfoot in a patient with preexisting neuropathy. In such instances, secondary signs of infection are crucial to determine the presence of osteomyelitis.

Neuroarthropathy with Superimposed Infection

In the presence of skin ulcerations, patients with preexisting neuroarthropathy commonly have osteomyelitis in comparison to patients without ulcers. The sensitivity of MRI in diagnosing osteomyelitis is limited in cases with preexisting neuroarthropathy and is usually used to determine the extent, rather than for diagnosis.

In a superimposed infection, there is gross soft tissue edema with fluid collections larger than expected for uncomplicated neuroarthropathy. Sinus tracts may develop from the collection leading to decompression. Disappearance of intra-articular loose bodies or subchondral cysts in a follow-up case of neuroarthropathy indicates superimposed infection.

The presence of "ghost sign" also indicates infected neuroarthropathy. Ghost sign refers to bones disappearing on T1-weighted (T1W) images due to gross T1 hypointensity and reappearing on the T2W and postcontrast images. On the contrary destruction of bones with absent ghost sign suggests uncomplicated neuroarthropathy.

Septic Arthritis

In diabetic patients, septic arthritis is a result of direct spread of infection from the soft tissue to the adjacent joint, rather than the hematogenous route. Hence, the frequently affected joints are adjacent to areas of callus formation/ulceration, viz. the ankle, subtalar, metatarsophalangeal, and interphalangeal joints. Midfoot septic arthritis shows features identical to midfoot neuroarthropathy.

On MRI, complex joint effusion with market synovial thickening and enhancement is often noted. Contiguous extension into a sinus tract may be seen. Periarticular soft tissue edema and subchondral marrow edema with marginal erosions are noted. Extension of marrow edema beyond the subchondral bone with marked T1 hypointensity suggests contiguous osteomyelitis.

Musculotendinous Complications

Infective tenosynovitis occurs adjacent to sites of ulceration and frequently involves the peroneal tendon and Achilles tendon. In the forefoot, flexor tendons are frequently involved. On MRI, septic tenosynovitis is seen as peritendinous enhancement with cellulitis with an adjacent skin ulcer.

Denervation of muscles may be seen due to peripheral neuropathy, which in acute phase is not picked up on imaging. In the subacute phase, diffuse muscle edema is seen, usually after 2–4 weeks of denervation. In chronic stages, there is muscle atrophy with fatty infiltration.

Myositis and pyomyositis are seen in association with infection of the adjacent soft tissues. Infective myositis presents as muscle edema and is indistinguishable from reactive myositis. Focal rim-enhancing lesions in a background of muscle edema and fascial enhancement are seen in pyomyositis.

CONCLUSION

Imaging of complications of diabetic foot is challenging and multimodality imaging remains the strategy of choice for accurate diagnosis and MRI plays a pivotal role in the evaluation of complications of diabetic foot.[4,5]

TAKE-HOME MESSAGES

- X-ray is a simple and reliable modality for early identification of foot complications in diabetes.
- MRI provides comprehensive details of soft tissue, bone and joints that aids in clinical decision making.
- MRI T2 weighted fat saturated sequence, T1 weighted and post contrast T1 weighted sequences should be asked for evaluation of diabetic foot complications.
- MRI is a very sensitive modality for early identification of Charcot foot and osteomyelitis.

REFERENCES

1. Lam DW, LeRoith D. The worldwide diabetes epidemic. Curr Opin Endocrinol Diabetes Obes. 2012;19(2):93-6.
2. Rosskopf AB, Loupatatzis C, Pfirrmann CWA, Böni T, Berli MC. The Charcot foot: a pictorial review. Insights Imaging. 2019;10(1):77.
3. Ranachowska C, Lass P, Korzon-Burakowska A, Dobosz M2. Diagnostic imaging of the diabetic foot. Nucl Med Rev Cent East Eur. 2010;13(1):18-22.
4. Gangadharamurthy D, Horwich P, Greenman RL. The Diabetic Foot—Imaging Options and Considerations. US Endocrinology. 2007;(2):75-8.
5. Daneshvar K, Anwander H. Diagnostic Imaging of Diabetic Foot Disorders. Foot Ankle Clin. 2022;27(3):513-27.

Common Diabetic Foot Problems Encountered

1. Gangrene

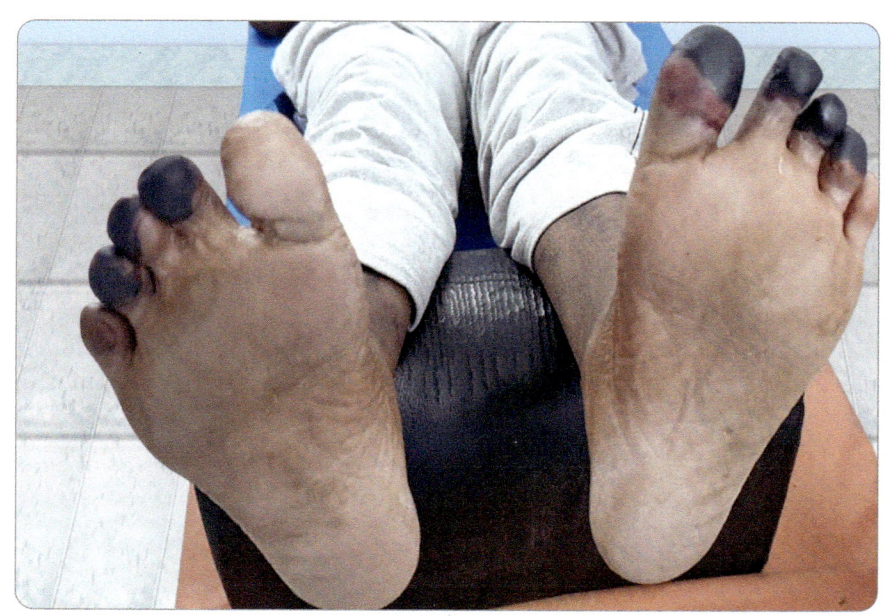

Gangrene is of two types: (1) Infective gangrene and (2) Ischemic gangrene. Infective gangrene needs early debridement, while ischemic gangrene needs early revascularization.

2. Small Muscle Atrophy

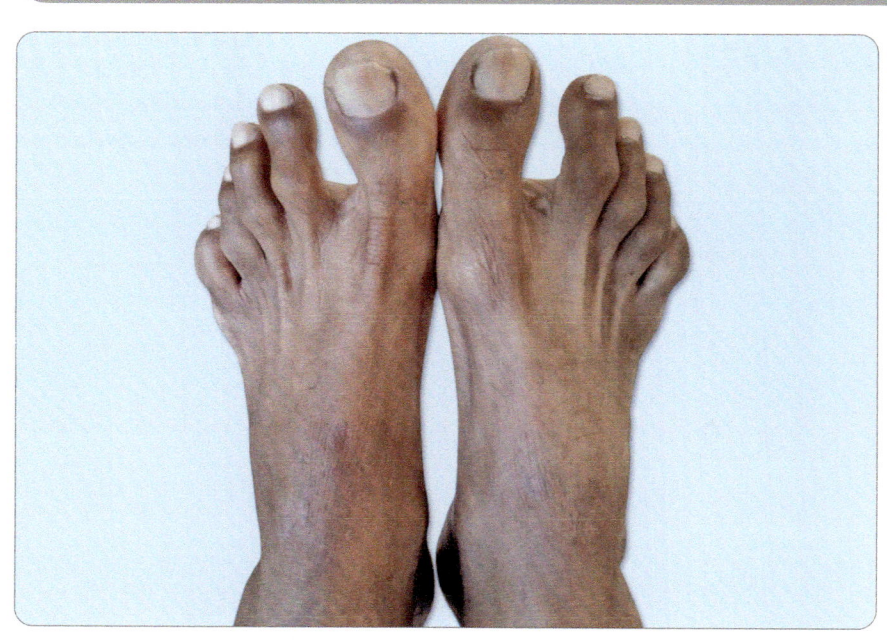

Small muscle atrophy can occur in distal symmetric polyneuropathy (DSPN) and it is mostly related to motor neuropathy. Atrophy of muscles is believed to be the main factor that is responsible for the development of an imbalance between the flexor and extensor muscles, which results in clawing of toes (as visible in this picture), prominent metatarsal heads, and the development of high plantar foot pressures that can lead to diabetic foot ulcer (DFU) in combination with DSPN.

3. Callus

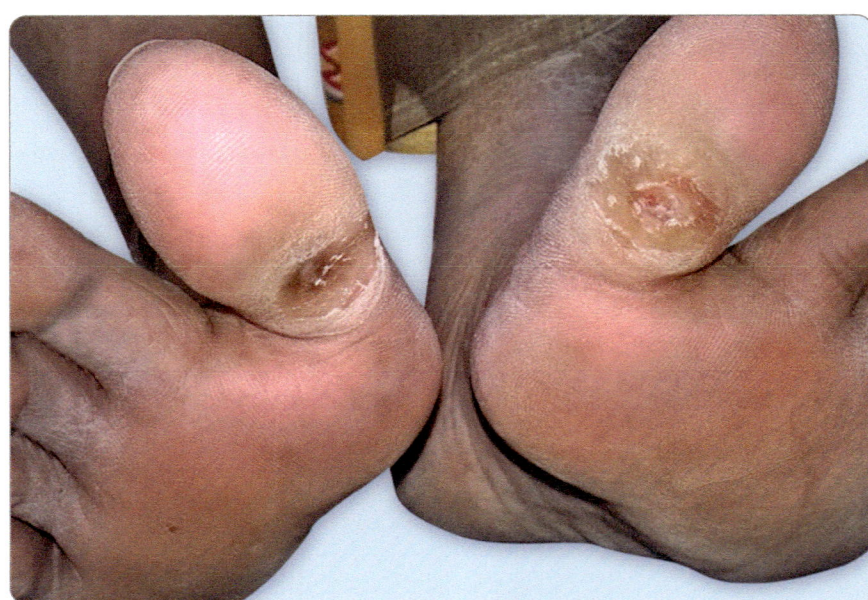

This photograph shows a bilateral callus at the head of the first metatarsophalangeal (MTP) joint. The cause for a callus is diabetic neuropathy and high pressure under the first MTP joint. The cells in the skin react to these factors by increasing keratinization and a callus is formed. The callus may break down and form an ulcer if proper offloading is not provided.

4. Dry Feet with Fissure

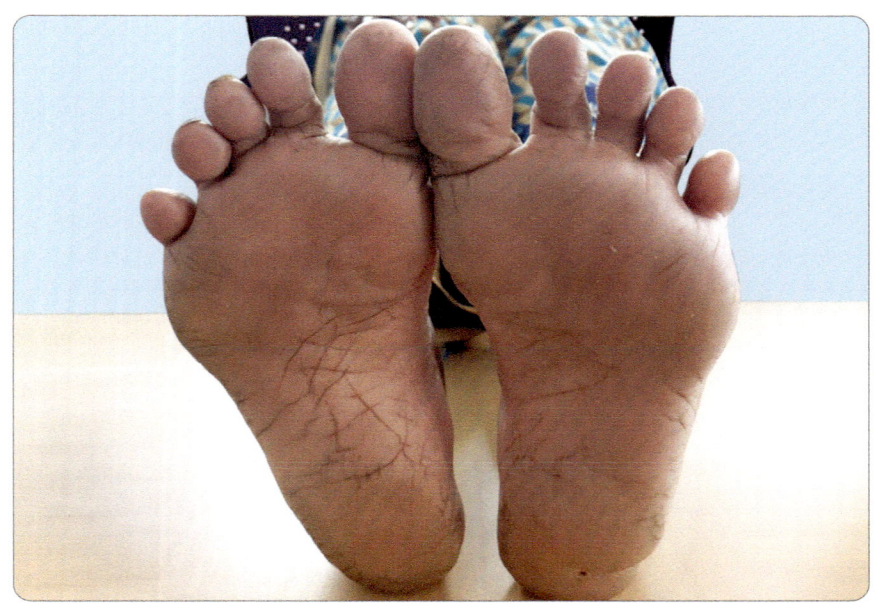

This picture shows dry feet and fissures. The autonomic neuropathy which accompanies DSPN often results in dry feet due to lack of proper sweating and moisture in the feet. Dry skin and fissures can be easily prevented by keeping the feet moisturized, avoiding walking barefoot, and wearing proper footwear.

5. Charcot Neuroarthropathy

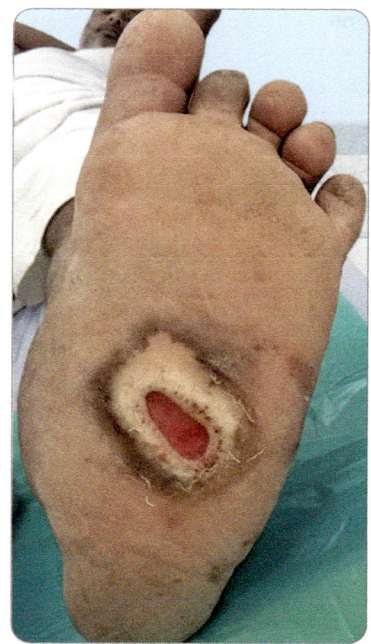

This photograph is a classic case of Charcot neuroarthropathy with a midfoot ulcer. The hallmark deformity which is clearly seen in this image is a collapse of the tarsal bones, which is referred to as a Rocker bottom deformity. An acute Charcot will need total offloading to reduce the inflammation and prevent the destruction of the underlying bones. A chronic Charcot foot with a mid-foot ulcer will need good wound care, callus debridement, and proper offloading to heal the ulcer.

6. Swelling of the Feet and Ankle

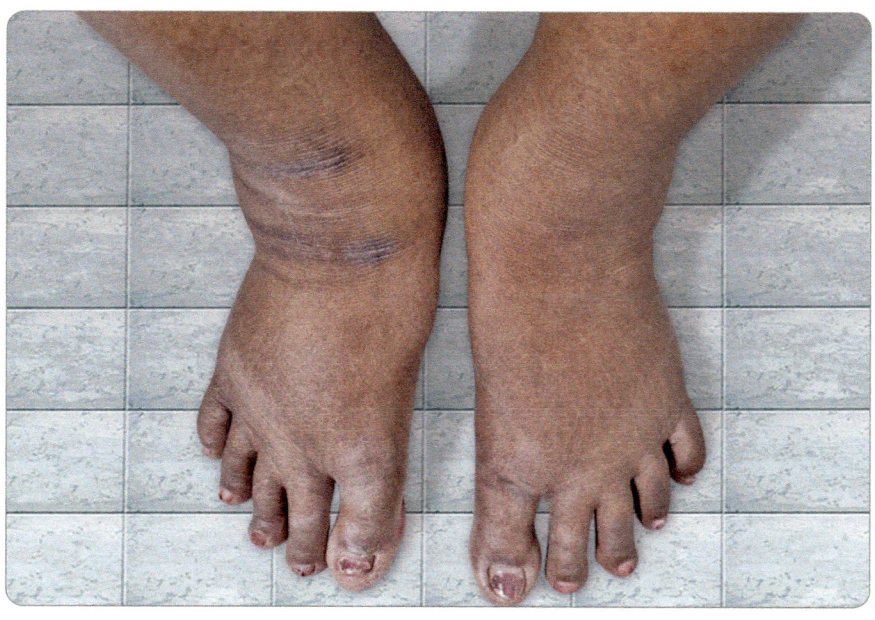

Swelling of the feet and ankles is often an early symptom of venous insufficiency. This is a condition where the venous return from the feet to the heart is impaired. Other common causes of painless swelling are diabetic neuropathy lymphedema, heart failure, hypothyroidism, chronic kidney disease, and chronic liver disease.

7. Curved Corners of the Toenail

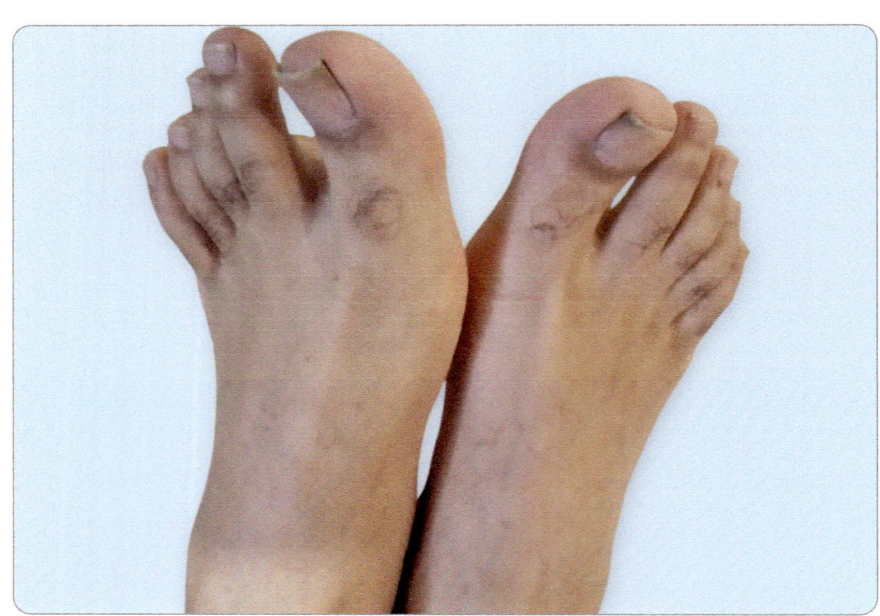

People with diabetes should take more care while trimming their nails. Toenails should not be cut with sharp scissors, blades, or knives as it may cause injury to toe in the insensate feet. The corners of the nails should be gently trimmed with a nail-filer. If the nails are very thick, then they can take help from a podiatrist also.

8. Hallux Valgus Deformity

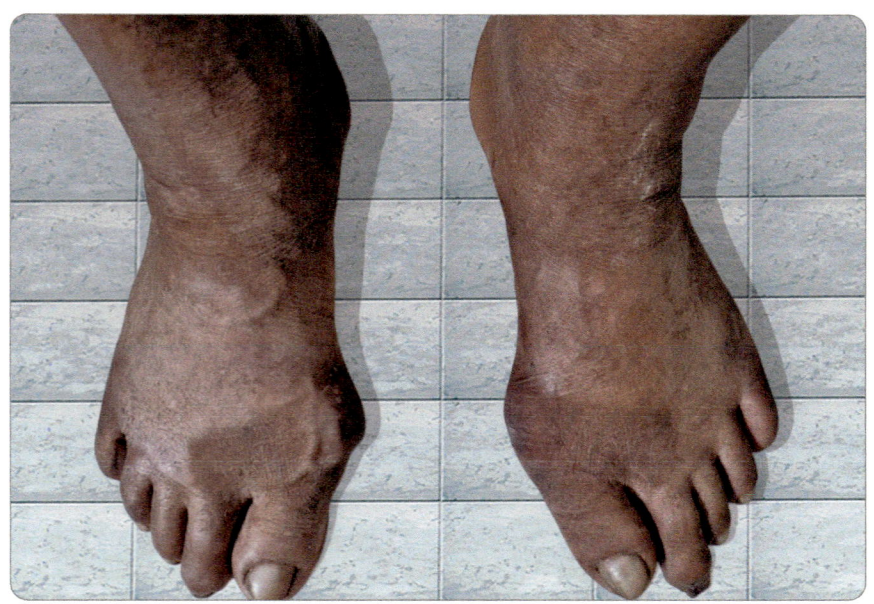

When the MTP joint (big toe joint) is subjected to continuous pressure, it can result in hallux valgus deformity. There will be lateral deviation of the MTP joint and abduction of the first meta bone. This often leads to the thickening of the skin on the bony prominence on the medial side, also known as "Bunion".

9. Flatfoot

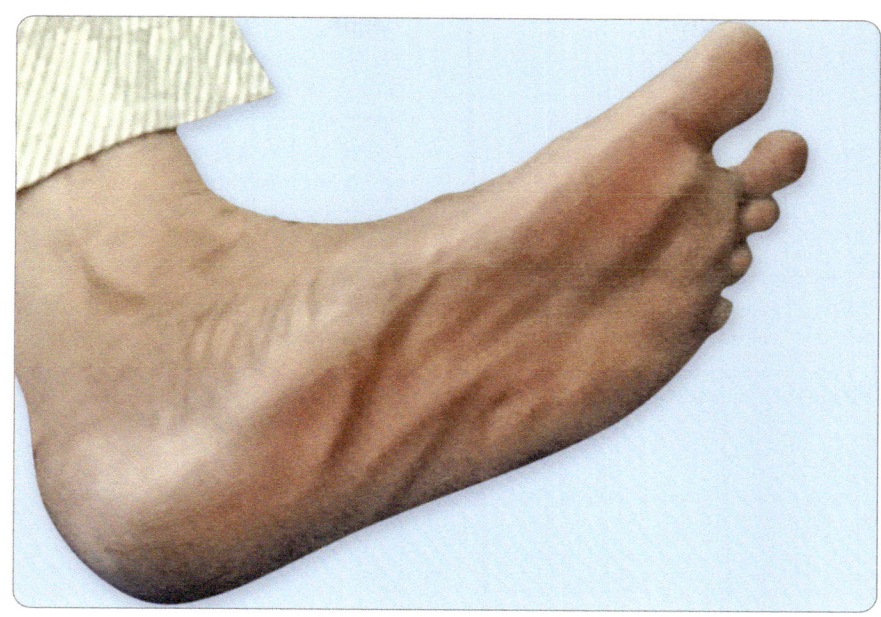

Flatfoot also known as pes planus flatfoot is characterized by the absence of the medial arch. Adults can develop flatfeet through injury, tight Achilles tendon, abnormal joint formation, continued stress on the foot and its arch, obesity, and diabetes. Such patients need a customized insole in the footwear and must avoid barefoot walking.

10. Onychomycosis

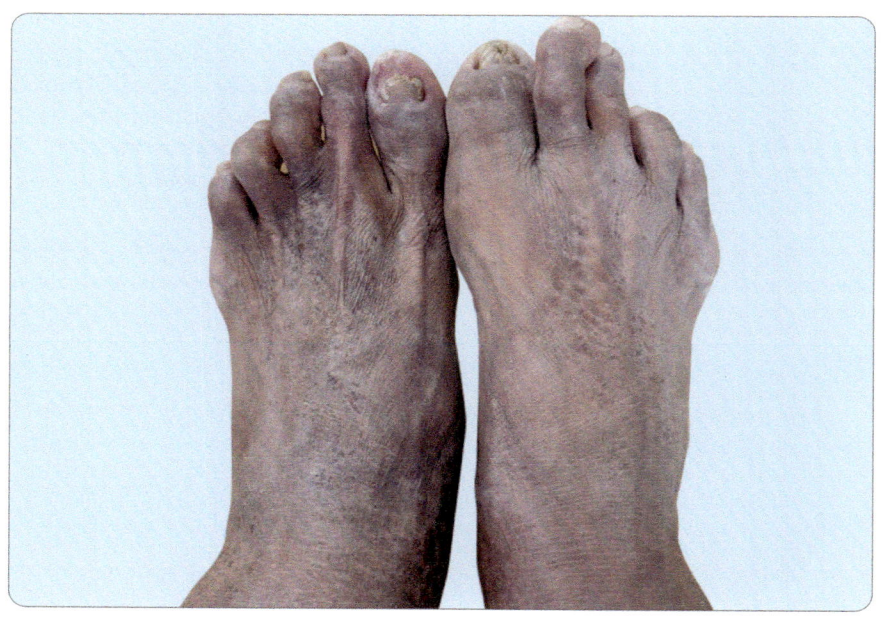

It is a fungal infection of the toenails. There are several situations that produce this condition in diabetes such as high blood sugars, keeping the feet wet for a long time, and wearing nonbreathable socks and footwear. Prolonged diabetes leads to the thickening of the nails and acceleration of subungual keratinization, which increases the probability of onychomycosis.

11. Toe Rings

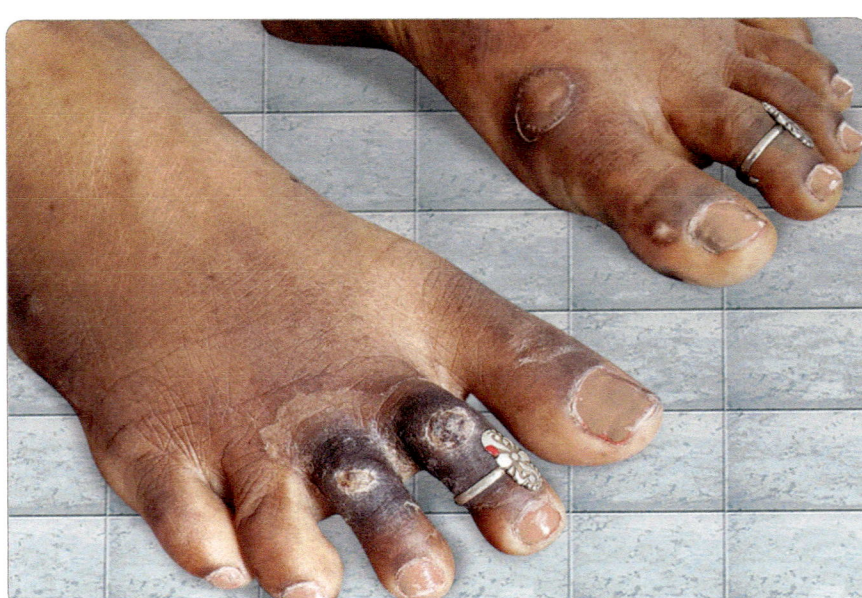

Toe rings are worn by some Indian women. In people with diabetic neuropathy and pedal edema such toe rings can decrease the oxygen and blood supply to the toe. If not removed and cleaned regularly, it can also lead to fungal infection due to dust and sweating resulting in ulceration.

12. Clawing of Toenails

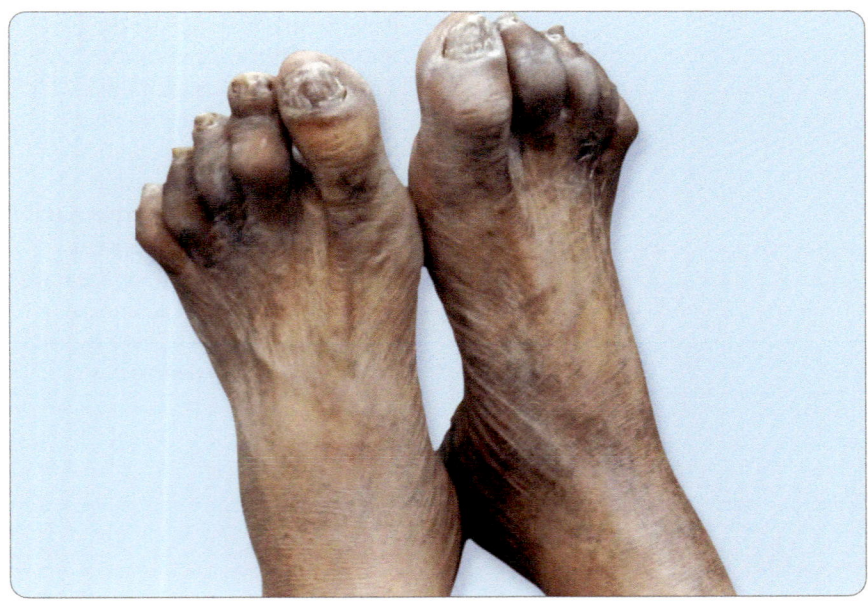

In claw toe deformity, a "Buckling Phenomenon" can be noted, which causes increased pressure on the dorsal hammer digit deformity as well as on the plantar metatarsal head leading to ulceration.

Common Diabetic Foot Problems Encountered 119

13. Below-Knee Amputation

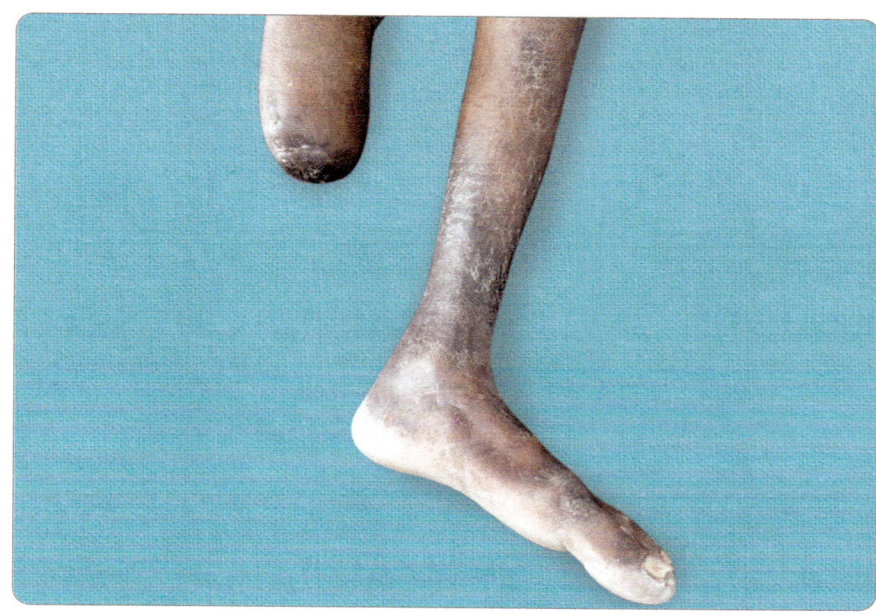

Most of the lower limb amputations in diabetes are caused due to neuropathy. Some are due to a neuroischemic condition. Management includes control of diabetes, infection, assessment of vascular status, and revascularization if necessary and active debridement.

14. Foot Examination in a Person with Diabetes

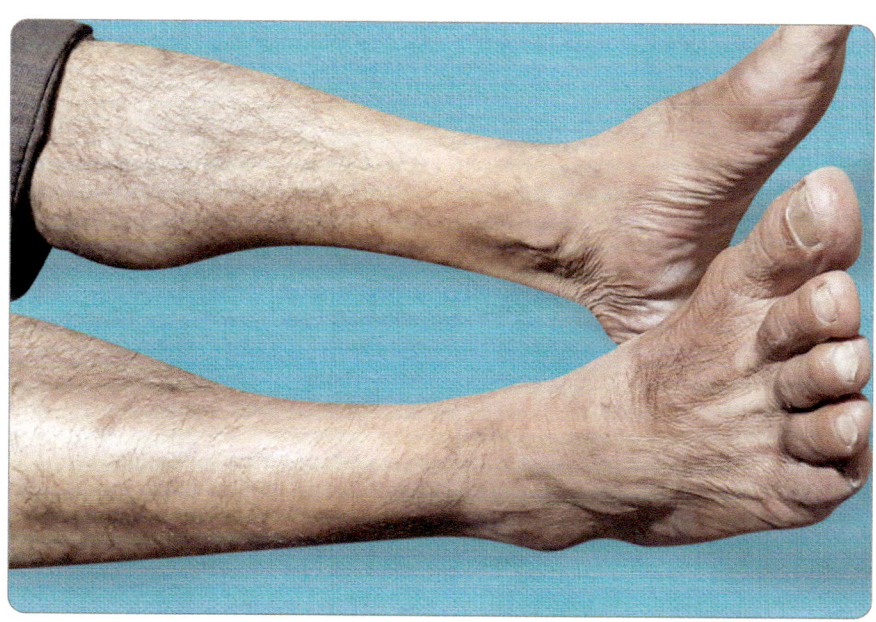

What should we look for?
- Any changes in skin color, dryness, thickness, or cracking
- Check for any fungal infection between the toes
- Look for the presence of a callus on the plantar aspect of the foot
- Any deformities like claw toes and Charcot foot
- Muscle wasting is seen in people with severe motor neuropathy.

15. Great Toe Amputee

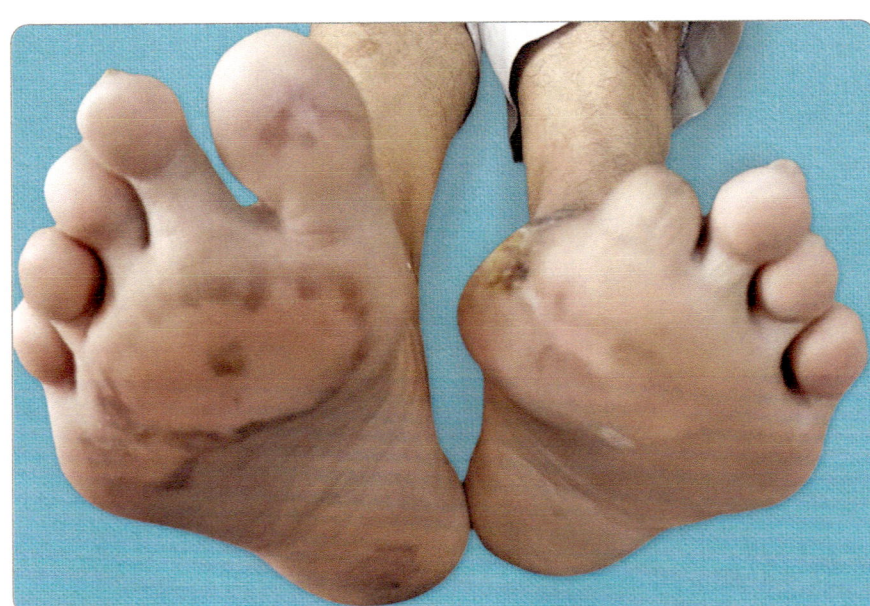

After a toe amputation, the pressure distribution of the foot is significantly altered and such patients need a customized insole to prevent ulceration.

16. Intertrigo

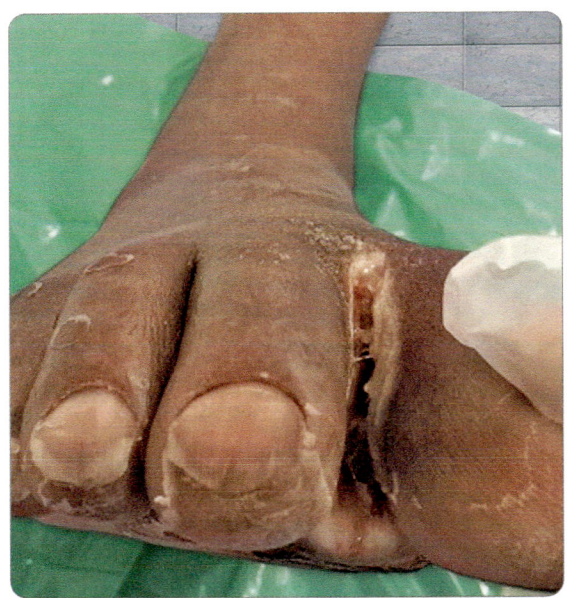

Intertrigo or fungal infection between the toes is found mostly in a hot and humid environment, where a person is more likely to sweat. It can also occur in people who wash their legs frequently and do not dry them completely, especially between the toes.

17. Healing of the Stump Wound

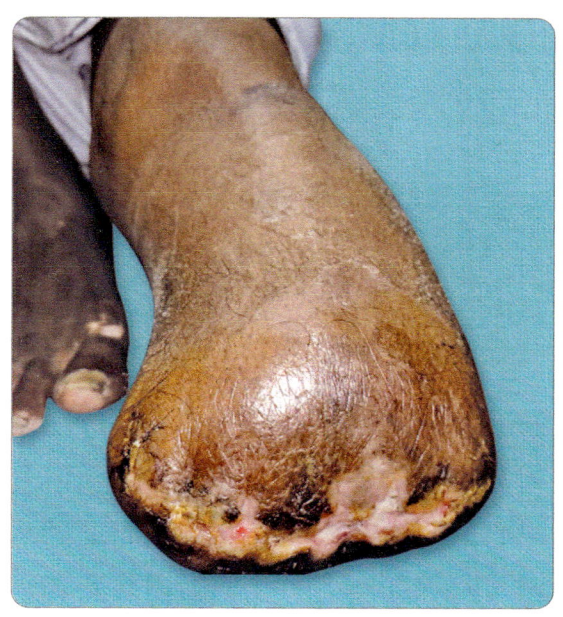

Sometimes the stump infection leads to a revision amputation. Peripheral arterial disease (PAD) as well as infection in the lower limb should be properly addressed to prevent infection of the stump after a major amputation is done.

18. Offloading of Foot Ulcer by Felted Foam Dressing

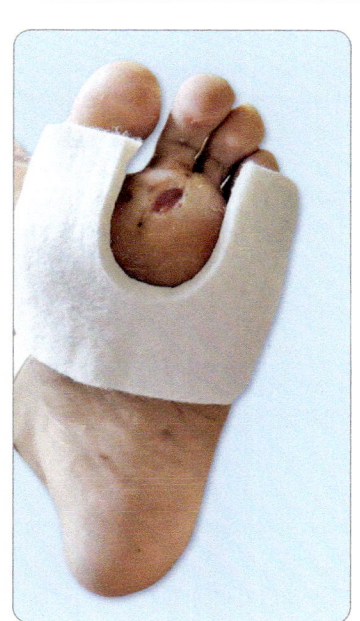

Off-loading devices are ideally used for the treatment of DFUs. The felted foam used along with other offloading techniques is useful to reduce or redistribute the plantar pressure and heal the ulcer.

19. Improper Footwear

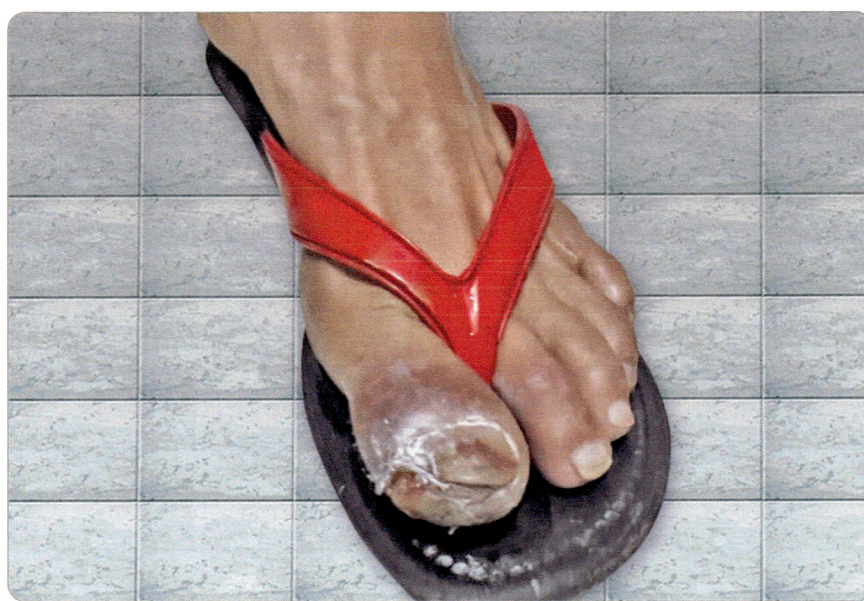

This picture shows improper footwear in someone with a diabetes-related foot ulcer and small muscle wasting (motor neuropathy). Avoid footwear without a counter like a *Chappal* as seen in this picture.

20. Diabetic Neuropathy

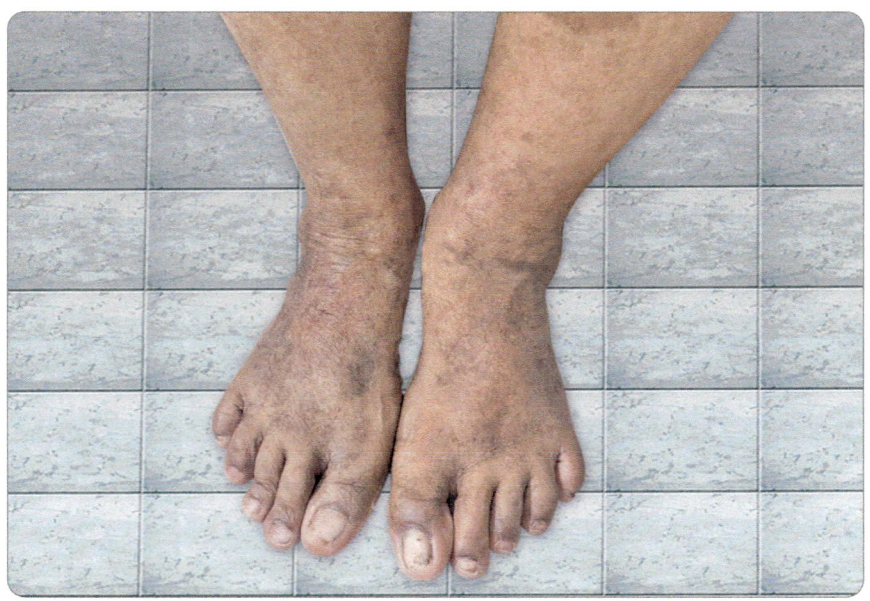

Diabetic neuropathy can cause loss of sensation in feet. Some people may present with symptoms of numbness, tingling, burning, or pain but some may be asymptomatic. Neuropathy can lower the ability to feel pain and temperature like heat or cold. If a person is unable to feel pain, he/she might not notice a small cut, blister, or sore. Early treatment is always recommended for a better prognosis.

21. Plantar Psoriasis

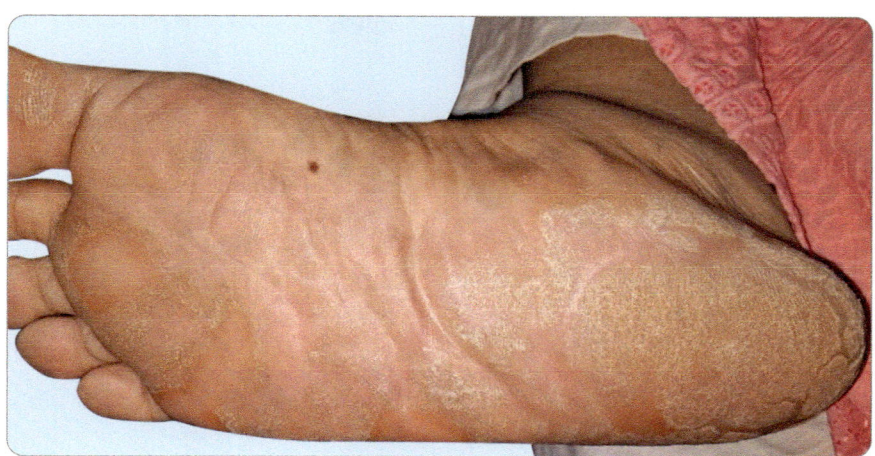

A chronic skin disease that occurs on the soles of feet is called plantar psoriasis. It causes thickening and discoloration of skin, which in turn can result in pain, bleeding, and cracking of skin. Plantar psoriasis is found to be associated with diabetes and it affects the physical quality as well as daily activities of patient's life. Topical steroids, emollients, and keratolytic agents are used for the treatment of mild psoriasis. However, severe cases require phototherapy or treatment with systemic drugs.

22. Screening for Sensory Loss with 10 g Monofilament

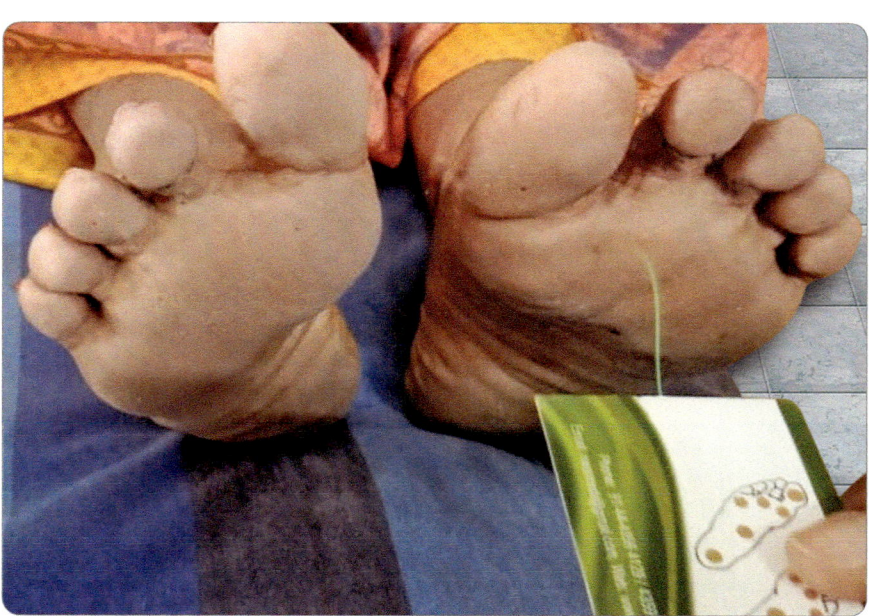

Peripheral neuropathy can be assessed by using a monofilament test. The Semmes–Weinstein monofilament test is used to assess loss of peripheral sensation (LOPS). A 10 g monofilament must be applied to the patient's hands to establish the sensation. Different sites must be chosen for the application of monofilament perpendicular to the skin surface to ensure that the filament bends on the application of force. It must not be applied directly on any foot ulcer, callus, or scar. The total duration of the procedure for each site must not exceed 2 seconds.

23. Ankle Callosity and Hyperkeratosis

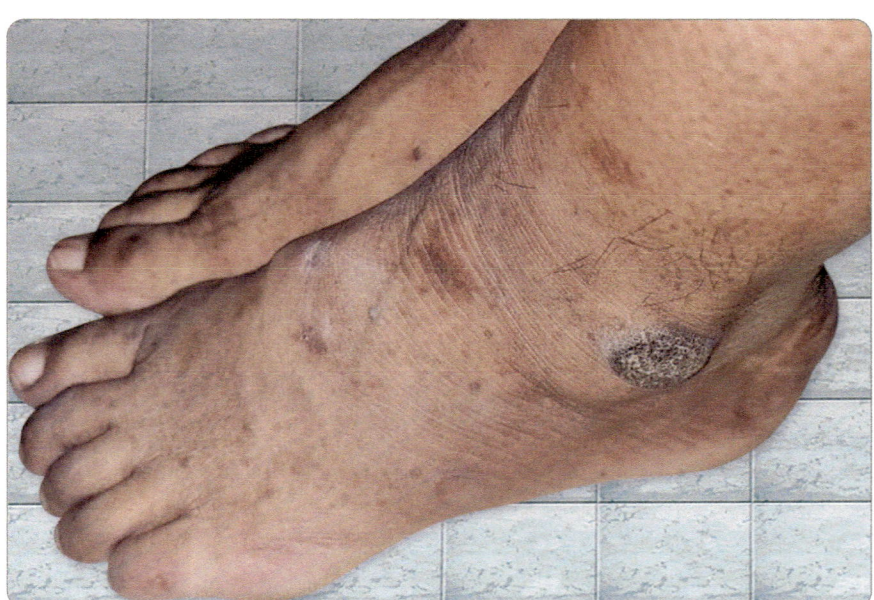

Ankle callosities are commonly seen among people living in developing countries like India because of continuous friction of the ankles, which they develop due to the habit of sitting on hard surface or in a crossed leg position. Localized hyperkeratosis and hypermelanosis along with roughening of skin is seen on clinical examination. Patients are usually asymptomatic and are referred only for cosmetic reasons.

24. Eschar

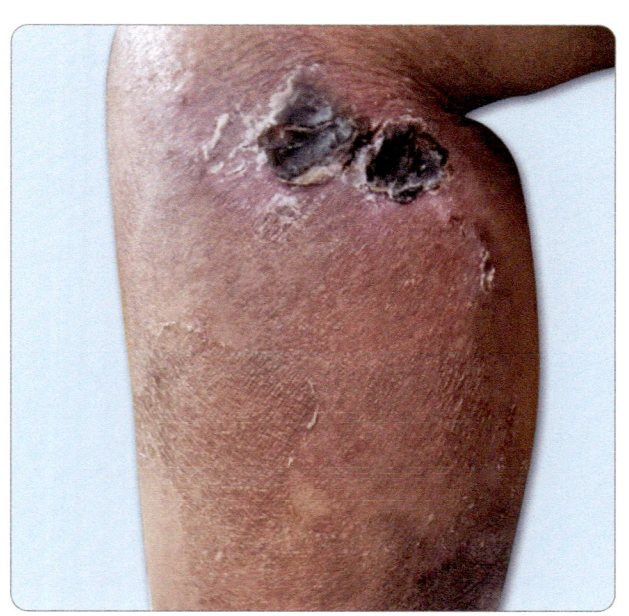

Dead and dried tissue sometimes gets accumulated within a wound, which can be called as Eschar. It usually occurs in the advanced stages of pressure ulcer wounds and blocks visibility to the underlying wound bed. It is very important to keep the skin dry and clean to avoid this condition. Debridement can be considered as an ideal treatment to remove the dead tissue.

25. Hallux Varus

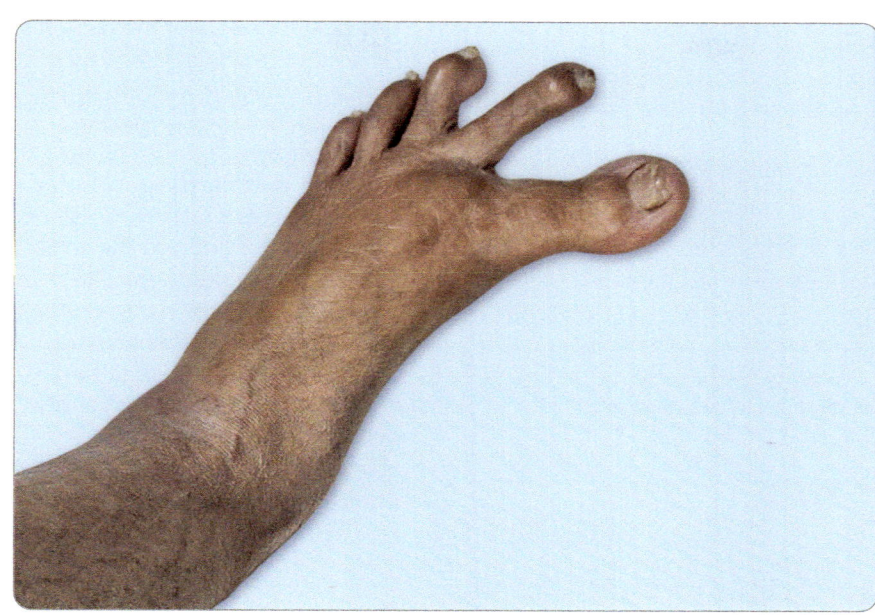

Medial bending of the big toe either due to surgery or due to trauma or any other systemic inflammatory conditions like rheumatoid arthritis or psoriasis is called hallux varus. Patient usually complains of pain due to the deformed toe because of inappropriate foot wear and difficulty in walking. Modification of the shoe with wide toe boxes is recommended in these patients. However, surgery is advised in severe cases.

26. Cellulitis with Blister

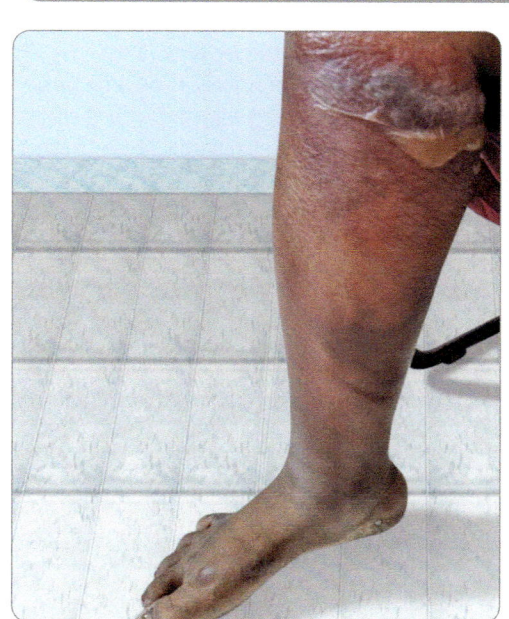

An infection in the deeper layers of skin caused due to *Streptococcus* and *Staphylococcus* infection is called cellulitis. A diabetic foot is highly susceptible to cellulitis. Neuropathy, a decrease in blood supply, and a diminished immune system are considered risk factors. It can lead to complications like sepsis and toxic shock syndrome. Mild infections require treatment with analgesics. However, severe cases of cellulitis in diabetes may require hospitalization.

27. Ankle-brachial Pressure Index Testing

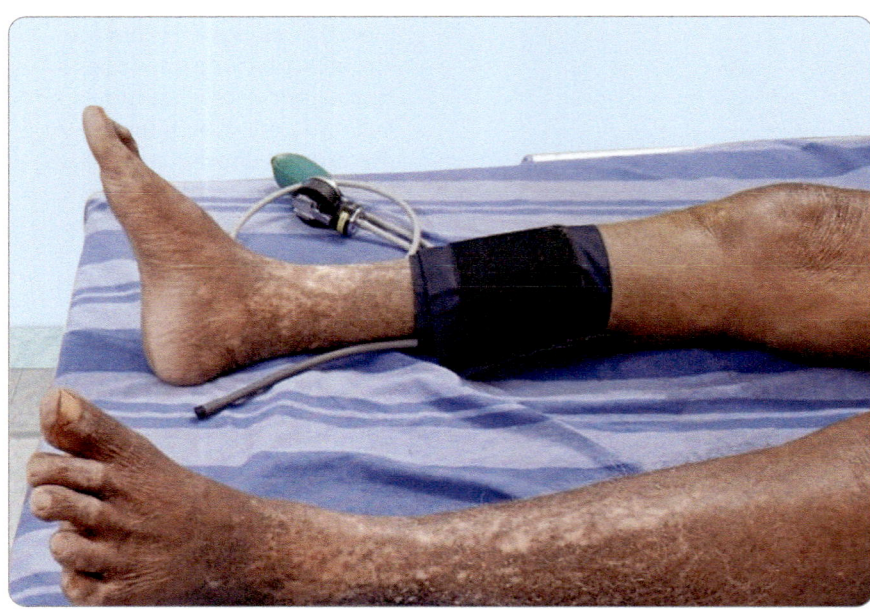

The vascular status of the patient's lower limb can be assessed by a simple yet reliable method called ankle-brachial pressure index (ABPI) testing.

Ankle-brachial pressure index is calculated as a ratio of the blood pressure in the artery in the ankle divided by the arterial blood pressure of the arm. If the resultant ratio appears to be less than 0.9, the patient is diagnosed to have PAD. This test helps us to identify patients who are at increased risk of developing PAD as well as cardiovascular events.

28. Probe-to-bone Test

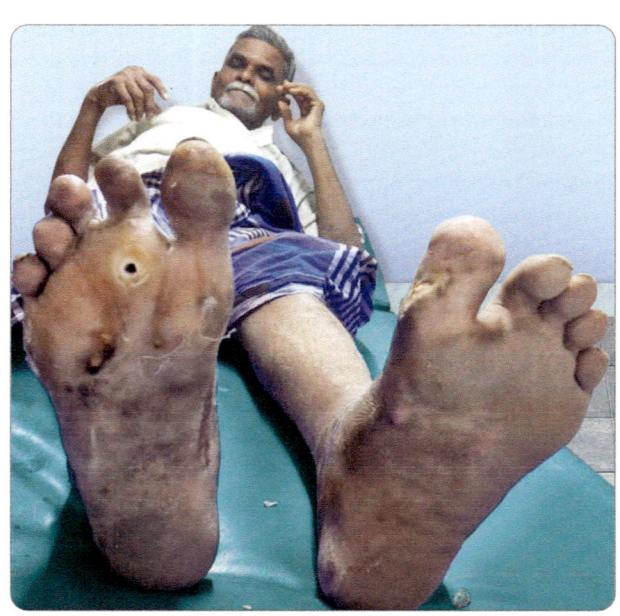

This test can be used to differentiate between osteomyelitis and any soft tissue infection. Probe-to-bone (PTB) test uses a blunt instrument to palpate bone through the ulcer, which is indicative of osteomyelitis. Neuropathic ulcers are best diagnosed using this test. PTB should be included in the evaluation and assessment of all DFUs in the primary stages itself.

Common Diabetic Foot Problems Encountered 127

29. Ingrowing Toenails

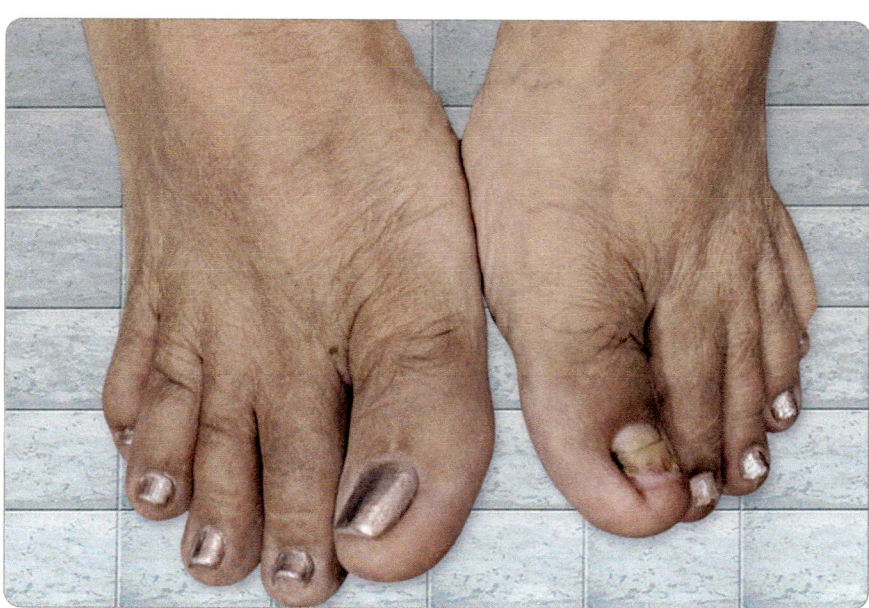

In this case, the edges of the toenails grow into the soft tissue of the adjacent nails. Teenagers with sweaty feet, elders whose toenails thicken with age, injury, and wearing inappropriate shoes can contribute to ingrowing toenails. This, in turn, can cause pain, swelling, and infection. Treatment includes self-foot care practices, applying topical antibiotics, and consulting the podiatrist in severe cases.

30. Offloading of Heel Ulcer

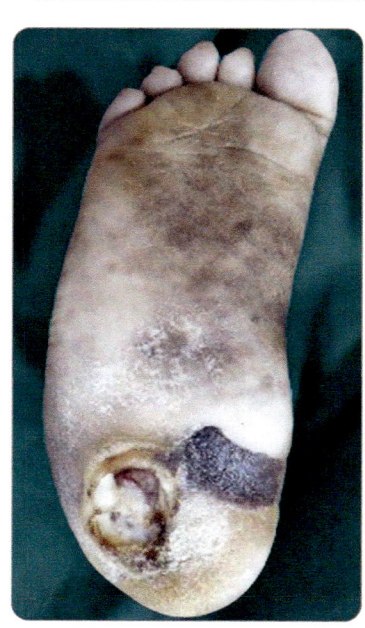

Heel ulcers are difficult to treat because of their anatomical location and little subcutaneous tissue making them more prone to pressure ulcers and difficult to heal. International Working Group on the Diabetic Foot (IWGDF) guidelines 2019 suggest that plantar heel ulcers can be effectively treated by using a knee-high offloading device or any other offloading intervention that can also be considered to reduce the plantar pressure.

31. Varicose Veins

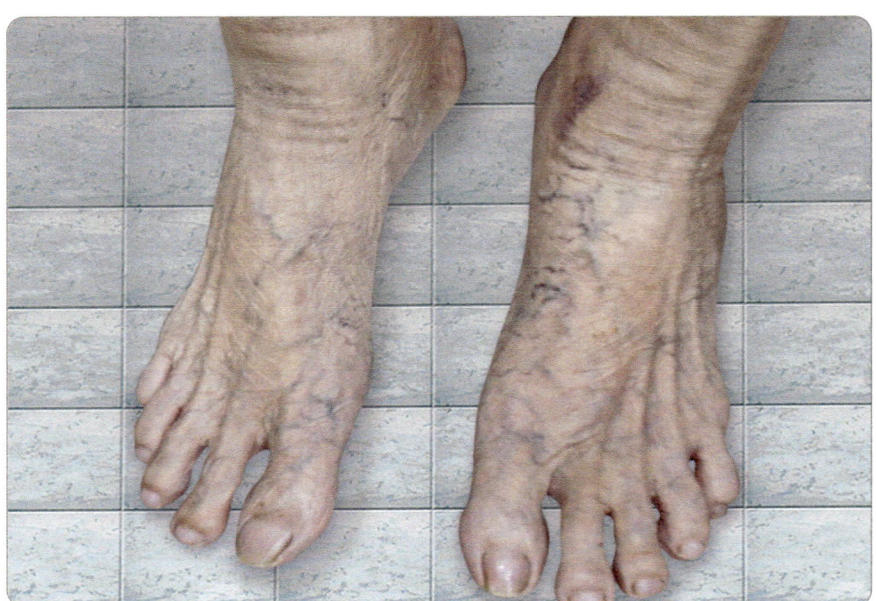

A common clinical condition in which veins of the legs become swollen and twisted caused by weak or damaged vein walls is called varicose veins. This causes the blood to pool, sometimes even flow backward, and get distorted due to an increase in the blood pressure of the veins. Prolonged sitting or standing, pregnancy, being overweight or obese, and smoking are considered some of the important reasons for varicose veins. Treatment includes lifestyle changes like being physically active and avoiding sitting or standing for prolonged periods. However, endovenous ablation and sclerotherapy are the treatment modalities advocated in minor cases and surgery is advised in severe cases.

32. Pitting Edema

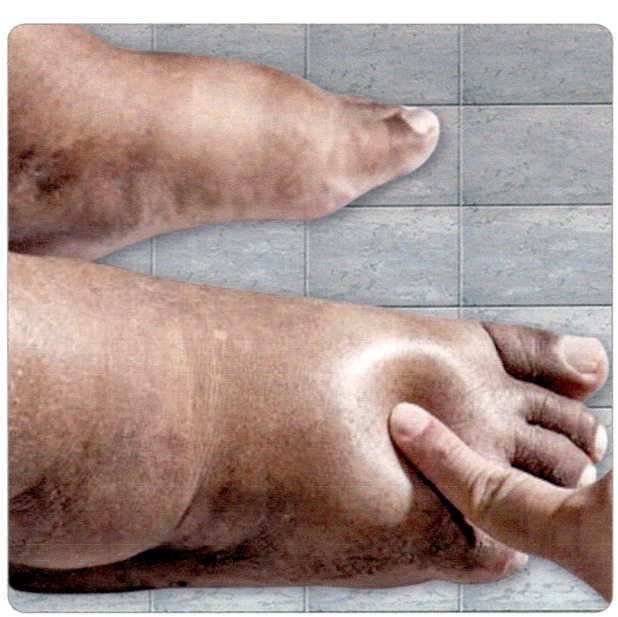

When excess fluids accumulate in the body, it can result in swelling. It is of two types: Pitting and nonpitting edema. This picture shows pitting edema, which indicates that when pressure is applied, an indentation or pit appears. Diabetes can cause fluid to accumulate in the legs because it can affect blood circulation.

Prolonged sitting or standing, obesity, low protein levels, and pregnancy are some of the other reasons, which can cause pitting edema. Mild cases might undergo spontaneous resolution or may require treatment by elevation of the leg. However, severe cases may require the help of diuretics. Compression stockings are advised in some chronic cases to increase blood circulation.

33. Classification of Ulcer on the Basis of Depth

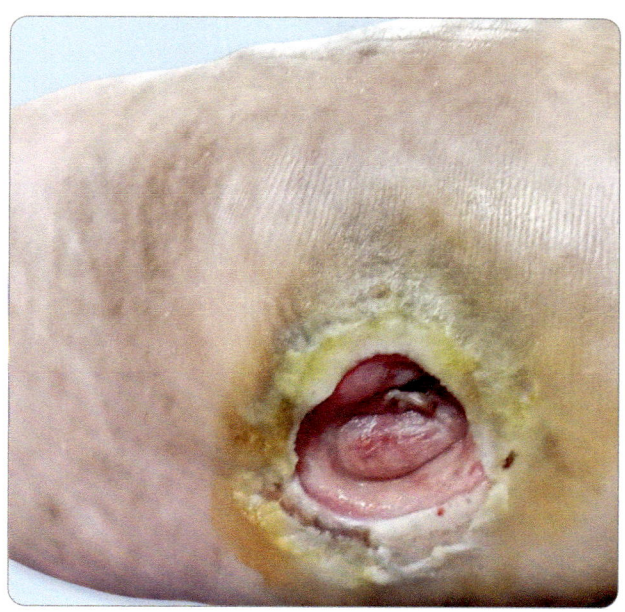

Wagner's classification of diabetic foot ulcers:
The depth of the ulcer, gangrene, or osteomyelitis in a patient can be assessed by using Wagner's system of classification for DFUs. It is a very simple system and has six grades (grades 0–5). The first three grades are related to the depth of the ulcer. Grade 3 shows bone involvement and grades 4 and 5 show the extent of gangrene (partial or complete).

34. Negative Pressure Wound Therapy

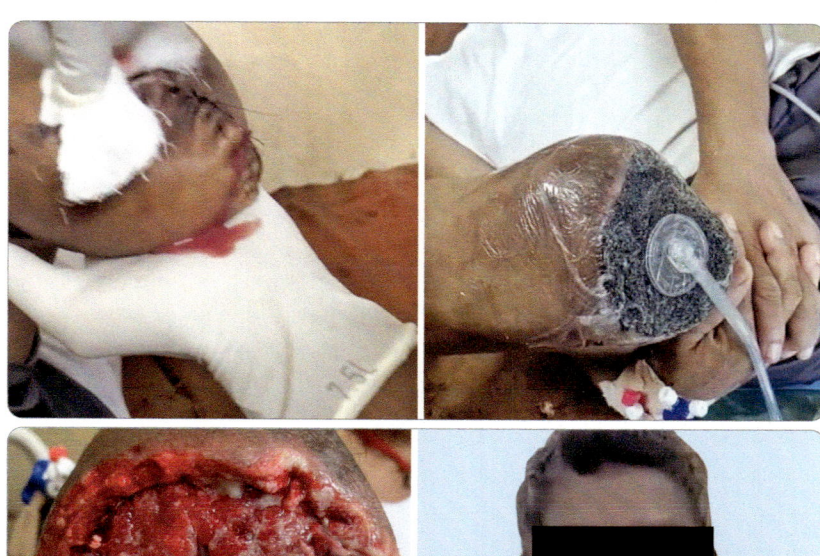

This wound therapy which is used to treat both chronic and complex foot ulcers in diabetes is otherwise called vacuum-assisted closure (VAC). This assists in wound drainage and also promotes granulation tissue formation as well as blood circulation. When other systems fail, this therapy helps in the removal of bacterial products, reduction of swelling, and closure of wounds.

This picture (on the top right) shows how negative pressure when applied with an air-tight adhesive covers the wound can promote granulation tissue formation and thereby assist in the postoperative management of DFUs (bottom left).

35. Hyperbaric Oxygen Therapy

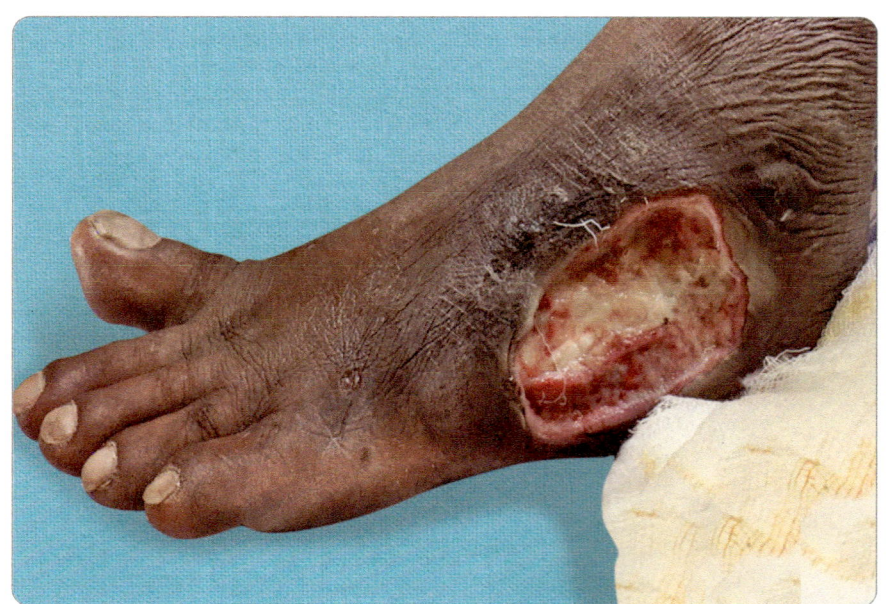

Hyperbaric oxygen therapy (HBOT) is used for the treatment of complex DFUs. In chronic wound infections, the tissue becomes hypoxic due to decreased oxygen supply, which hinders the healing process. In this therapy, the patient is subjected to 100% oxygen at higher atmospheric pressure. HBOT enhances the rate of ulcer healing by promoting the formation of new blood vessels and thereby helps to decrease amputations.

36. SINBAD Classification

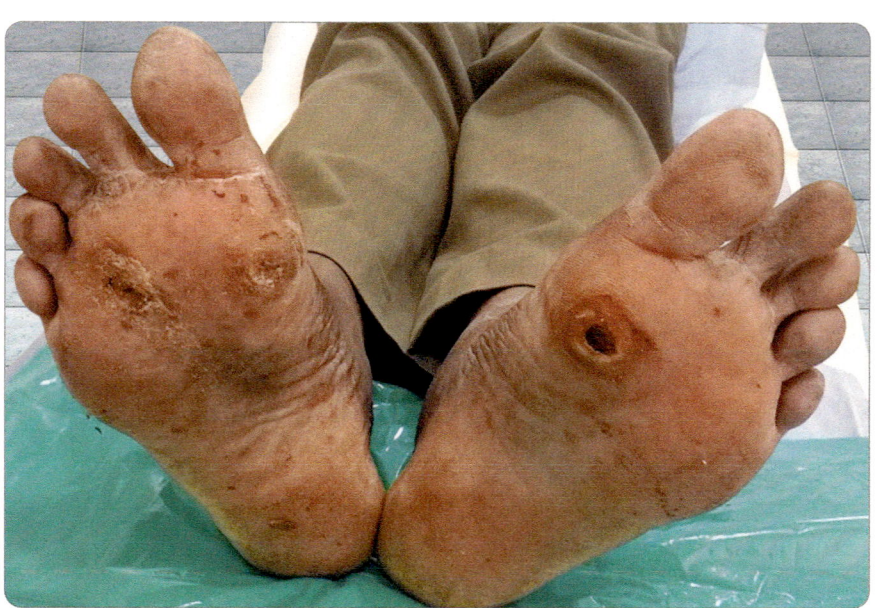

A simple classification that analyses the Site, Ischemia, Neuropathy, Bacterial Infection, Area, as well as Depth of Diabetic foot ulcer is called the SINBAD classification. This system uses a binary method (0 indicates absent and 1 indicates present) with six essential criteria for examination of the foot ulcer. The simplicity of the system enables it to predict the healing time.

37. Dry Skin

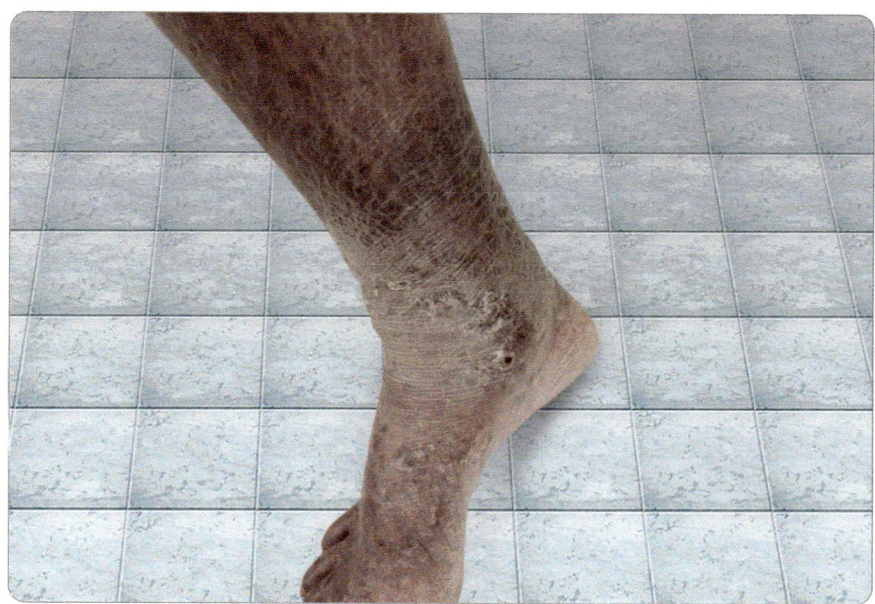

Dry and itchy skin can occur in people having diabetes due to neuropathy. In diabetic neuropathy, the body loses its ability to control moisture. This, in turn, poses a major problem as it causes bacteria to enter the bloodstream through the open cracks and fissures, which consequently ends up in infection.

38. Onychauxis

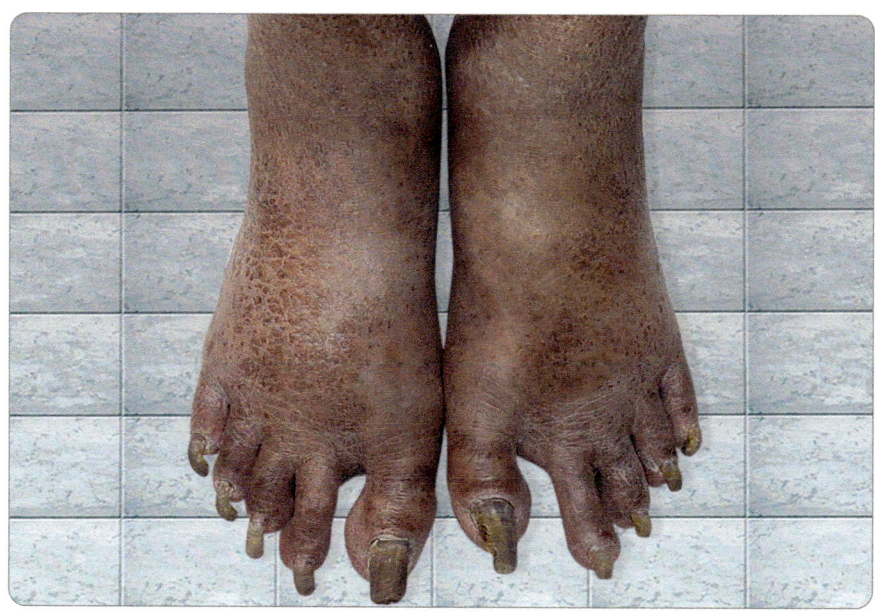

Any thickening, overgrowth, or discolorization of nails can lead to onychauxis. Some of the causes which can lead to onychauxis are age, fungal infection, trauma causing alterations to the nail bed, and systemic conditions such as diabetes, psoriasis, cancer, and rheumatoid arthritis. Trimming or filing of nails and wearing appropriate footwear are recommended to prevent this condition.

39. Wet Gangrene

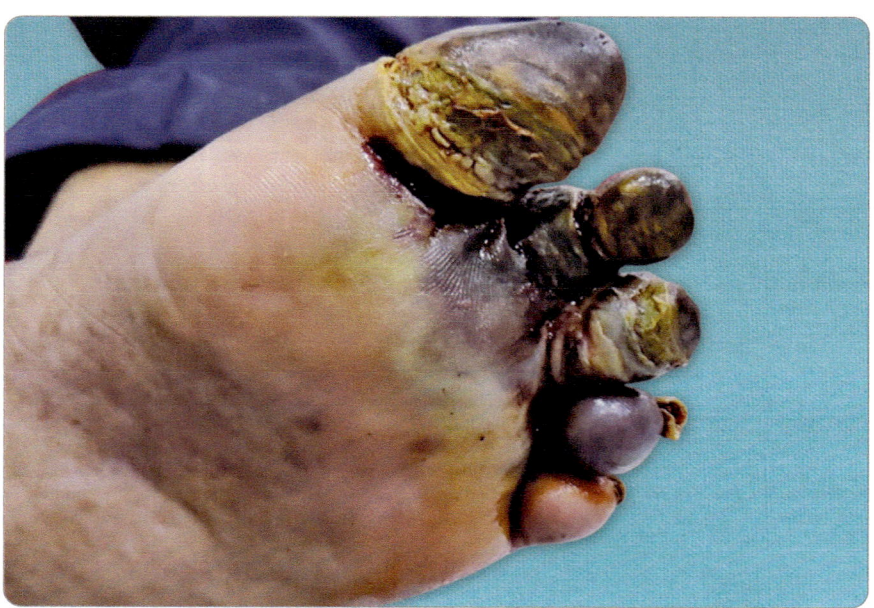

Wet gangrenes are common in diabetes due to trauma and the subsequent infection spreads rapidly if not treated adequately. Symptoms include swelling, discharge, and the development of blisters and the tissue becomes necrotic because of improper blood supply or infection. The ideal recommended treatment of choice remains surgical debridement along with glycemic control supplemented with analgesics and antibiotics, if necessary.

40. Body and Mind

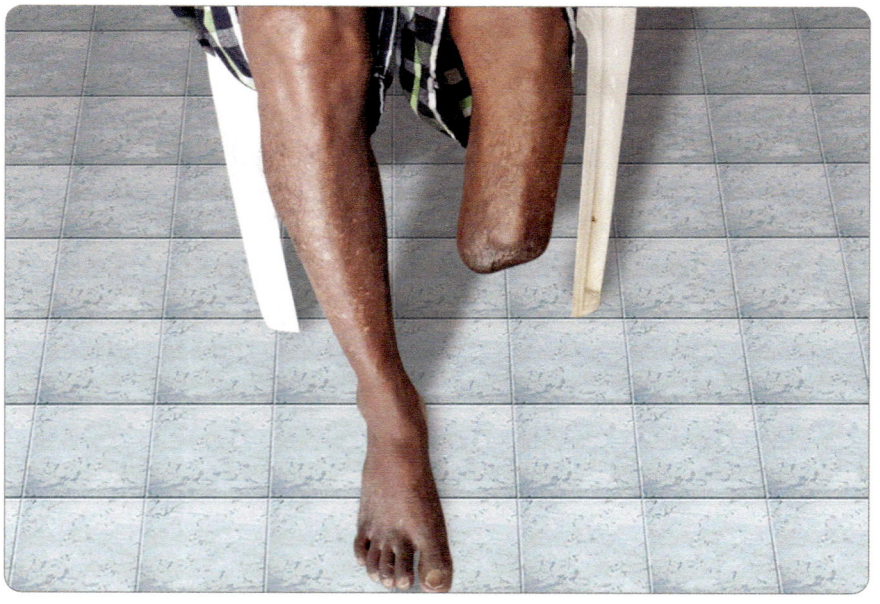

Rehabilitation of both the body and the mind gains paramount importance in restoring the normal physical and mental health of the patient. An amputation can psychologically affect a person because it can lead to symptoms of depression and anxiety and can even cause suicidal tendencies.

Successful rehabilitation requires appropriate management of pain, exercises for muscle strength, re-establish the lost function to an extent with the help of a prosthesis, and educating the patient's family encouraging them to provide emotional support.

41. Offloading for Charcot Foot

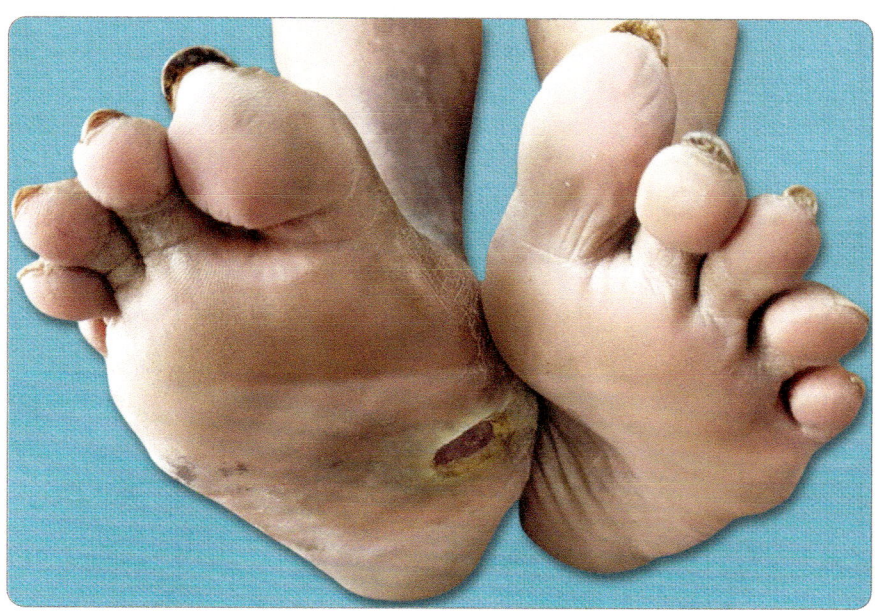

Charcot arthropathy is a rather serious complication of diabetic foot affecting the bones, soft tissues, and joints caused due to neuropathy wherein the patient is unable to perceive injuries resulting in consequential deformities.

Charcot restraint orthotic walker (CROW) and *pneumatic walker* are some of the common offloading methods used for the treatment of Charcot foot. CROW is an effective Charcot offloading device used to prevent the development of foot ulcers and reduce pain. A pneumatic walker can be described as a boot that restricts the movement of the foot during walking, thereby increasing blood circulation and decreasing friction.

42. Biofilm

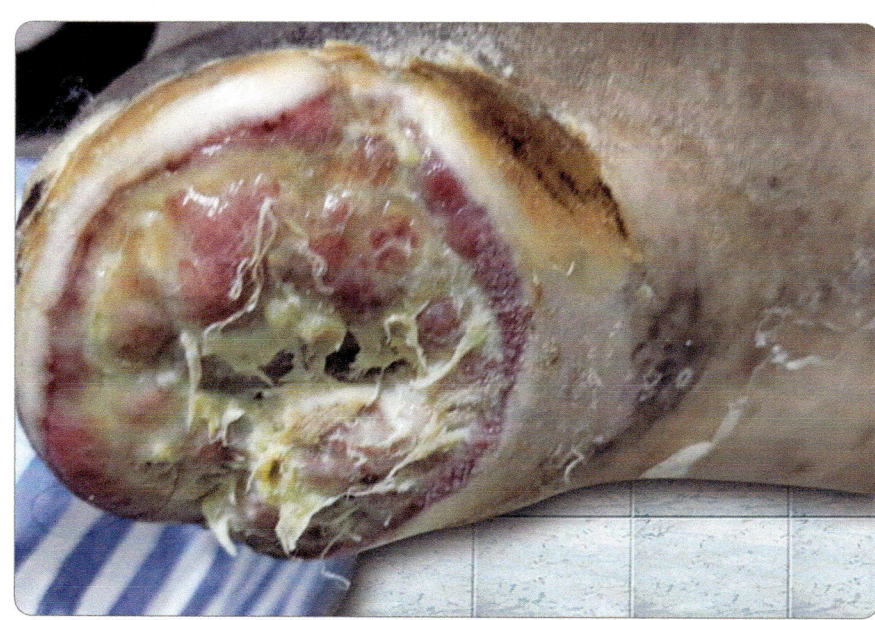

When microbial cells are implanted in a matrix composed of extracellular polymeric substance (EPS), which is made of nucleic acids, lipids, polysaccharides, and proteins, the bacteria adhere to either the biotic or abiotic surfaces, which is called biofilm. These biofilms are present in both acute and chronic wounds giving mechanical protection to bacteria, thereby preventing the percolation of antimicrobial agents into them. Recurrent infections occur in biofilm infections because the immune response of the host becomes weakened. Biopsy of tissues is the ideal recommended method to expose the biofilm and sharp debridement is the treatment of choice advocated to remove the biofilm.

43. Slough

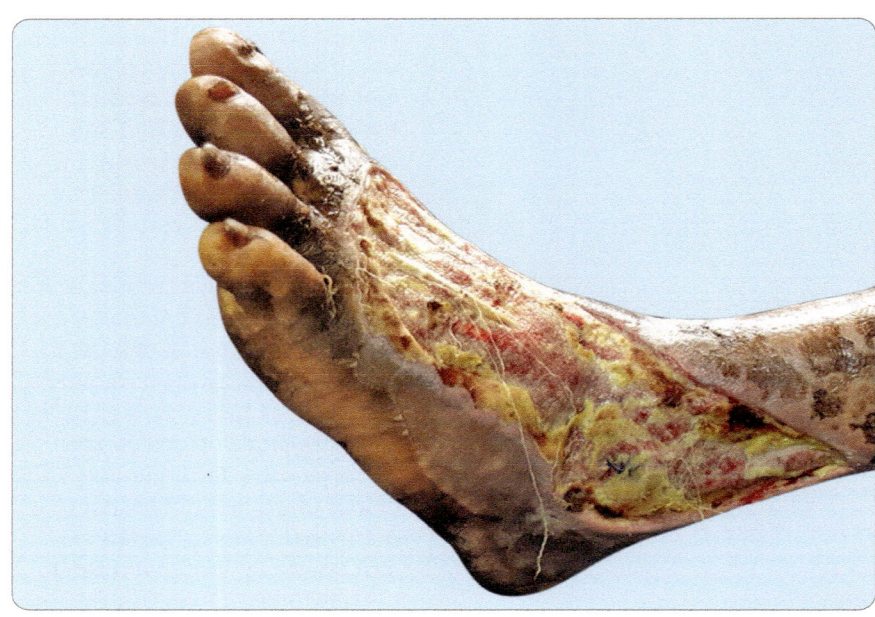

Wound healing produces slough, which consists of fibrin, microbes, living and dead cells, and white blood cells. This yellow, fibrinous material covers the wound completely making it strenuous for surgeons to gain accessibility to the wound, thereby delaying the process of wound healing. Removal of the slough is accomplished by autolytic, conservative, or surgical methods of debridement.

44. Granulation Tissue

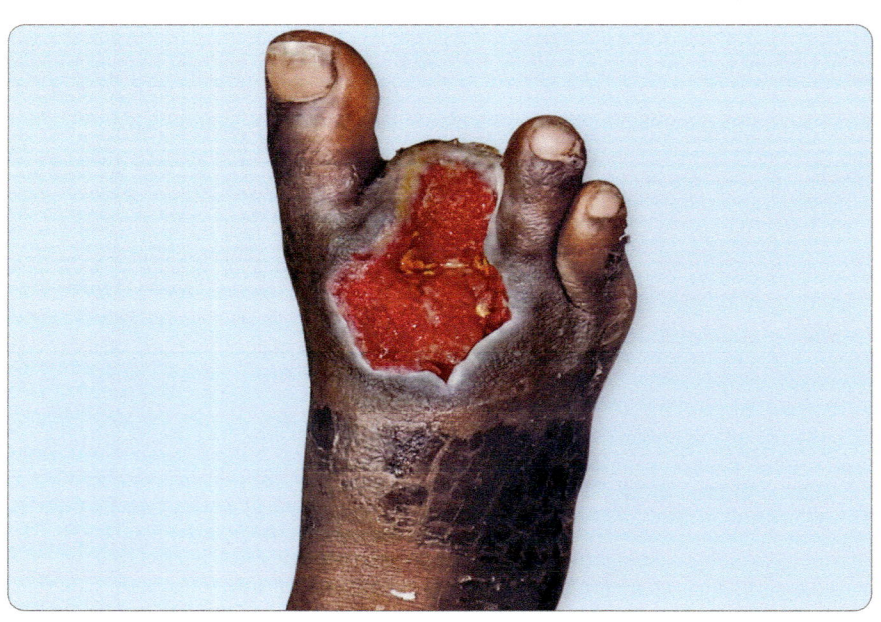

Healing of wounds occurs either by primary or secondary intention. The presence of healthy granulation tissue is suggestive of good wound healing. It is painless, appears pink to red, and is also soft when palpated.

45. Importance of Vascular Assessment

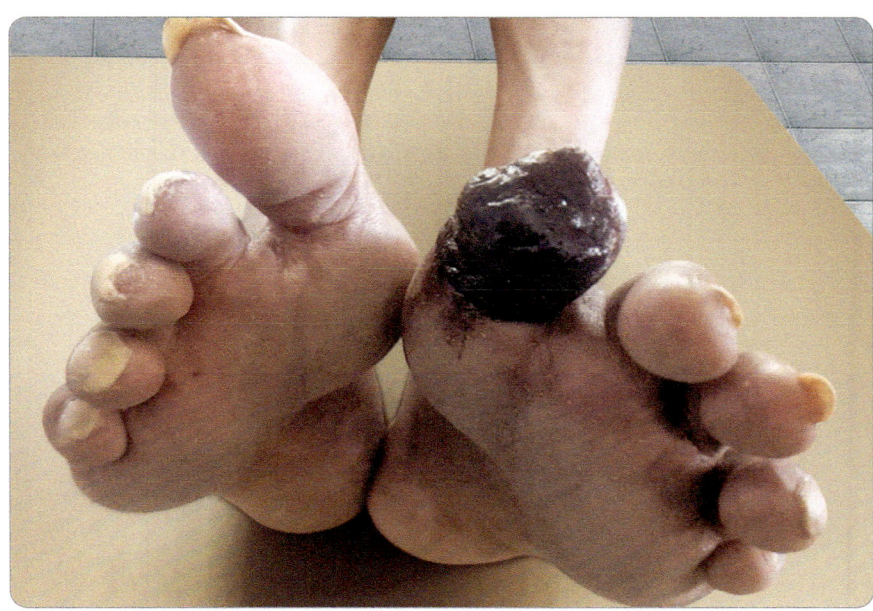

It is imperative to understand that assessment of vascular status is very important in patients with foot ulcers, infection, or necrosis associated with diabetes. ABPI, MR angiogram, and arterial color Doppler are the various methods that can be used for vascular assessment. It helps us to identify patients with either normal or improper circulation that can decide the treatment of choice. The ideal recommended procedure of choice for those with normal circulation appears to be surgical debridement or stabilization of bone. Similarly, if amputation is to be avoided revascularization is ideally advocated. Digital subtraction is one of the recent methods, which helps us to acquire excellent image quality of the microvessels.

46. Skin Grafts

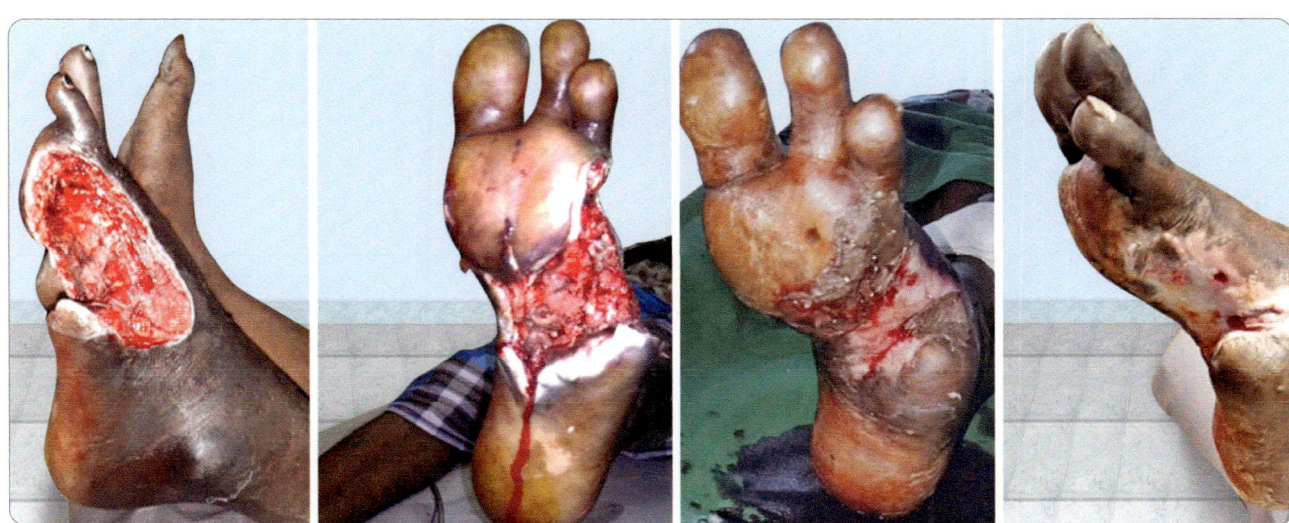

In diabetes, reconstruction of the lost skin can be replaced with the help of skin grafts because the wound sometimes remains open for a longer time in spite of adequate treatment. The skin that is to be replaced is best placed on the wound bed to ensure appropriate contact between the graft and the wound bed. An appropriate dressing has to be placed over the donor as well as the recipient site to prevent any possible infection.

47. Necrotizing Fasciitis

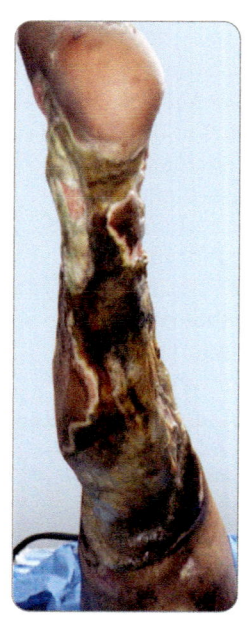

It is a rare, inflammatory disease that occurs when bacteria breach the skin and enters the body. People with a decreased immunity are at a higher risk of developing this condition, which is also known as flesh-eating disease. The patient experiences severe pain, ulcers, fever, and other signs of infection. Prompt diagnosis is necessary because this disease can cause rapid destruction of tissues. Antibiotics as well as early and aggressive surgery remain the treatment of choice to prevent complications.

48. Toenail Injury

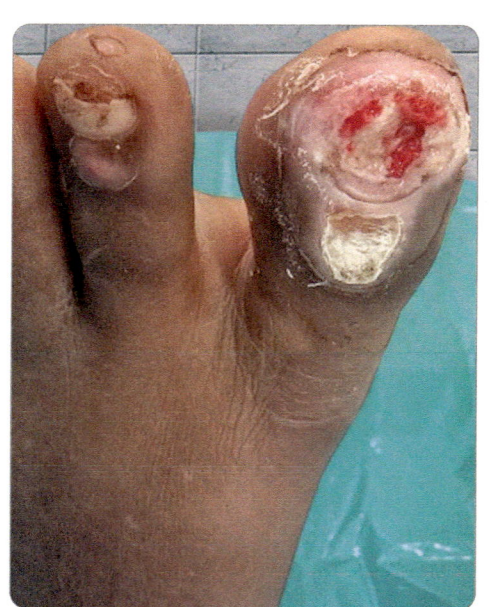

Toenail injuries occur due to injury to the toenails during physical activities, sports, or accidents. Patients may develop subungual hematoma when the blood collects under the injured toenails. Treatment depends upon the intensity of the pain. Conservative treatment like trimming or filing of broken nails and changing the dressing of the wound regularly is advised when the patient does not experience pain. In severe cases, complete drainage of the wound and surgical removal of the toenail is advised.

49. Osteomyelitis

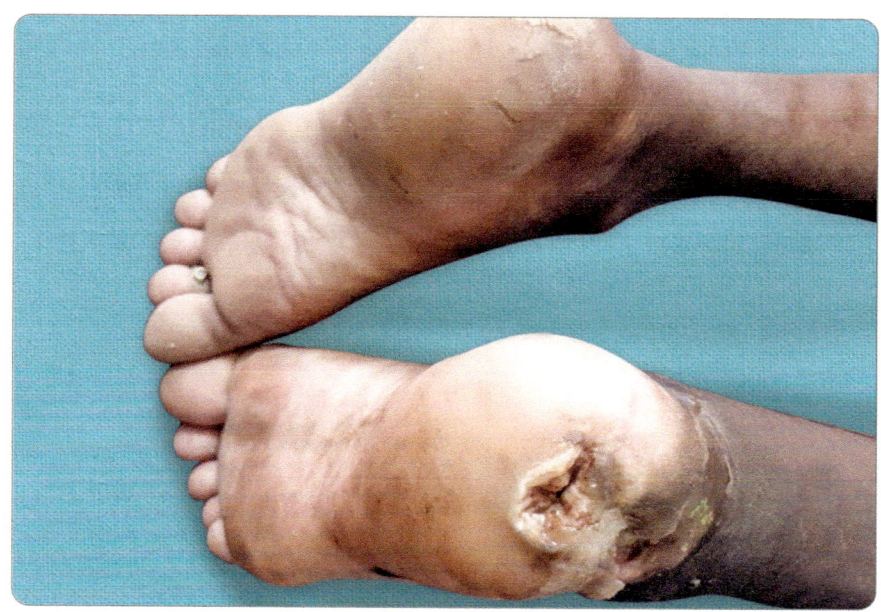

When any soft tissue infection spreads into the bone in a person with a DFU, one should suspect osteomyelitis. The forefoot has a 90% risk of getting affected by osteomyelitis followed by mid-foot and hind-foot (5% each). The probe-to-bone test (PTB) and depth of the ulcer are considered two important criteria for the diagnosis of osteomyelitis. However, the gold standard for diagnosis is always the bone biopsy test. Antibiotics and aggressive surgery remain the first line of treatment after early diagnosis to prevent any risk of amputations.

50. Eczema

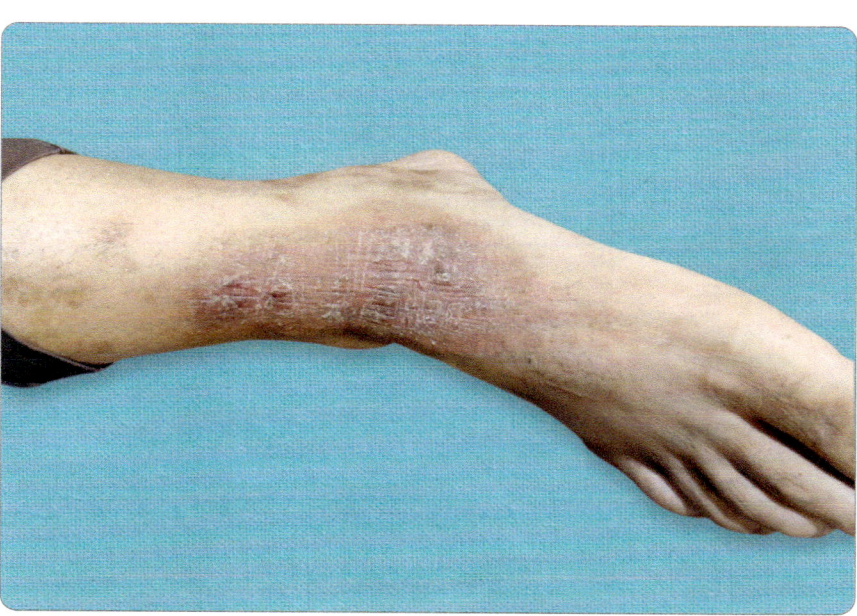

Eczema is a skin disease characterized by inflammation of the skin along with the development of blisters and itchiness. The patient can develop contact dermatitis, stasis dermatitis, or dyshidrotic eczema. The most common type appears to be contact dermatitis, which is present on the dorsum of the feet. Dyshidrotic eczema can occur either on the plantar surface of the feet or between the toes. Eliminating the allergen and use of topical steroids are the ideal recommended treatment of choice for eczema.

51. Cracked Heels

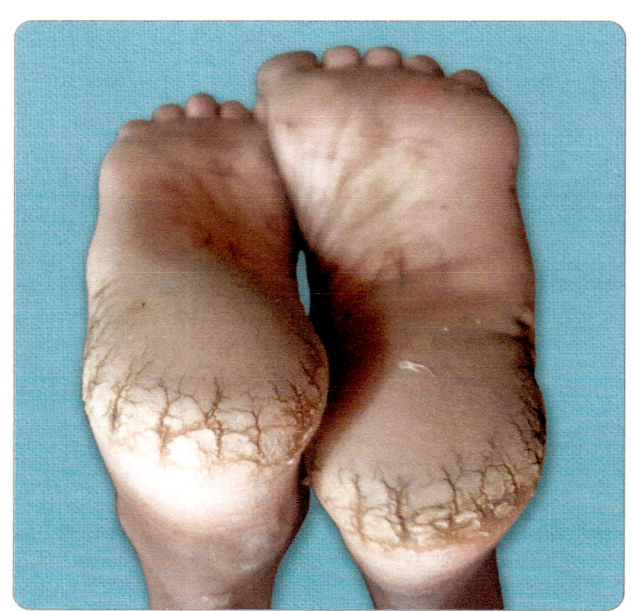

This picture shows dry and cracked heels, which occur because of damage to sweating nerves in diabetes (autonomic neuropathy). This condition occurs due to lack of sweating. This can be prevented by applying a moisturizing cream after a bath. Wearing appropriate shoes also help because cracked heels, if left untreated can result in infection.

52. Amputation of Foot

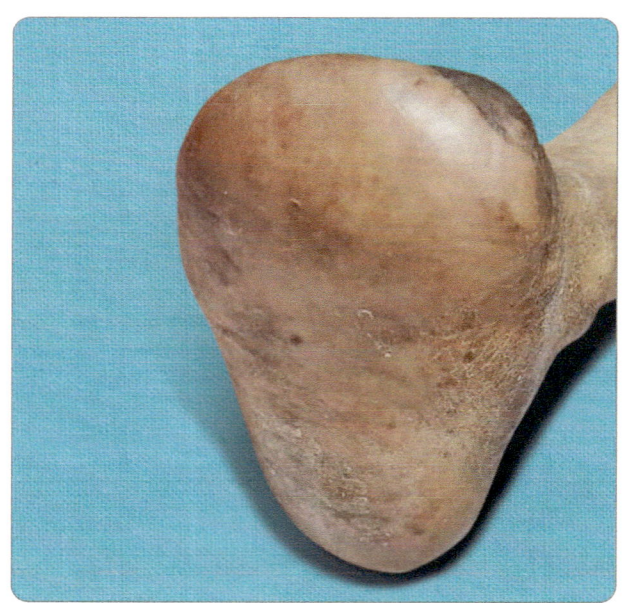

Amputation of the foot is often done when there is an infection of the forefoot/toes. If vascularity is reduced, revascularization should be done before amputation. At times, amputation of the foot may be possible instead of below-knee amputation.

Common Diabetic Foot Problems Encountered 139

53. Bilateral Great Toe Amputee

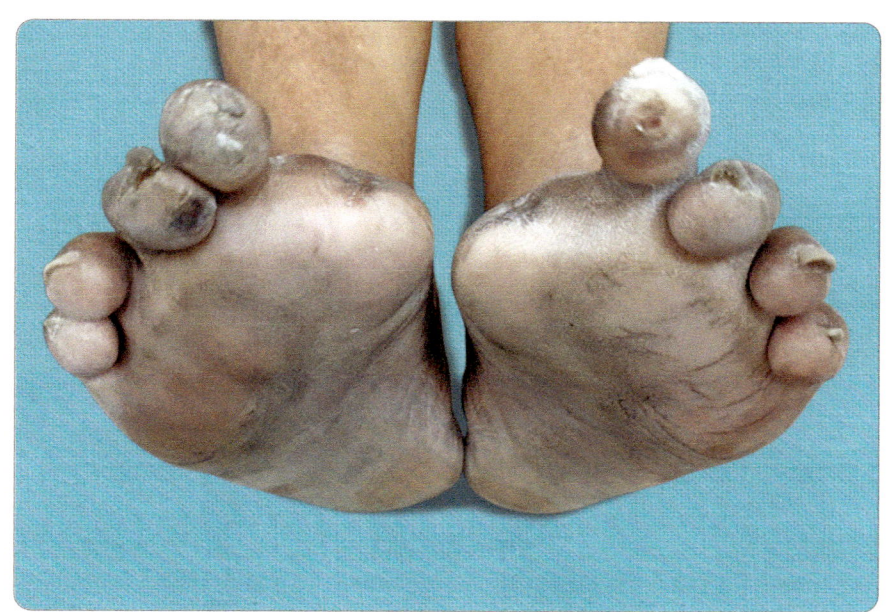

This photograph shows bilateral great toe amputation with an ulcer in the second toe on the left foot and the second and third toes on the right foot. X-ray of both feet is necessary to find out the extent of bone involvement and ankle–brachial index is necessary to find out if there is adequate blood supply for both feet.

54. Maceration of Feet Due to Keeping the Feet Wet for a Long Time

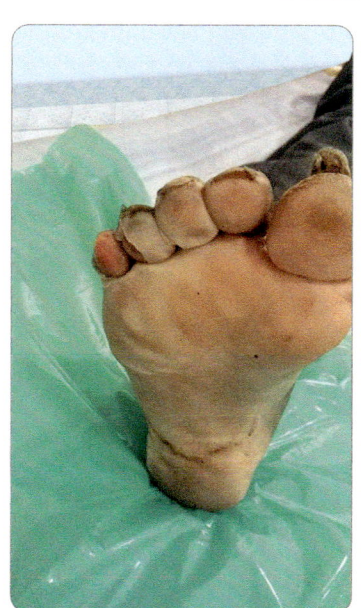

In diabetes, one should avoid keeping the feet wet for a long time due to maceration, especially if there are insensate feet. When the skin becomes moist, it becomes soft and breaks down leading to maceration of the feet. This, in turn, is considered a potential reason for the invasion of microorganisms.

55. After Removing the Macerated Skin

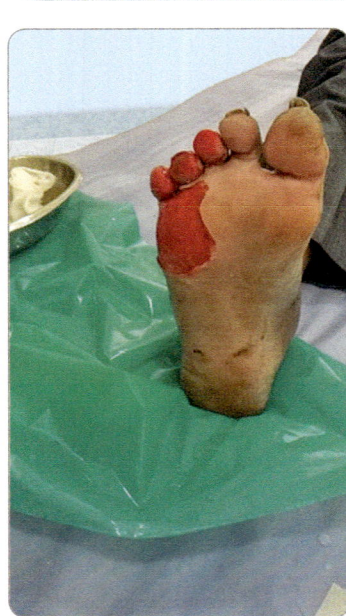

Adequate removal of macerated skin is often recommended. If left untreated, macerated skin can pave way for microbial invasion and infection. This, in turn, can cause pain and delayed wound healing.

56. Angiosome

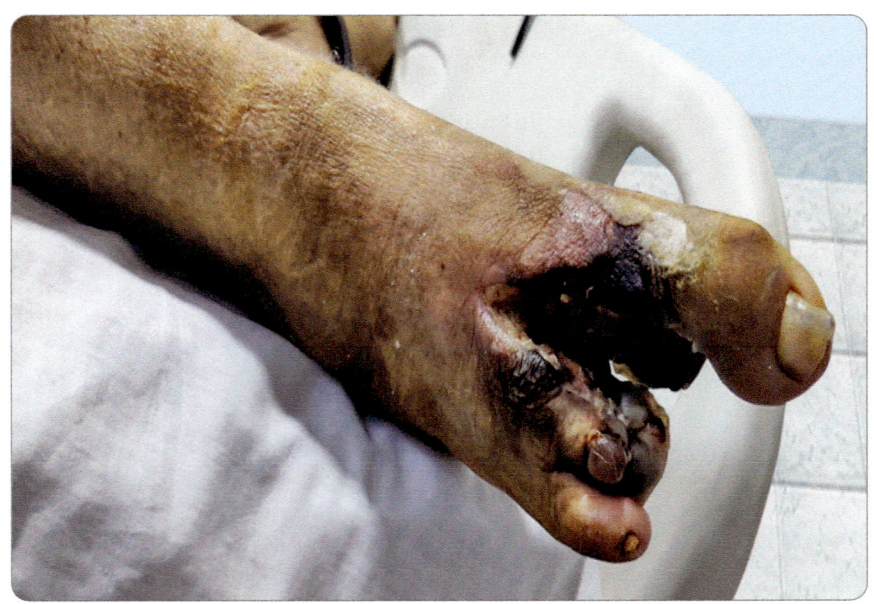

This picture shows a wound in the area of the dorsalis pedis artery. There is a need to reestablish circulation to ensure adequate wound healing. In any gangrenous wound, revascularization of the source artery can reduce the healing period as well as decrease the rate of amputations.

Common Diabetic Foot Problems Encountered   141

57. Partial Gangrene of the Toe

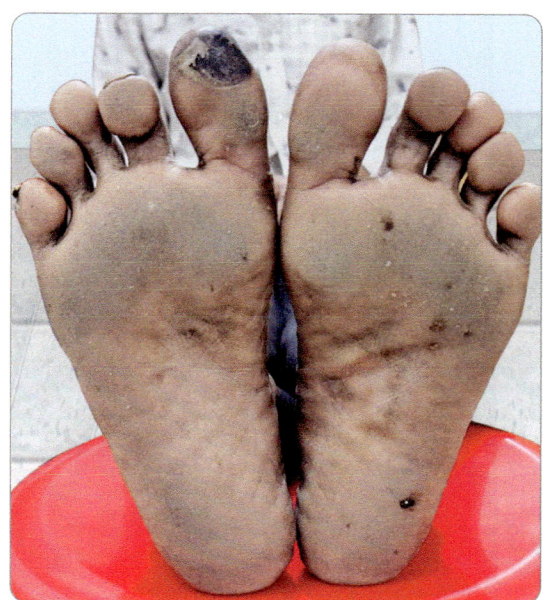

This picture shows partial gangrene of the toe. The blood supply should be ascertained by an ankle–brachial index/color Doppler/digital subtraction angiography. The decision to amputate the toe can be taken only after that. Once peripheral arterial disease is excluded, it could be a neuropathic wound due to barefoot walking.

58. Cellulitis of Left Leg

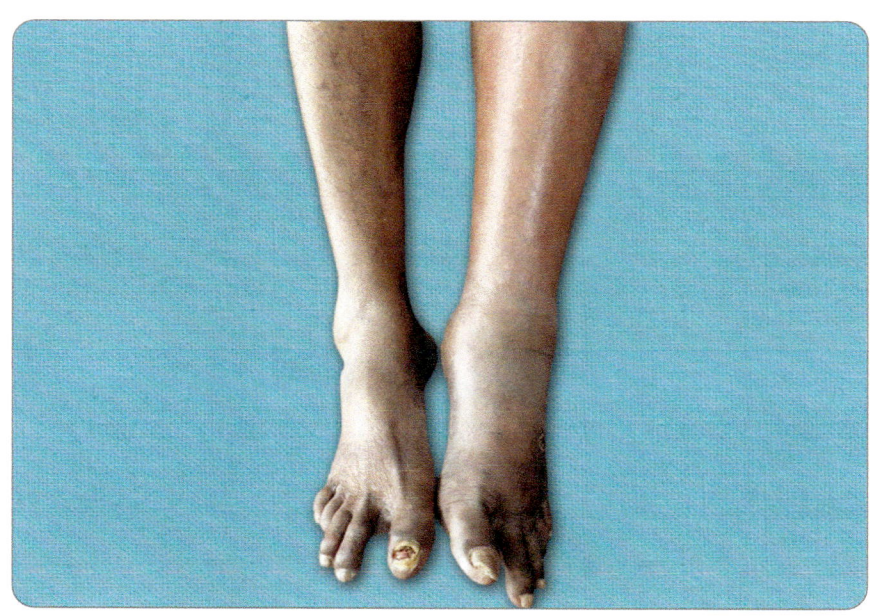

Cellulitis is a condition characterized by infection of the deep layers of skin and presents with swelling, redness, and pain in the affected area. A thorough clinical history and local examination are essential for a diagnosis of cellulitis. Treatment requires the use of the most appropriate antibiotics based on the severity of the infection.

59. Recurrent Pressure Ulcers

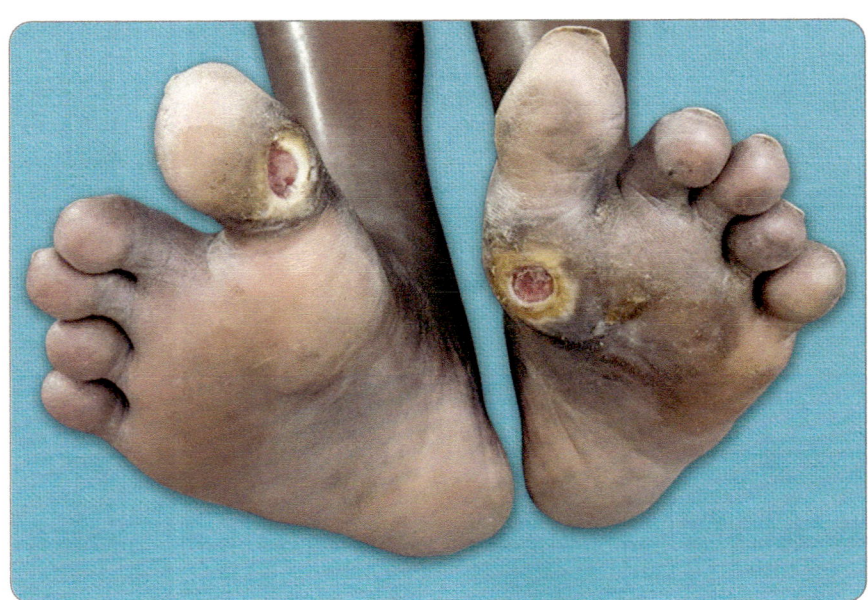

Recurrent pressure ulcers occur due to walking barefoot, which is a common practice seen in India. The use of inappropriate footwear is also considered one of the major reasons for these pressure ulcers. The reason for the occurrence of pressure ulcers could be attributed to neuropathy and poor blood circulation seen in people living with diabetes. This can be easily avoided by using proper footwear while walking.

60. Self-treated Callus

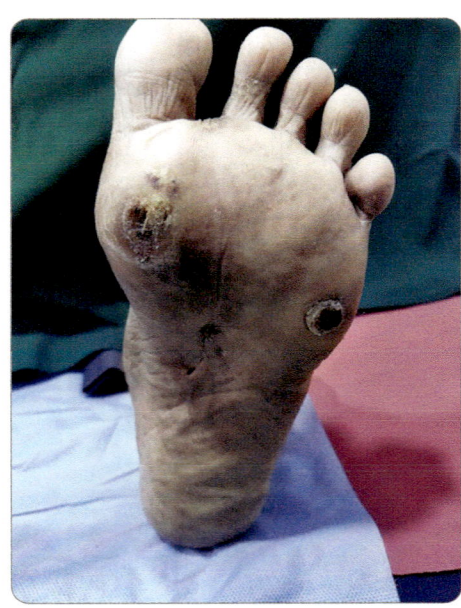

Callus is a thick, hard covering over the skin that develops in response to persistent pressure. This is a case of self-treated callus where the local application of turmeric paste is visible over the medial and lateral aspects of the diabetic foot. The margin of the callus has been removed and now it is with a visible thick hardcover prevalent in the center.

61. Abscess in the Right Leg with Typical Neuropathic Feet

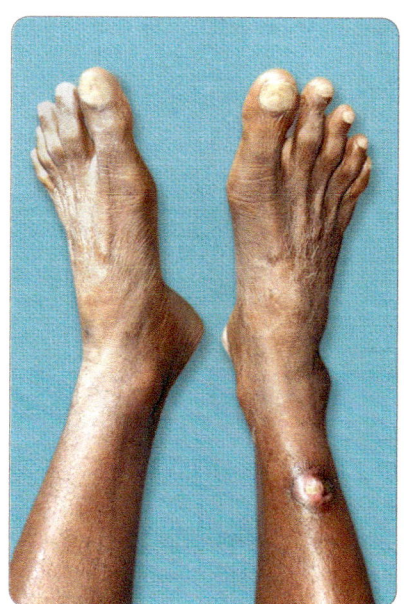

The abscess is surrounded by cellulitis and has to be dealt with surgically if needed. Proper foot examination must be taught to the patient.

62. Hammer Toes

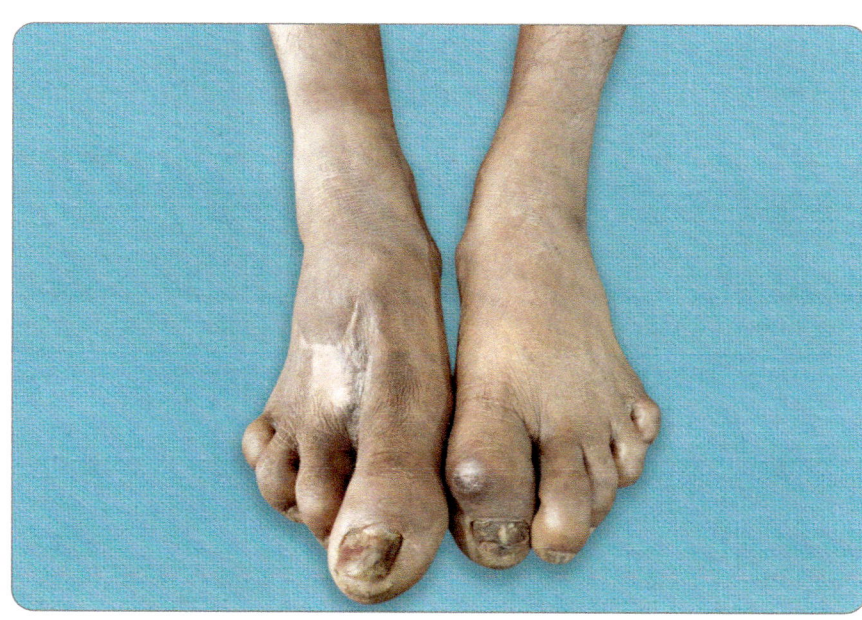

The most important reason for hammer toes in diabetes appears to be the use of inappropriate footwear. Narrow, short, ill-fitting shoes are considered to be a major cause of the development of hammer toes. They can be surgically corrected. Corrective surgeries are considered the treatment of choice in cases of recurrent ulcers and when conservative treatment fails.

63. Unilateral Pedal Edema

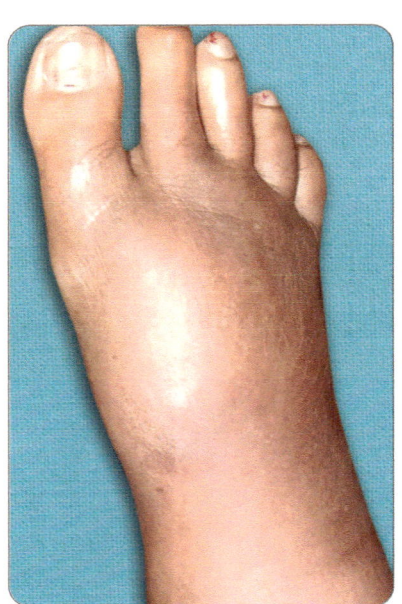

The etiology could be Charcot foot, chronic venous insufficiency, cellulitis, etc. The management will depend upon etiology.

64. Diabetic Dermopathy

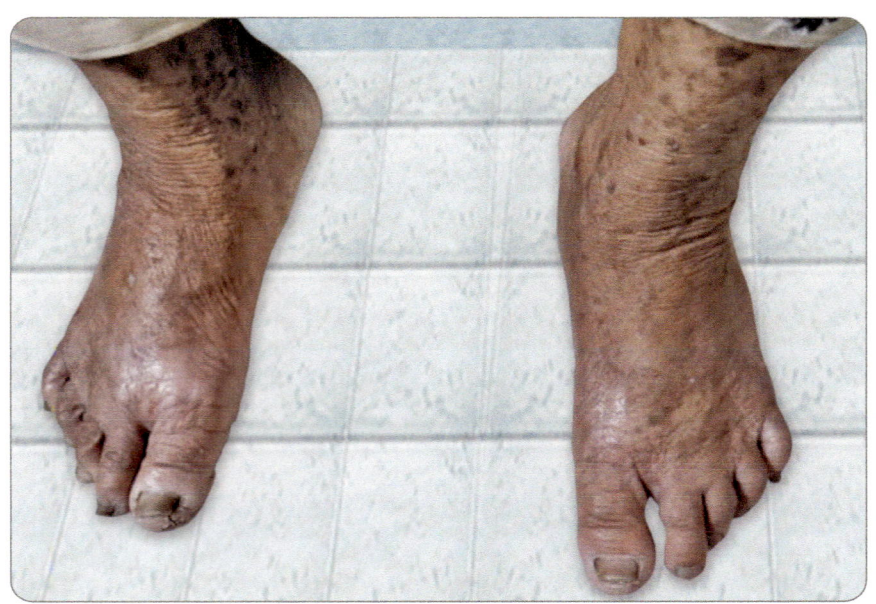

Diabetes can induce changes in microvessels, which can cause skin problems. This is called as "diabetic dermopathy." In such cases, the skin becomes light brown with oval or circular patches. This condition is considered harmless and usually does not require any treatment. Proper foot care advice should be given.

65. Diabetic Foot Infection

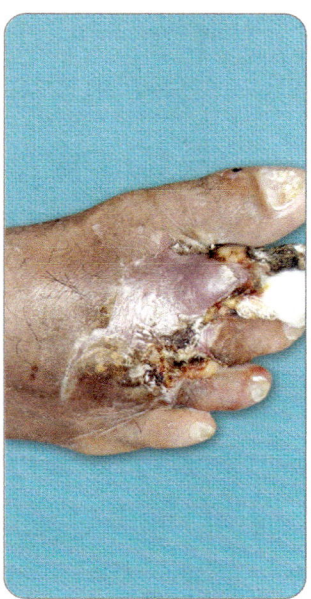

A radiograph of the foot is needed to rule out bone involvement. Evaluation of the foot for peripheral arterial disease is necessary. This type of lesion needs active surgical debridement and antibiotics.

66. Prick Injury

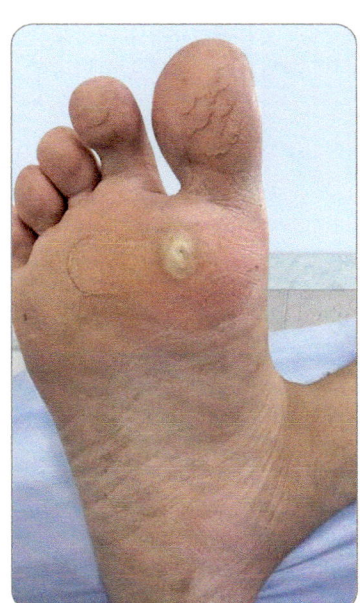

Diabetic neuropathy damages the nerves in the feet, which can cause loss of sensation. This is a case of prick injury where the patient is not able to perceive the injury due to diabetic neuropathy, which when left untreated can result in infection. Proper foot examination should be advised for people with diabetic peripheral neuropathy.

67. Callus Debridement

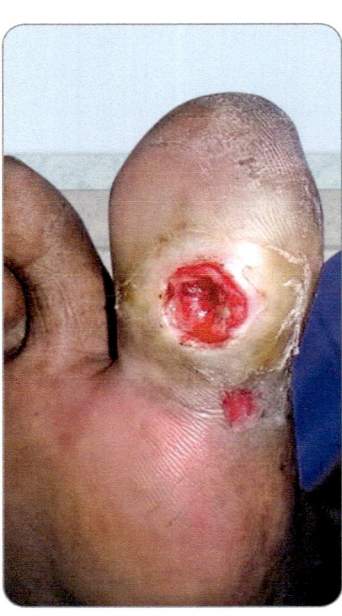

Callus develops on pressure points in diabetes due to the practice of walking barefoot or without appropriate footwear. Callus debridement usually requires the surgical removal of all the thick and dead tissue completely followed by proper dressing and offloading. An X-ray of the foot is needed to rule out bone involvement. Proper foot examination should be advised.

68. Callus in the Forefoot

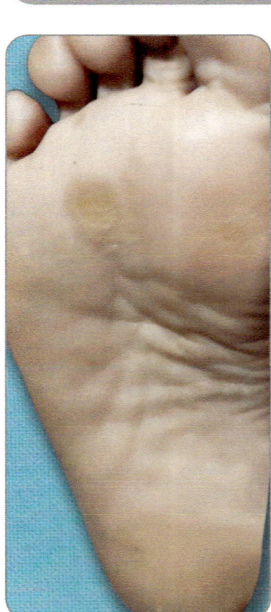

The callus is usually seen in the first metatarsophalangeal joint. However, the pressure points may vary depending on gait. One should not forget the use of proper footwear in preventing these conditions.

69. Wound with Healthy Granulation Tissue

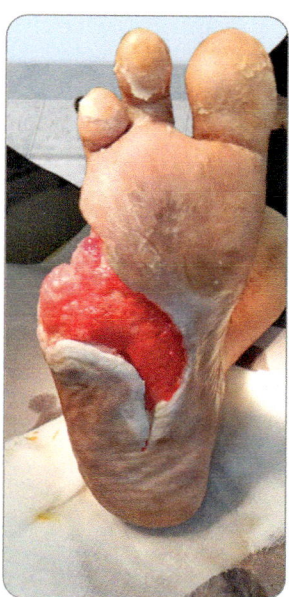

This picture shows a large wound with healthy granulation tissue with the loss of the last two toes. Negative pressure wound therapy which is also known as vacuum-assisted closure can help us in reducing the swelling as well as the size of the wound.

70. Diabetic Foot Ulcer in the Heel Region—Heel Wounds are Difficult to Heal

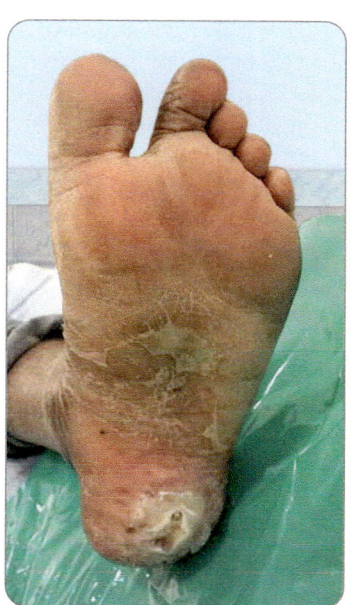

This picture shows a foot ulcer in the heel region of a patient with diabetes. The skin surrounding the ulcer looks macerated. This occurs when the area is exposed to moisture for a long time. Maceration of the skin can retard the healing of the wound and can make the skin more vulnerable to infection. The macerated skin feels soft and also appears lighter in color.

71. Sausage Toe/Dactylitis

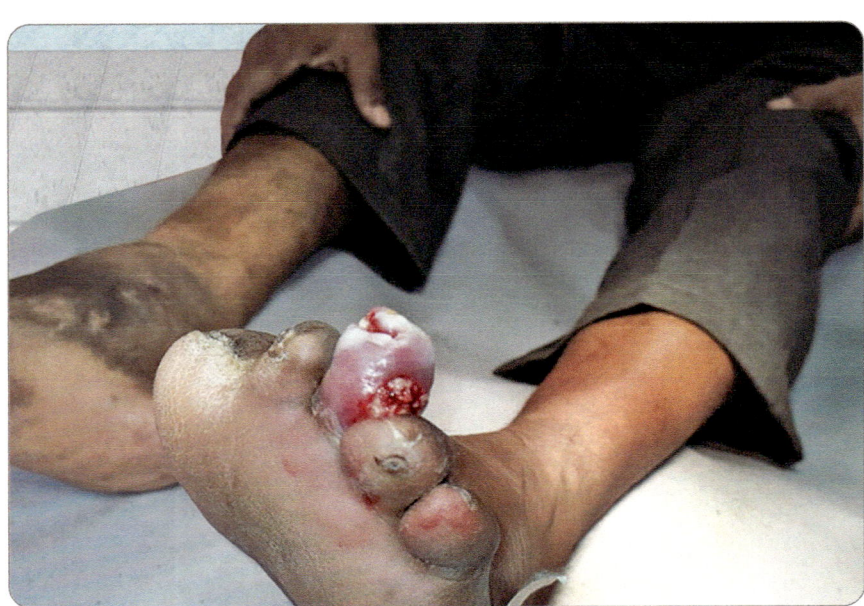

Dactylitis is a condition in which toes become red, swollen, and painful giving the appearance of sausage. Hence, it is otherwise called as "sausage toes." In patients with diabetic neuropathy, this clinical presentation of a swollen, red toe is highly suspicious of osteomyelitis. This can cause difficulty in walking. Diagnosis is by taking an X-ray and removing the infected bone and offloading.

72. Amputation of Second, Third, and Fourth Toes on the Right Foot

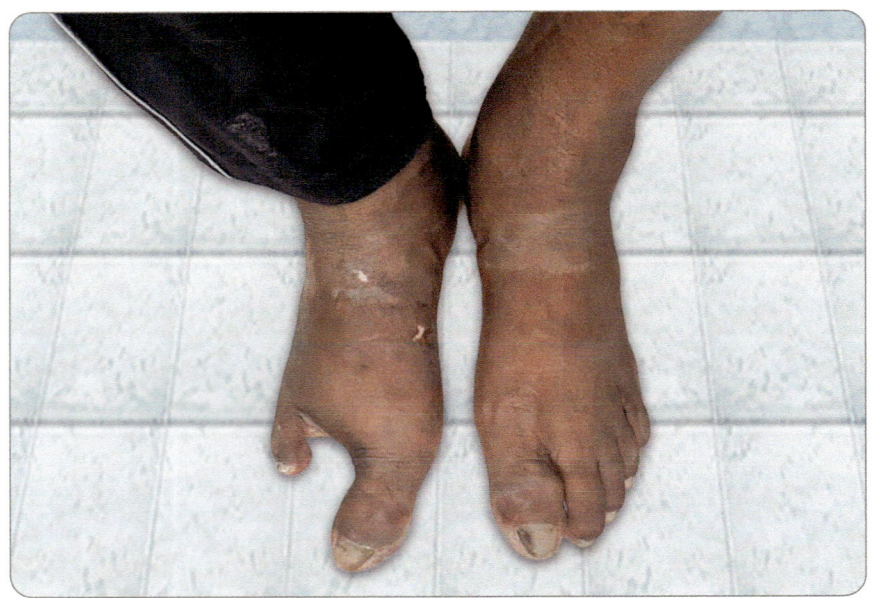

Amputation could have been the result of a diabetic foot infection, which has been treated well leaving only two toes on the right foot. It is important to plan proper offloading due to changes in the biomechanics of the right foot. The contralateral foot is also susceptible to amputation due to neuropathy ± peripheral arterial disease.

73. Loss of Skin Elasticity in Autonomic Neuropathy

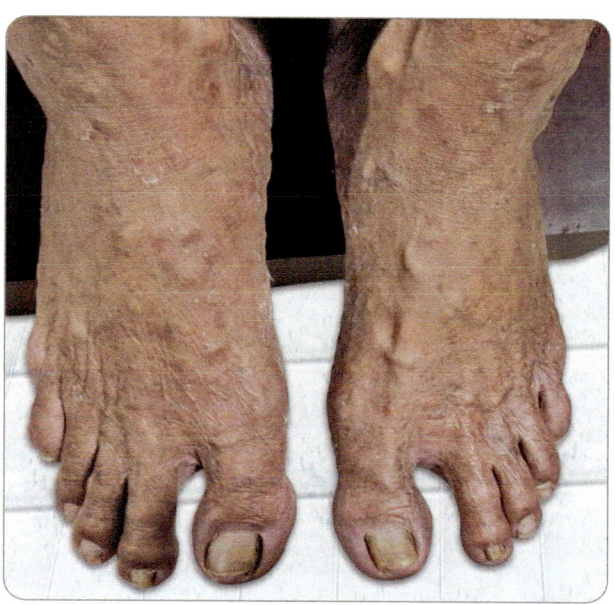

Autonomic neuropathy is very commonly seen in people living with diabetes. It is characterized by dry, flaky skin due to a decrease in sweating and loss of skin elasticity, which occurs due to its inability to resist sheer pressure. Wasting of muscles is also prominently seen.

74. Diabetic Foot Ulcer on the Medial Aspect

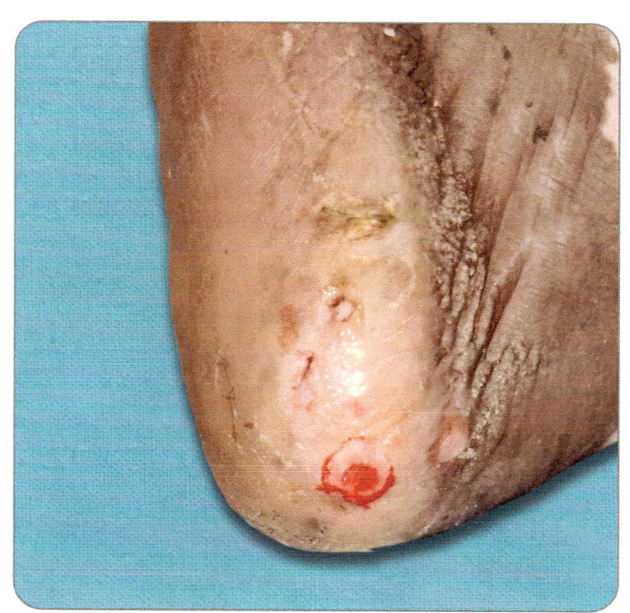

This picture shows an ulcer on the medial aspect of the foot. The surrounding skin appears dry. The underlying bone condition should be investigated and the foot should be examined for peripheral arterial disease. Treatment requires the use of antibiotics and appropriate dressing for the foot ulcer along with offloading.

75. Diabetic Ulcer in the Forefoot Region

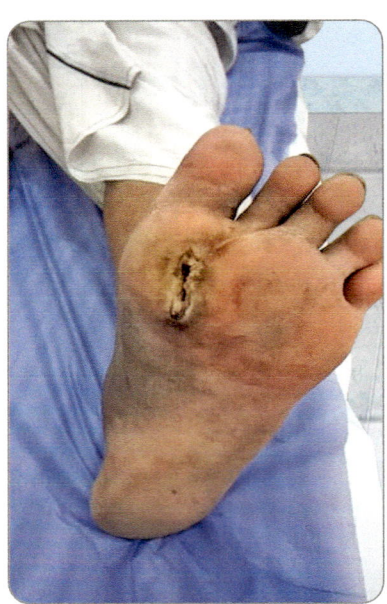

This picture shows a forefoot ulcer involving the head of the first metatarsal bone. The patient requires an assessment of neuropathy along with radiographs of the foot to rule out osteomyelitis. The vascular status of the feet should also be evaluated. Treatment requires debridement of the ulcer followed by proper offloading.

76. Foot Examination using A Biothesiometer

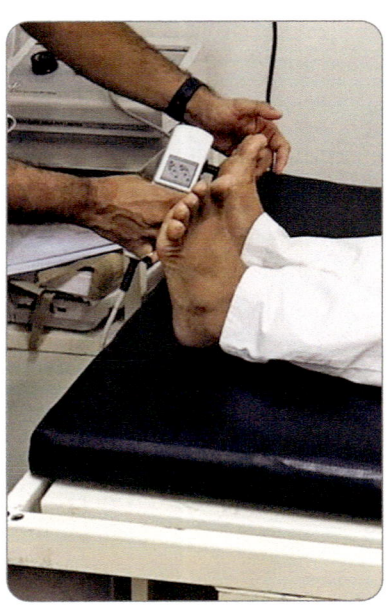

The examination of the foot can be done using a biothesiometer. It is a simple, noninvasive handheld device that can be used to measure vibration perception threshold. The strength of the vibration is gradually increased until the vibration sensation is perceived by the patient. The probe is connected to a monitor and the resultant values are recorded. If the value is more than 25 Volts, it is considered to be predictive of future ulceration.

77. Skin Lesions on the Plantar Aspect of the Foot

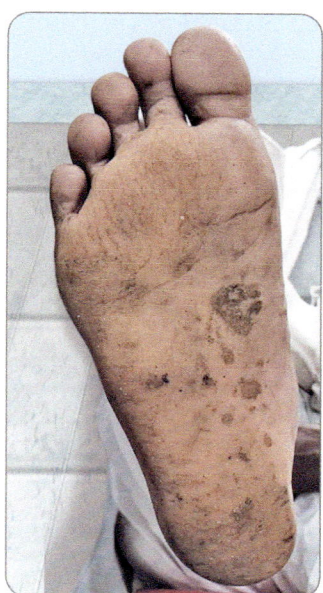

Skin lesions are very common, especially in people with diabetic peripheral neuropathy. Therefore, proper foot care is important in all people with diabetes.

78. Interdigital Infections

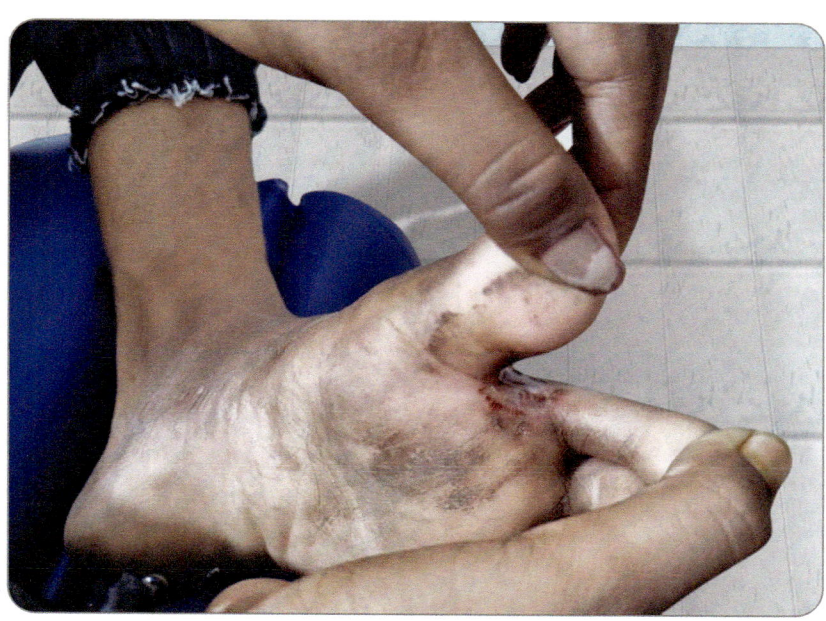

Interdigital fungal infections are very common in people with diabetes. They can cause inflammation and the development of fissures creating a break in the continuity of the epidermis of the skin of feet. This can pave way for bacterial infections. It can present clinically with redness, itching, and signs of inflammation. Toe separators which are made of silicone and placed between the toes are recommended for these patients. Good foot hygiene practices like wiping dry between the toes is therefore important.

79. Plantar Foot Ulceration in a Person with Deformities

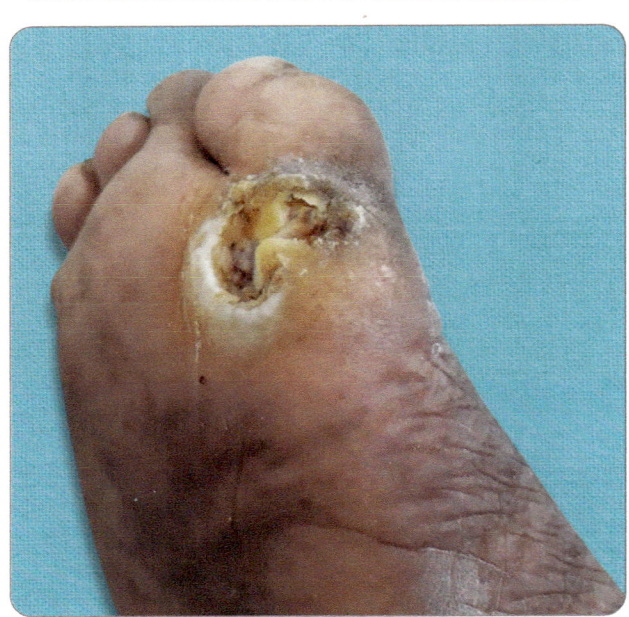

Foot deformities lead to altered biomechanics and such people need customized footwear. This ulcer needs proper offloading. Callus debridement is recommended all around the ulcer and an X-ray of the foot is required to rule out osteomyelitis.

80. Treatment of Cellulitis

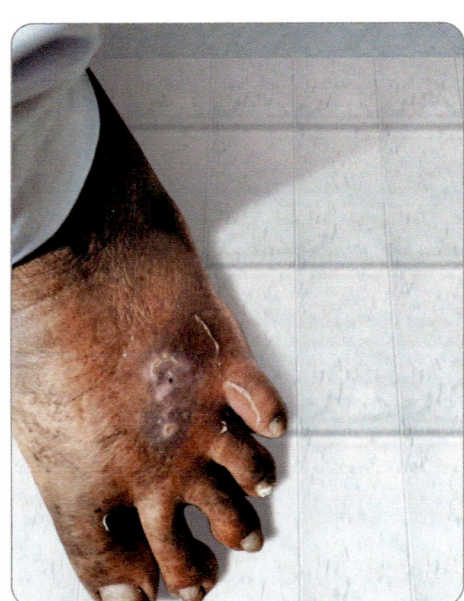

This condition is characterized by a marked swelling that is soft and tender to the touch. In some cases, it is associated with systemic symptoms like fever. Elevation of the limbs helps to reduce swelling. Treatment involves elevation of the limb and antibiotics either in oral or intravenous routes depending on the severity of the infection.

81. Importance of Foot Exercises in Diabetic Neuropathy

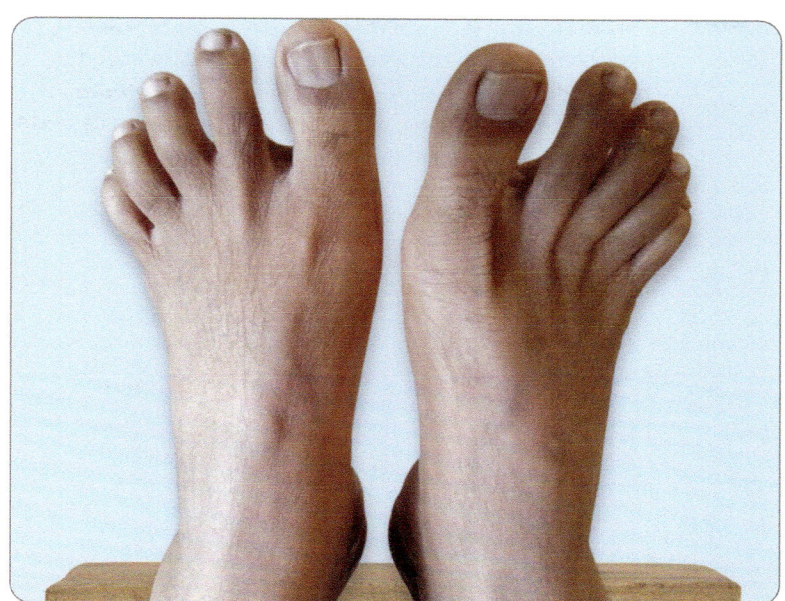

Wasting of muscles is very common in neuropathy affecting the feet. Foot muscle exercises will aid in reducing the altered biomechanics in such feet.

82. Recurrent Pressure Ulcer after Amputation

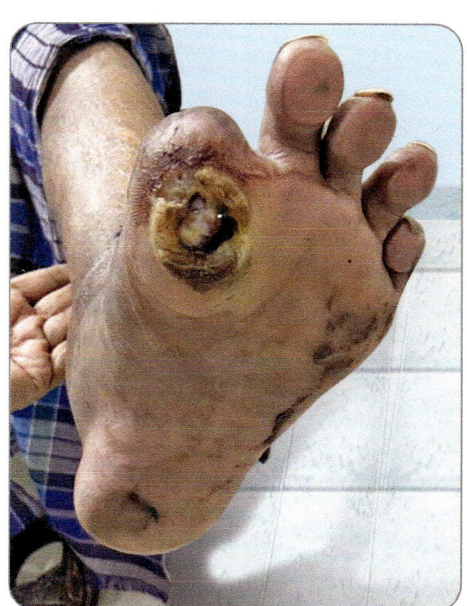

In a patient with diabetes, these pressure ulcers can be seen after amputation due to unequally distributed pressure while walking. This condition occurs either when proper offloading is not done after amputation or if the prescribed offloading footwear is not used regularly.

83. Left Foot Charcot with an Ulcer

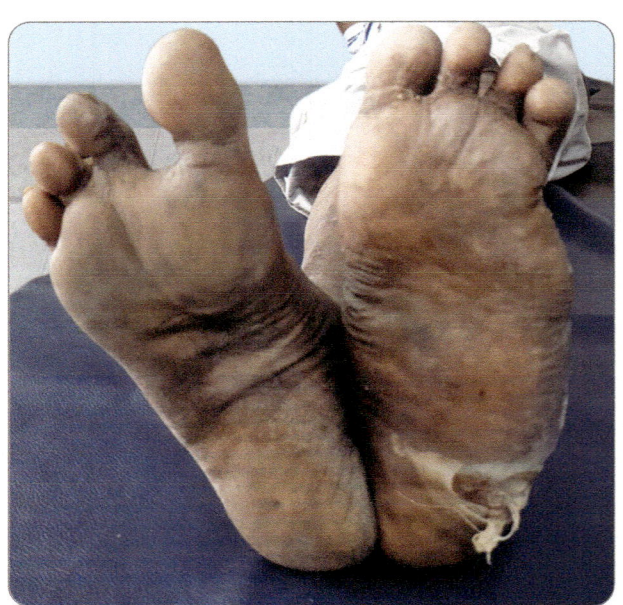

Charcot foot is a serious dreadful complication seen in people living with diabetes and peripheral neuropathy. Treatment involves surgical debridement along with appropriate offloading of the joint. Surgical correction of Charcot is indicated in patients with recurrent plantar ulcers.

84. Intertrigo

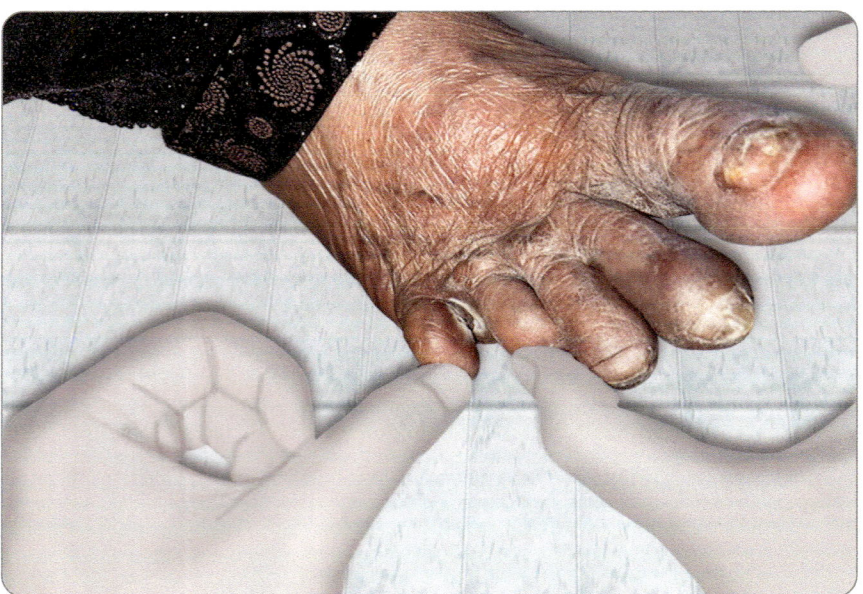

This condition is very common among old people who are unable to keep the interdigital space dry. Treatment comprises prescription of oral antifungal drugs and topical application of dusting powder. It is best advised to keep the area dry and clean.

85. Skin Diseases in the Feet Like Psoriasis

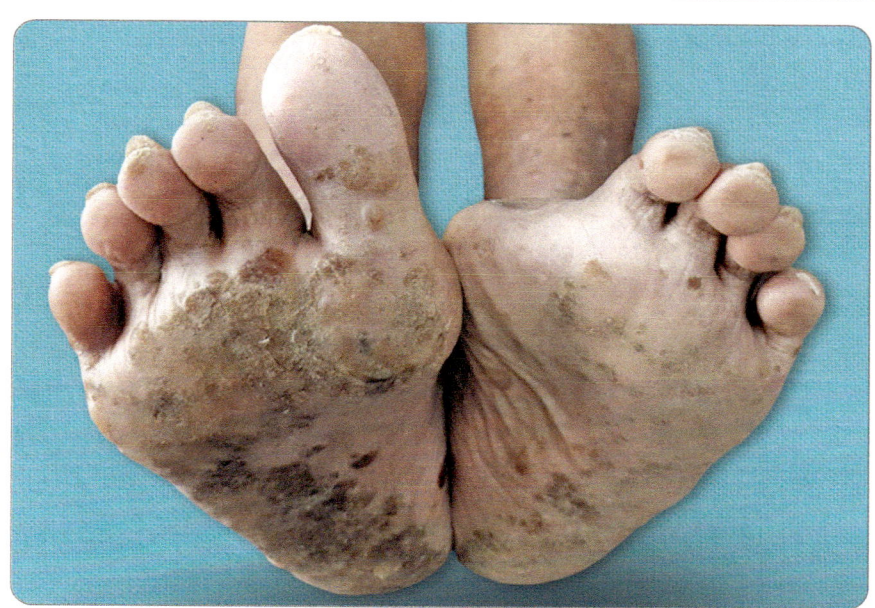

In people living with diabetes, skin diseases are quite common. Dry skin is one of the most common conditions seen in diabetes. One should not forget to rule out other skin diseases like eczema and psoriasis.

86. Exostectomy (Resection of Bony Protrusion)

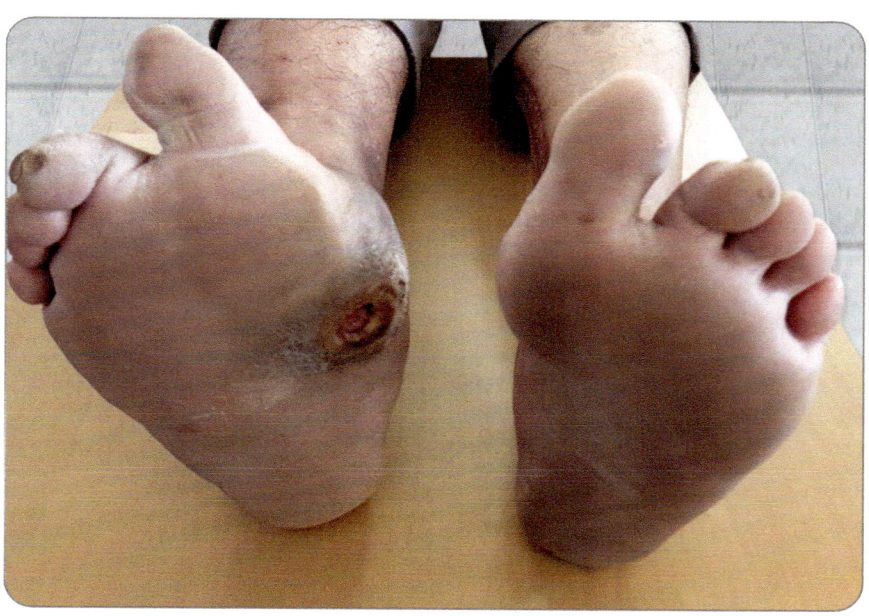

This picture exhibits a case of recurrent ulcer in a mid-foot Charcot. Exostectomy (resection of bony protrusion) is considered in such cases. This procedure is indicated in a person with an ulcer which can cause a bony prominence in a stable foot and can prevent infections like osteomyelitis. Ideal management requires a multidisciplinary approach comprising a team of diabetologists, surgeons, and orthopedic surgeons who can work in coordination to resolve such cases.

87. Right Foot Infection from the Stump of the Great Toe up to the Heel

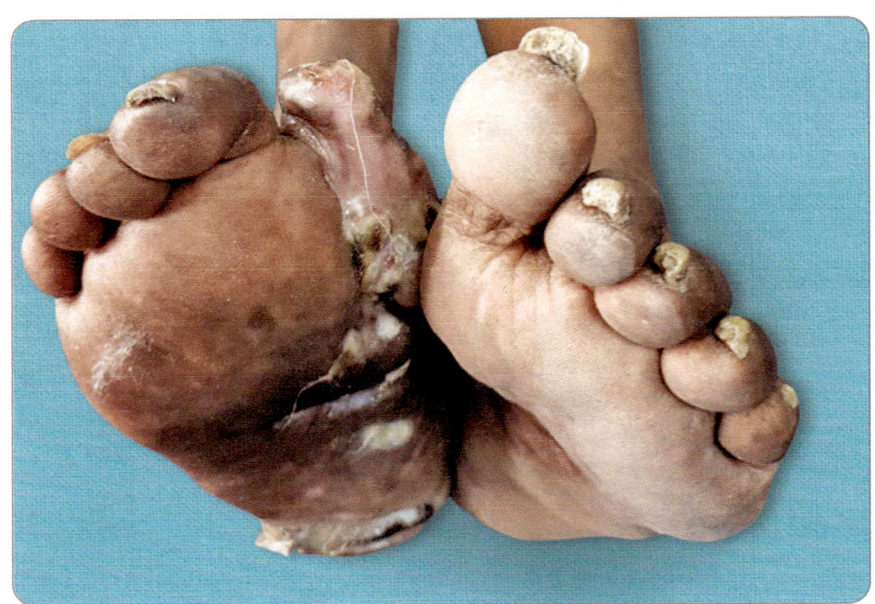

This picture shows a right foot infection starting from the stump of the great toe and extending up to the heel of the patient. The infection spreads all along the fascial plane and it requires complete debridement along with necessary antibiotics to treat the condition.

88. Bilateral Bunion

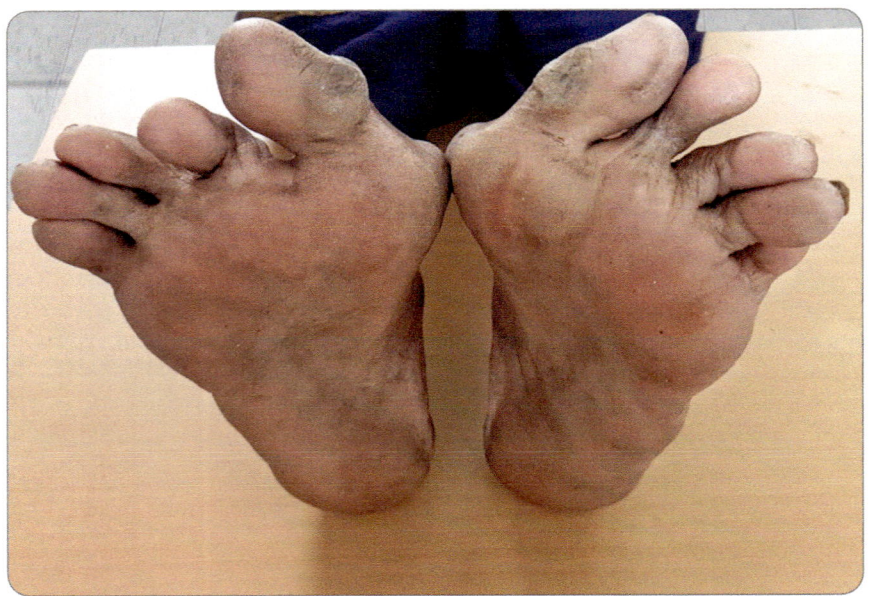

This is a case of bilateral bunion with multiple calluses. This condition occurs due to improperly distributed foot pressure. Bunionectomy is the surgical procedure indicated to correct bunions. A small portion of bone is removed and the alignment is corrected. This procedure also helps us to repair the soft tissue surrounding the big toe.

89. Heel Ulcer Over Tendon Achilles

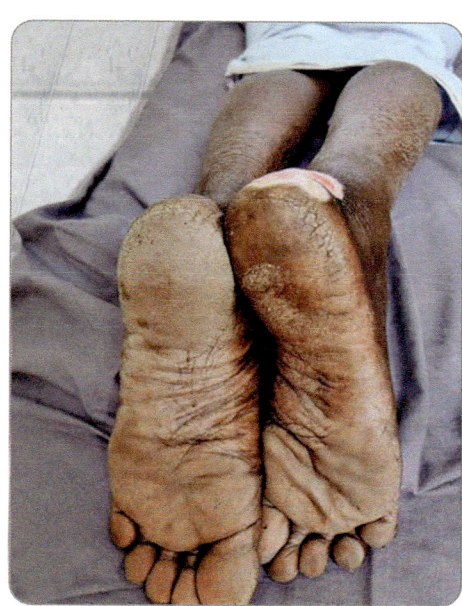

This picture shows a heel ulcer over the tendon Achilles (TA). Care must be taken not to cause damage to the TA.

90. Pus Discharge from Abscess Over the Lateral Malleolus

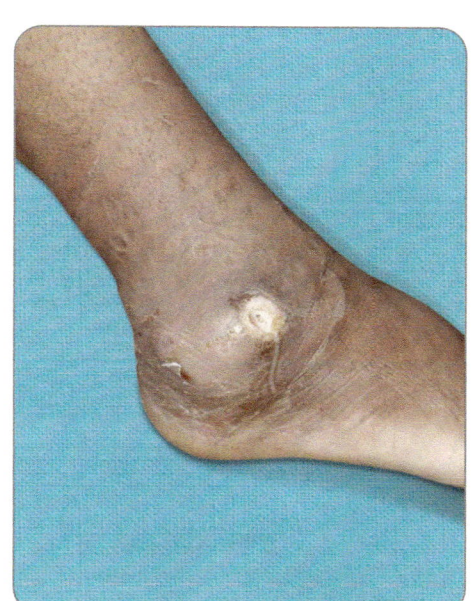

This is a case of abscess over the lateral malleolus where prominent pus discharge can be seen. Radiographs of the ankle joint must be taken to rule out osteomyelitis. Treatment comprises surgical debridement of the infected bone along with intravenous administration of antibiotics for 2–6 weeks.

91. Friction Blister

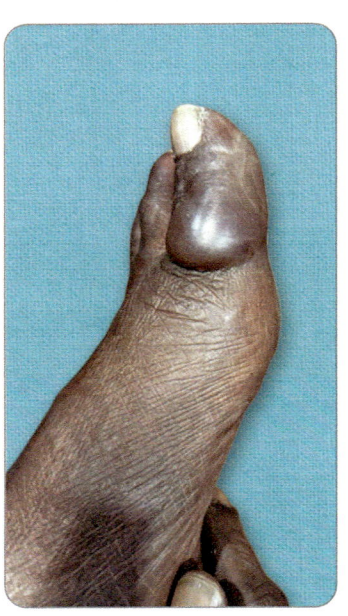

This condition usually occurs due to prolonged friction and irritation to the skin as a consequence of wearing tight footwear. These blisters usually contain clear fluid, which accumulates below the outermost skin layer. In mild cases, it can resolve with the development of callus but the ideal treatment involves drainage of the fluid and wearing appropriate footwear.

92. Monofilament

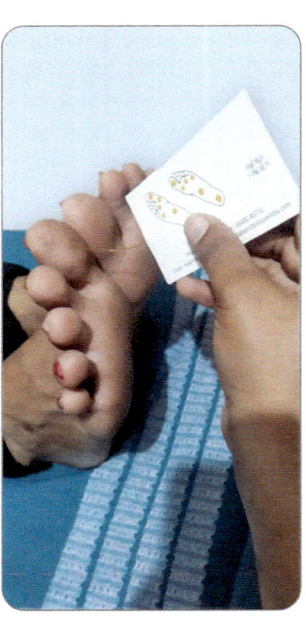

A monofilament is used to test the loss of protective sensation (LOPS) in a person with diabetic neuropathy. The patient is asked to close his eyes and the monofilament is held perpendicular to the skin for a few seconds. The tip of the monofilament is placed at specific areas of the foot until it bends and is then gradually removed. This test is quick, inexpensive, simple, and easy-to-use to detect the loss of LOPS.

93. Ulcer Over the Base of the Great Toe

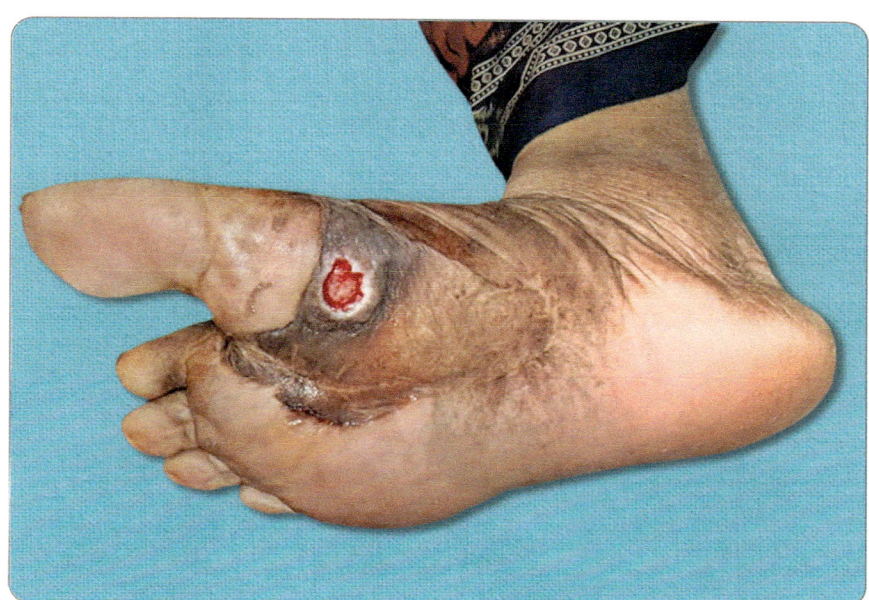

This picture shows an ulcer over the base of the great toe where skin grafting was done previously. This condition might occur in certain cases even after appropriate offloading has been done. In such cases, surgical offloading procedures like resection of the head of the metatarsal and Achilles tendon lengthening are considered good options.

94. Deformed Nails in Fungal Infection

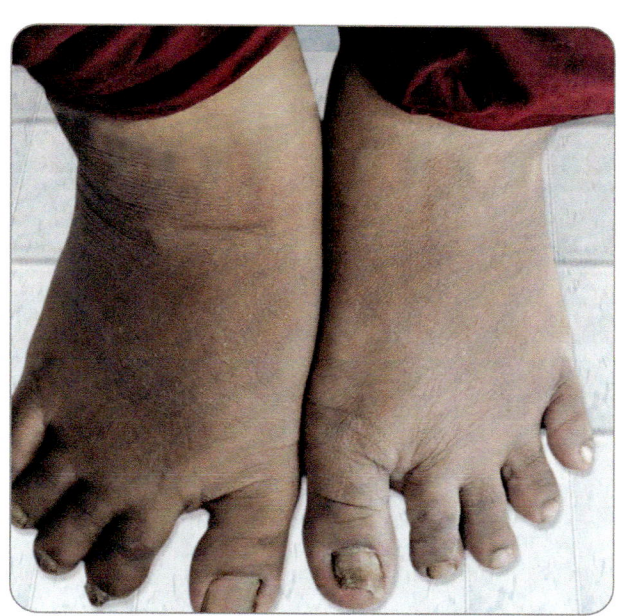

In a patient with diabetes, the nails can be deformed, thick, discolored, or can become fragile due to fungal infection. One should not forget to rule out systemic conditions such as thyroid, iron, vitamin B12, and biotin deficiencies. This condition can be easily prevented by following some simple measures such as maintaining clean, dry, and short nails and using antifungal powders or sprays.

95. Examination of Peripheral Pulses

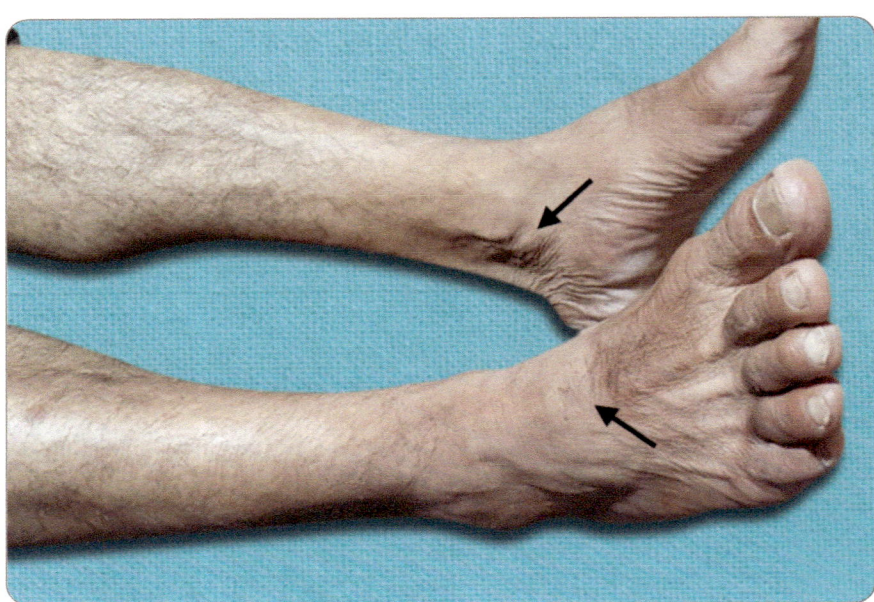

It is important to examine the peripheral pulses of a patient with diabetes. The dorsalis pedis artery can be palpated on the dorsal surface of the foot distal to the bony prominence of the navicular bone. The pulsation of the posterior tibial artery can be palpated behind the medial malleolus of the foot. Absent dorsalis pedis as well as posterior tibial artery are considered to be major predictors of vascular diseases in people with diabetes. Their assessment plays a very significant role to classify patients based on their risk and treat them accordingly.

96. Ischemic Wound of the Forefoot with Extensive Necrosis or Gangrene

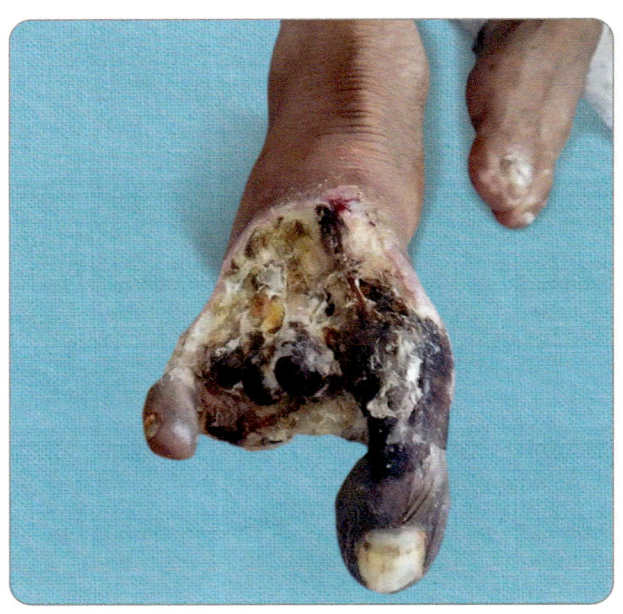

This is a clinical picture of an ischemic and necrotic wound in the forefoot region. In such cases, before starting with debridement of the wound it is important to assess the vascular status of the foot followed by revascularization if required. If left untreated, it can result in even amputation of the foot.

97. Clawing of Toes

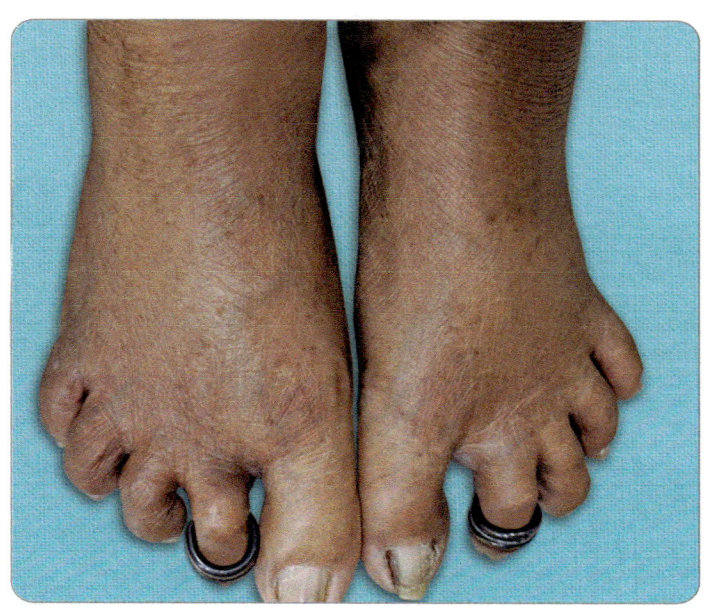

In patients with diabetic neuropathy, and in patients who walk regularly with toe grip footwear this condition is seen. The continuous pressure can increase the susceptibility of developing calluses over the tip of the toes. Toe rings can also be removed in such cases.

98. Middle Toe Amputee with an Ulcer Over the Dorsum of the Foot

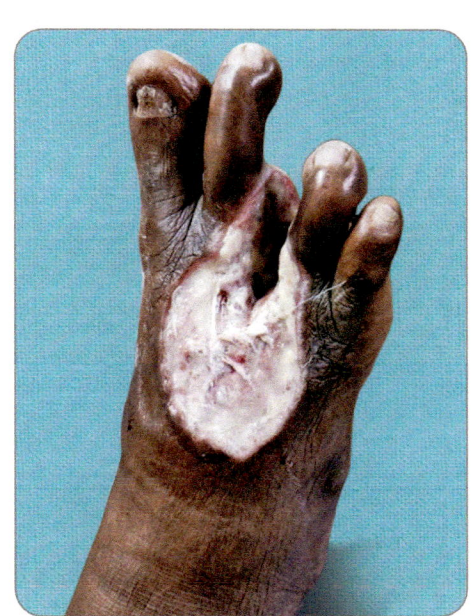

This picture shows a middle-toe amputee with a nonhealing, pale-looking unhealthy ulcers present over the dorsum of the foot. It becomes imperative to monitor the glycemic status, and levels of albumin and hemoglobin in the blood. Surgical debridement of the wound along with vascular assessment is recommended in such patients.

99. Skin Prone to Infection Due to Aging

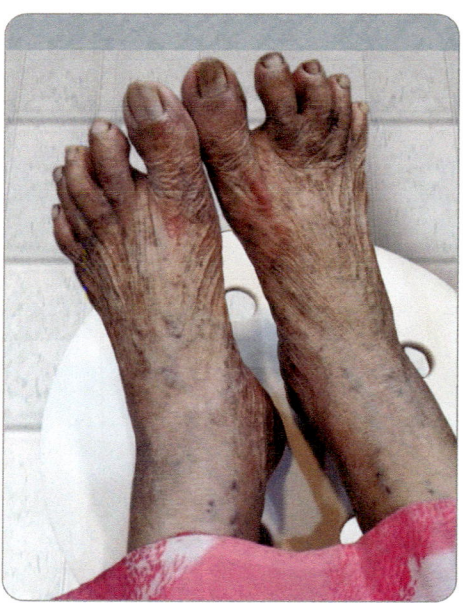

In a patient living with diabetes, due to loss of subcutaneous tissue and decreased elasticity of the skin, the skin becomes more prone to infection. In some cases, mild abrasion can also lead to infection. It is recommended to keep the skin dry after bathing. A good moisturizer is indicated to prevent skin from drying. Bare foot walking has to be avoided completely.

100. Midfoot Infected Callus

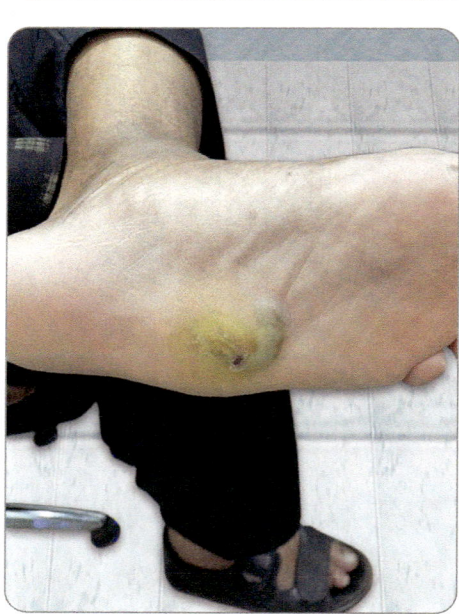

This picture shows a callus in the midfoot region with pus collection in the area surrounding the callus. Radiograph should be taken to rule out any underlying bone involvement, which is to be followed by debridement. Complete offloading has to be done to ensure adequate wound healing.

INDEX

Page numbers followed by *f* refer to figure and *t* refer to table.

A

Abscess 50, 143
Achilles tendon 112, 117
   lengthening, percutaneous 25
Alginate 26, 69, 70
American College of Cardiology 19
American Diabetes Association 18
   modified 62*t*
American Heart Association 15, 18
Amoxicillin 24
Amputation 15*f*, 51, 138, 148
   causes of 14
   diabetes-related 16
   levels of 15
   types of 15
Angiogram 18, 38
   postprocedure 21*f*
Angiography 18
Angiopathy, diabetic 6
Angioplasty 20*f*, 42*f*, 79
Angiosome 38, 39, 140
   concept of 38
   revascularization 40
   territory 43*f*
Ankle 35*f*, 39*f*
   callosity 124
   exercises 81
   joints 84
Ankle–brachial
   index 18, 38, 68, 76, 84, 139
   pressure index 126
      testing 126
Anterior perforator artery angiosome 39
Anterior tibial artery 20*f*, 39, 43*f*-46*f*, 48*f*, 77
   angiosome 39
Antibiotics 136
   sustained local delivery of 72
   systemic 90
Antiplatelet agents 19
Artery, infrapopliteal 19*f*, 42*f*
Atherectomy 21
Atherosclerosis 25
Auscultation 38

B

Balloon angioplasty 21*f*
Below-knee amputation 76, 119, 138
Big toe joint 116
Biofilm 133
   removal of 71
Blister 125
Body 132
Bone
   abnormalities 51
   biopsy 50
   complications 111
   destruction 86*f*
   infection of 106
   marrow edema 85*f*, 109*f*
   normal 51
Bony fragmentation 108*f*
Bony protrusion, resection of 155
Buckling phenomenon 118
Buerger exercises 81
Bunion 116

C

Calcaneal bone involvement 29*f*
Calcaneal sequestrum 55*f*
Calcaneocuboid joint 84
Calcaneum 30*f*
   plantar aspect of 41*f*, 108*f*, 110*f*, 111*f*
Calcaneus 84
Callus 50, 114, 146, 162
   debridement 146, 152
   formation 108
Cardiovascular system 76
Cefoperazone 24
Ceftriaxone 24
Cellulitis 28*f*, 50, 109, 125, 141, 143
   treatment of 152
Cephalexin 24
Cerebrovascular accident 96
Charcot foot 7, 24, 29*f*, 51, 52, 61, 64, 84, 87, 88, 88*f*, 133, 144, 154
   acute 65*f*
   deformity 51
   radiographic features of 52*f*
Charcot neuroarthropathy 12, 83, 84, 86-88, 115
   acute 84, 87
   bilateral 84
   chronic 84, 87
   classification of 83
   development of 83
   pathophysiology of 83
Charcot neuro-osteoarthropathy 83
Charcot restraint orthotic walker 26, 64
Chennai urban population study 17
Chopart–Lisfranc joint 87
Clavulanate 24
Claw toe deformity 59*f*, 118
Clindamycin 24
Computed tomography 18, 50, 86*t*, 106
   angiography 18, 38
Coronary artery disease 96
C-reactive protein 24
Critical limb-threatening ischemia 14, 38
   diagnosis of 38
   risk factors of 38
Cuneiform bone, intermediate 59*f*

D

Dactylitis 148
Deformity 83
Denosumab single-dose injection 87
Dermatitis, contact 137
Dermatological examination 9, 12
Diabetes mellitus 1, 3, 6, 11, 17-19, 76, 84, 90, 93, 94, 96, 98, 102, 103, 106, 111, 125
   epidemiology of 1
   prevalence of 1, 14
Diabetic foot 7, 24, 27*f*, 38, 62*t*, 76, 106
   amputation, risk factors for 15
   complications of 106-108, 112
   examination of 61
   infection 4, 6, 11, 11*f*, 24, 50, 105, 106, 145
      diagnosis of 24, 50
      epidemiology of 1, 3
      incidence of 1
      management of 61, 24, 68
      prevention of 4*f*
      radio imaging of 50
   management of 61
   pathogenesis of 6
   prevention of 61
   problems 113
   ulcer 1, 11, 14, 15*f*, 22, 26, 61, 113, 147, 149
      depth of 130
      infected 90
      nonhealing 65*f*, 72*f*
      risk factors of 4*t*
      Wagner's classification of 129
   wounds, complex 24, 25
Diabetic shoe 63*f*

Digital subtraction 135
    angiogram 19f, 24
Direct revascularization 38, 41
Distal phalax 25
Distal venous arterialization 48f
Doppler ultrasound 18, 38
Dorsal midfoot 108f
Dorsalis pedis artery 22f, 46f, 77
    angiosome 39
Dorsum 35f
Doxycycline 24
Drainage 25
Dressing material 70t, 74
    types of 70
Dry feet 114
Dry skin 131
Duplex ultrasound 18
Dyshidrotic eczema 137
Dyslipidemia 38

E

Eczema 137
Edema
    periarticular 85
    pitting 128
Electronic baropodogram 62, 63f
Endothelial nitric oxide synthase 83
Endovascular revascularization 39
    interventions 19
    techniques 21
Epidermal growth factor 73
Epithelial edge advancement 69
Erosion 51
Erythrocytes 90
European Society of Cardiology 18
European Wound Management
    Association 69
Exostectomy 155
Exostoses 51
Extracellular matrix 73
Extracellular polymeric substance 133

F

First metatarsophalangeal joint 146
Fissure 114
Fixators, external 25
Flatfoot 117
    deformity 59f
Flexor
    digitorum longus 25
    hallucis longus 25
    tendons 25, 27f, 112
Foams 70
    dressing 71f
Foot 39f, 107f
    amputation of 11, 138
    and ankle
        computed tomography scan of 86
        swelling of 115
        asymmetrical swelling of 85f, 107f

charcot neuroarthropathy of 83, 84, 87, 88
deformities 52, 152
dorsum of 32f, 43f
examination of 119, 150
exercises 81, 153
infection 156
    risk factors for 3
lateral radiograph of bilateral 108f
maceration of 139
magnetic resonance imaging of 84, 108f
plantar aspect of 43f, 151
three compartments of 32f
ulcer 11, 15, 135, 147
    complex 129
    diabetes-related 122
    offloading of 121
    over dorsum of 161
X-ray of 86
Forefoot 112, 146
    ischemic wound of 160
Fracture 83, 86f
    pathological 30f
    traumatic 51
Fragmentation 51
Friction blister 158
Fungal infection 117, 131, 159

G

Gangrene 32f, 109, 113, 129, 160
    infective 113
    ischemic 113
Ghost sign 112
Granulation tissue 21f, 44f, 49f, 134
Great toe
    amputation, bilateral 139
    amputee 120
    plantar surface of 46f
    reduced inter phalangeal joint space of 99
    stump of 156
    ulcer over base of 159
Growth factors 73

H

Hallux
    valgus deformity 116
    varus 125
Hammer toe 143
    deformity 37f
Healthy granulation tissue 147
Heart disease, ischemic 76
Heel
    bilateral 108f
    cracked 138
    plantar aspect of 110f
    ulcer 71f, 127, 157
        offloading of 127
    wounds 147
Hemoglobin, glycated 76, 90

High-arched foot 59f
Hydrocolloid 69, 70
Hydrofiber 26, 69
Hydrogel 26, 69, 70
Hyperbaric oxygen therapy 130
Hyperglycemia 38
Hyperkeratosis 124
Hypertension 38, 76, 90
    medications 19
Hypothyroidism 103

I

Ilizarov fixator 25
Imipenem 24
Immunopathy 6
Incision 25
Infection 51, 69
    bacterial 130
Infectious Disease Society of America 68
Infective necrotic wound 29f
Inflammation control 69
Infrapopliteal disease 41f
Ingrowing toenails 127
Insulin-like growth factor 73
Interdigital fungal infections 151
Interleukin 83
International Diabetes Federation 1, 2f, 6, 11
International Working Group on Diabetic Foot 4, 18, 127
    guidelines 4f, 26, 74
    offloading guidelines 66
    wound healing guidelines 74
Intertrigo 120, 154
Ipswich touch test 12
Ischemia 130

J

Joint
    abnormalities 51
    complications 111
    interphalangeal 56f, 84, 98
    intertarsal 84

K

Keller arthroplasty 25
Kidney disease, chronic 18, 90
Knee 35f
    pain 64

L

Laser technology 22
Lateral calcaneal artery 41f
    angiosome 39
Lateral plantar artery angiosome 39
Left ventricular ejection fraction 76
Leg 35f
Leukocytes 90

Leukocytosis 24
Levofloxacin 24
Linear fixators 25
Linezolid 24
Lithoplasty, intravascular 22
Lower extremity
   amputation 1, 15t, 62
   ischemia 15
Lower limb amputations 15f, 119
   reduction of 14

M

Macerated skin 140
   adequate removal of 140
Magnetic resonance
   angiography 18, 38
   imaging 24, 50, 52, 84, 85f, 86t, 106, 108
      role of 52
   spectroscopy 87
Marrow edema 86f, 110f, 111f
Medial calcaneal artery 41f
   angiosome 39
Medial cuneiform, fragmentation of 108f
Medial plantar artery 46f
   angiosome 39
Medical therapy 87
Meropenem 24
Metatarsal bones 51
Metatarsal head resection surgery 25
Metatarsophalangeal joint 62, 77, 84, 98, 114
Metronidazole 70f
Mid foot
   bones 86f
   collapse 86f
   swelling 108f
Middle toe amputee 161
Monocytes 90
Monofilament 158
   test 98
Motor neuropathy 113, 122
Multiple tarsometatarsal dislocations 109f
Multiple vessel calcification 81
Muscles
   atrophy of 113
   denervation of 112
   substantial necrosis of 15
   wasting of 153
Musculoskeletal examination 10, 12
Musculotendinous complications 112
Myositis 112

N

Nanofibers 73
Naviculocuneiform joint 84
Necrotic wound 160
   infection 29f, 32f, 54f
Necrotizing fasciitis 35f, 50, 74f, 136
Negative pressure wound therapy 73, 74, 129

Nephropathy 6
   diabetic 11
Neuroarthropathy 106, 107, 111, 112
   chronic 109f
Neurological examination 9, 12
Neuropathic feet, typical 143
Neuropathy 3, 6, 15, 50, 79, 122, 130
   autonomic 149
   diabetic 26, 122, 145, 153, 161
   peripheral 61, 123
Neurotraumatic theory 83
Nontraumatic lower limb amputations 14
Nuclear scan 86, 106

O

Obesity 38
Onychauxis 131
Onychocryptosis 12, 117
Optimum wound care, principles of 68, 68f
Orthotics
   indispensable role of 61
   use of 61
   walkers 68
Osteomyelitis 15, 25, 30f, 50-52, 99, 106, 107, 111, 112, 129, 137, 150, 152
   contiguous 112
   diagnosis of 52, 107
Osteopenia 51, 83
   periarticular 107f, 108f
   subchondral 52
Osteophytes 51
Osteoprotegerin 83

P

Pedal
   arch angioplasty 20
   edema, unilateral 144
   osteomyelitis 107
   plantar loop technique 20
   pulsations 76
Peg insoles 63
   use of 64f
Pencil and cup appearance 52
Peptide, calcitonin gene-related 83
Percutaneous deep venous arterialization 20
Percutaneous needle flexor tenotomy 25
Periarticular marrow edema 109f, 110f
Periosteal reaction 51
Peripheral artery
   disease 11, 14, 17, 24, 25, 38, 62, 68, 121
      characteristics of 17
      early detection of 17
      management of 17
      prevalence of 17
   occlusion 15
Peripheral pulses, examination of 160
Peripheral sensation, loss of 123
Peripheral vascular disease 3, 6, 15, 17

Peroneal artery 39
   angiosomes 39
   branch of 41f
Peroneal tendon 112
Piperacillin 24
Plain balloon angioplasty 20, 20f
Plantar
   artery
      filling of 21f
      nonopacification of 19f
   foot ulceration 152
   heel ulcers 127
   loop technique 20f
   pressure 121
   psoriasis 123
   vein 22f, 48f
      arterialization of 22f
Platelet-derived growth factor 73
Pneumatic walker 64, 65f
Polyacrylate 72f
Polyester mesh 69, 70f
Polyneuropathy, distal symmetric 113
Polyurethane 26
   film 70
   foam 71f
Poor glycemic control 6, 11
Positron emission tomography 50, 86, 107
Postdebridement foot 42f
Posterior tibial artery 21f, 39, 41f, 44f-47f
   angiosomes 39
   distal segment of 20f
   medial plantar artery branch of 46f
   occlusion of 48f
   plain balloon angioplasty of 20f
Post-transplant amputation 44f
Pressure ulcers, recurrent 142, 153
Prick injury 145
Probe-to-bone test 24, 50, 126
Protective sensation, loss of 7, 12, 50, 62, 158
Pseudomonas aeruginosa 69
Psoriasis 155
Pus discharge 157
Pyomyositis 112

R

Radiography 50
Raised erythrocyte sedimentation rate 24
Random blood sugar 90
Removable cast walker 26
Research Society for Study of Diabetes in India 6
Respiration rate, normal 76
Retinopathy 6, 15
Revascularization
   indirect 39
   surgical 39
Rocker-bottom foot 84

S

Sausage toes 148
Save feet and keep walking campaign 6, 7

Sclerosis 52
    subchondral 51
Sclerotherapy 128
Semmes–Weinstein monofilament test 62
Sensory loss, screening for 123
Septic
    arthritis 112
    gangrene 15
Shoe-bite ulcer 71*f*
Shoes, modifications of 68
Silicon adhesive border 71*f*
SINBAD classification 130
Single-photon emission computed tomography 86
Skin
    disease 123, 155
    elasticity, loss of 149
    graft 28*f*, 36*f*, 72*f*, 135
    hypertrophic 25
    lesions 151
    macerated 140
    prone 162
    ulcerations 112
Small muscle
    atrophy 113
    wasting 122
Soft tissue 19*f*
    complications 108
    defect 55*f*
    infection 50, 52, 106
        deep-seated 24
        severe 15
    inflammation 108
Sonography 50
Split-thickness skin grafting 31*f*, 34*f*
Staphylococcus
    aureus 69
    infection 125
Stasis dermatitis 137
Statins 19
Streptococcus infection 125
Subcutaneous tissue 162

Subtalar joints 84
Sulbactam 24
Superficial femoral artery 41*f*
Surgery 107
    prophylactic 25

T

Talocalcaneal joint 52
Talonavicular joint 84
Tarsal bones 109*f*
Tarsometatarsal joint 84
    dislocation 59*f*, 107*f*
Tazobactum 24
Tendon achilles 157
Tenosynovitis, infective 112
Tenotomy procedure 25
Three-minute foot examination 11, 12*f*, 13
Tibial artery, posterior 19*f*, 21*f*, 39, 41*f*, 44*f*-47*f*
Tigecycline 24
Tissue
    debridement 69
    loss, severe 39
Toe
    brachial index 18
    clawing of 161
    gangrene 25
    partial gangrene of 141
    rings 118
Toenail
    clawing of 118
    curved corners of 116
    fungal infection of 117
    injury 136
Total contact cast 26, 64, 65*f*, 87*f*
Total leukocyte count 90
Transcutaneous oxygen pressure 24
Transforming growth factor
    alpha 73
    beta 73
Transverse tarsal joint 15
Tumor necrosis factor alpha 83

U

Ulcer 50, 108*f*, 109
    classification of 129
    depth of 129
    development 88*f*
    diabetic 105, 150
    neuropathic 126
    nonhealing 15, 21*f*, 27*f*, 46*f*, 70*f*, 72*f*, 55*f*, 96, 110*f*, 111*f*
Ultrasound 50

V

Vacuum-assisted closure 69, 73, 129, 147
    application of 74*f*
Vancomycin 24
Varicose veins 128
Vascular examination 10, 12
Vasculitis 25
Vasculopathy 6
Vessel, ischemia of 25
Vibration perception threshold 12, 78, 90
Visual impairment 11
Vitamin D supplementation 87

W

Wagner's classification 129
Wet gangrene 15, 132
Wound 147
    dressing 68, 72
    granulating 74*f*
    healing 40, 134
    images 91, 96, 98, 102, 104
    infection 58*f*
    ischemic 160
    nonhealing 43*f*, 56*f*
        ischemic 47*f*
    postdebridement picture of 33*f*
    postoperative 30*f*
    preparation 26